GASTROENTEROLOGY IN THE TROPICS AND SUBTROPICS

A Practical Approach

•

DAVID A.K. WATTERS
Professor of Surgery
University of Papua New Guinea

CLEMENT F. KIIRE
Associate Professor of Medicine
University of Zimbabwe

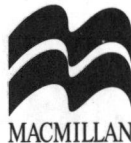

MACMILLAN

First published 1995 by
MACMILLAN EDUCATION LTD
London and Basingstoke
*Associated companies and representatives in Accra, Banjul,
Cairo, Dar es Salaam, Delhi, Freetown, Gaborone, Harare,
Hong Kong, Johannesburg, Kampala, Lagos, Lahore, Lusaka,
Mexico City, Nairobi, São Paulo, Tokyo*

ISBN 0–333–59343–X

10	9	8	7	6	5	4	3	2	
05	04	03	02	01	00	99	98	97	96

Printed in Hong Kong

A catalogue record for this book is available from the
British Library.

Cover illustration courtesy of WHO/UN photograph

Contents

Contributors

S.K. Acharya MD, DM
Department of Gastroenterology and Nutrition,
All India Institute of Medical Sciences, New Delhi,
India

C. Bem MBBS, FRCS, MD
30 Foxglove Avenue
Leeds, LS8 2QR
UK

F.J. Branicki MBBS, DM, FRCS, FRACS
Department of Surgery,
University of Queensland,
Royal Brisbane Hospital,
Australia

S. Chung MD, FRCS (Ed), MRCP (UK)
Department of Surgery,
Chinese University of Hong Kong,
Prince of Wales Hospital, Shatin, Hong Kong

C.P. Conlon MD, MRCP
Infectious Diseases Unit,
Nuffield Department of Medicine, Level 7,
John Radcliffe Hospital,
Oxford, OX3 9DU, UK

V. Gathiram MD, FCP (SA)
Department of Medicine,
University of Natal,
PO Box 17039, Congella 4013,
Durban,
South Africa

M. Gracey MD, PhD, FRACP
Aboriginal Health Policy and Programmes Branch,
Health Department of Western Australia,
Perth,
Australia

G.P. Hadley MB, CHB, FRCS
Department of Paediatric Surgery,
Medical School
University of Natal, Durban 4001,
South Africa

A.D. Harries MA, MD, FRCP, DTM&H
Department of Medicine, College of Medicine,
Private Bag 360, Chichiri,
Blantyre 3,
Malawi

C. Holcombe MD, FRCS
University of Liverpool,
PO Box 147,
Liverpool, UK

O.J. Jacob MS
Department of Surgery, University of Papua New Guinea,
PO Box 5623, Boroko,
Papua New Guinea

M. Kew MD, DSC, FRCP
Department of Medicine, University of the Witwatersrand,
Johannesburg, 2193 South Africa

S. Nundy MA, MB, MChir (Cantab), FRCS (Eng), FRCP (Edin)
Department of Gastrointestinal Surgery, All India Institute of Medical Sciences,
New Delhi 110029, India

G.B.A. Okelo MD, FRCP, DTM&H, FAAS, FTWAS
Department of Medicine,
University of Nairobi, PO Box 19676,
Nairobi, Kenya

S.J. O'Keefe MD, MSc, FRCP
Gastrointestinal Clinic, Department of Gastroenterology, Groote Schuur Hospital,
Observatory 7925, Cape Town, South Africa

I. Segal MBChB, FCP (SA)
Department of Medicine, University of the Witwatersrand,
Johannesburg, 2193, South Africa

A.A. Simjee MBChB, FRCP
Department of Medicine, University of Natal, PO Box 17039
Durban, South Africa

B.N. Tandon MD, FAMS
Pushpawati Singhania Hospital and Research Centre for Liver and Digestive Diseases,
c/o All India Institute of Medical Sciences, New Delhi 110029, India

J.D. Vince MB, CHB, MD, FRCP (Ed)
Department of Clinical Science,
University of Papua New Guinea,
PO Box 5623, Boroko,
Papua New Guinea

A. Wyman MD, FRCS (Eng)
Department of Surgery, Chinese University of Hong Kong, Prince of Wales Hospital,
Shatin, Hong Kong

Foreword

Most of the poorer and developing countries of the world are located in the tropics and subtropics and this book has been written with these countries in mind. The widening gap between richer and poorer countries is at least as visible in health (or lack of health) and health services as anywhere else. Medical progress and its sequelae of increasing clinical specialisation and costly technology have brought limited benefits to patients in poorer countries where lack of skills and material resources have greatly limited incorporation of new techniques into clinical services.

In these countries clinical skills remain paramount for diagnosis and management. Investigations available are often those upon which clinicians the world over relied to support their clinical judgement thirty and forty years ago and which served them and their patients well at that time. New technology has reduced awareness of the value of clinical skills in diagnosis; they together with relatively simple tests receive scant attention in many current medical books and journals.

Diseases, notably infections and nutritional disorders once common everywhere and still common in many developing countries, have become exotic in developed countries and deserving only of presentation at clinical meetings and small-print mention in large tomes.

Thus a single body of medical literature can no longer serve the needs of developed and developing countries equally and there is a growing need to supplement existing literature with specific publications in response to the special needs of the developing world. The best publications will be written by clinicians working in these countries, who are familiar with the day-to-day problems and pressures that are inevitable in under-staffed and under-resourced medical services. These clinicians are professionals who can extract from the depth and breadth of global medical knowledge that which is vital for competence in their health workers under their circumstances. They have sufficient experience to know how to provide the best possible care despite difficult conditions, are up to date in their field, and can recognise new knowledge or technology that is relevant for use within their resources. In this book the authors and contributors bring together just this combination of 'hands-on' experience and knowledge in the field of gastroenterology.

This book is not intended as a specialist text for gastroenterologists but as a practical book to help all clinicians trying to solve gastrointestinal problems for their patients; the organisation of the material under major symptoms reflects problems as they present. In line with the authors' objectives, common problems are covered. Problems of developing countries receive greater emphasis; management is geared to be feasible within a range of resources. Sound up-to-date medical concepts are a requirement for first class health care for all countries, so that basic sciences are included when necessary for understanding. The essentials stand out and non-essentials are excluded.

I can see this text supporting busy embattled clinicians – not only doctors but para-medical workers and nurses – at the bedside solving immediate problems. Under less pressurised conditions medical students and all clinical workers will discover that their lack of 'high-tech' resources need not prevent them providing first-class professional care to virtually all their patients providing there is good management of their scarce resources and that they themselves have highly tuned clinical skills.

The authors and publisher of this book deserve congratulations and gratitude for responding to the special needs of tropical and subtropical countries; the inhabitants of these countries will be the better served as their clinicians gain confidence from the wisdom and guidance contained in this book.

Antonia Bagshawe
Menzies School of Health Research
Darwin, Northern Territory, Australia.
Formerly Professor of Medicine
University of Zambia

Introduction

Maiduguri, Northern Nigeria, August 16th

A 40-year-old man presents with chronic epigastric pain. In every clinic there are so many patients with epigastric pain. Most of them appear relatively well. How should these be assessed and who should be endoscoped? And in the tropics, what is the role of surgery for the treatment of recurrent duodenal ulcer? Should *Helicobacter pylori* be eradicated before planning definitive surgery?

Mbale, Uganda, August 16th

A 38-year-old Ugandan male presents with diarrhoea, weight loss and malaise for 3 months. In his local health clinic he has been unsuccessfully treated with antibiotics. Recently he has also complained of a sore throat and pain when swallowing. He is the 23rd such patient this month. How should he be investigated in a busy outpatient department in a country where HIV infection is so prevalent? What can be done to relieve his suffering?

Rabaul, Papua New Guinea, August 16th

A 2-day-old neonate born in a remote village is transferred from a health subcentre with abdominal distension and failure to pass meconium. There is no anal orifice but a small amount of meconium is discharging from the introitus.

Madras, India, August 16th

A young adult villager is transferred with abdominal pain, weight loss and vomiting. There is a mass in the right iliac fossa. Does he have abdominal tuberculosis and will he require surgical intervention?

London, England, August 16th

The doctor studying tropical medicine pauses in the library to wonder which gastrointestinal cancers are common in sub-Saharan Africa. Is he likely to see many colorectal carcinomas when he goes to work in a mission hospital in the Northern Province of Zambia? And how common is appendicitis in urban centres in tropics? How will he cope with acute surgical emergencies such as sigmoid volvulus?

Hong Kong, August 16th

A 62-year-old lady presents with painful obstructive jaundice. Shortly after admission she develops rigors and becomes shocked. She obviously needs resuscitation but when should she have an ERCP?

Bangkok, Thailand, August 16th

Three patients are admitted with acute right upper quadrant pain. One is jaundiced. All have gallstones on ultrasonography. How should they be managed and what is the role of laparoscopic cholecystectomy in countries with a high incidence of gallstones?

Gastrointestinal disease is prevalent throughout the tropics and subtropics. The pattern of disease is usually different from that in the Western countries where most textbooks are written. Management protocols described in such textbooks may not be appropriate in tropical countries, particularly where the ability to investigate is limited and resources are scarce. This may be true even for 'Western' gastrointestinal diseases, which are on the increase in many parts of the tropics, particularly in urbanised populations.

We hope that those who read this text will find a practical approach to the management of gastrointestinal disease, whether medical, surgical or paediatric. We hope that if you practise in countries as varied as Zimbabwe, India, Malaysia, Brazil or Papua New Guinea you will find you can manage your patients with the resources you have available whether they present with jaundice, epigastric pain, an abdominal mass, dysphagia, diarrhoea, or are born with some frightening congenital malformation.

David A.K. Watters
Clement F. Kiire

Acknowledgements

We especially thank Mrs Vaporo Rei-Kondolo (Port Moresby) and Mrs P. Gwese, Ms D. Matipano and Ms M. Dziruni (Harare) for much work in retyping manuscripts and sending numerous faxes across the world through somewhat unreliable and sometimes disconnected phone lines. We thank Dr Ponifasio Ponifasio for help with redrawing figures and illustrations on the computer. We also thank Drs E. Brown, A. Seaton and P. Dewan for their comments on certain chapters. The Beit Trust, the Papua New Guinea Cancer Relief Society and SmithKline Beecham Pharmaceuticals made publication possible by agreeing to advance purchase copies of the book for distribution in the tropics. We thank them for their generous support. We also appreciate the support of our loved ones who put up with so much while we were burning the midnight oil and watching the sun rise over computer screens.

1

The Organisation of a Gastrointestinal Unit and Services in a Developing Country

The setting up of a gastrointestinal service in a Third Word situation requires a suitable environment, a wide range of instruments, competent operators and assistants. Many hospitals and clinics have developed highly sophisticated facilities. The facilities needed in an individual clinic or hospital depend upon the anticipated workload and procedures and diseases encountered. However, since endoscopy procedures vary enormously in complexity, a number of details must be taken into consideration when an endoscopy unit is being set up.

In discussing this subject, it is important to remember the following: gastrointestinal endoscopy instruments are high-technology sophisticated instruments that require careful handling and experienced care. The actual instruments that are purchased will depend on the needs in any particular area. But once purchased, the care of these instruments must be in the hands of someone who values them and has the experience to look after them. Thus, at the outset this subject needs to be addressed even though it is further discussed in this chapter. There are four options which we believe are available as regards the person whose ultimate responsibility is the care of endoscopy instruments:

1. a nominated medical officer,
2. gastrointestinal unit nurse/s,
3. specialist gastrointestinal unit technician,
4. hospital technician looking after specialised instruments in different departments.

We do not favour option (1) since doctors, especially in the Third World situation, have many duties that would not allow them to give the gastrointestinal (GI) instruments the care that they deserved. Similarly, option (4) is probably not suitable as this person's services are going to be competed for by different departments and also there will be the problem of 'Jack of all Trades, Master of None'. Option (3) is ideal but unlikely to be possible for cost reasons in a Third World situation and so option (2) is the most appropriate situation in these circumstances. Acquisition of the experience needed is discussed below but it has been found that despite having trained in the nursing field, GI nurses/ attendants prove to be very capable, conscientious and able in caring for and having responsibility of GI instruments. However the person is chosen, he or she will be referred to below as 'the assistant'.

Administration of the endoscopy unit

The overall administration of the endoscopy department will need to be shared between the endoscopy assistant and the medical staff with major decisions usually being taken by the latter. Much of the day-to-day administration, however, will be left to the assistant and her expertise will be reflected in the efficiency of the unit.

To carry out these duties well she will need a degree of technical awareness and an ability to plan ahead to ensure that all essential items are available when required. Successful administration is largely a personally developed skill relying on an adequate knowledge of the aims and requirements of the department and on an ability to get to know other workers within the hospital. The assistant should then know the right person to contact when something needs to be done. The main headings for departmental administration are:

1. stores and equipment,
2. records,
3. training.

Stores and equipment

For proper efficiency, adequate stores of all materials used within the department must be obtained and kept up to date. To find that the unit is suddenly short of disinfectant, paper towels, drugs and other important items can cause a major problem. To avoid this, the assistant should identify all departmental items that will require regular re-stocking and make a full list in a suitable 'stock book'. The book should also indicate the date on which the last delivery of any particular item was made together with the quantity supplied. Periodically the stock list should be consulted and the store cupboard checked to determine whether adequate quantities are available in order for fresh supplies to be obtained in good time. By working in this way the assistant will soon be able to identify those items with a rapid turnover and ensure that her stock is up to date. She must, of course, be familiar with the local procedure for ordering her requirements from the main hospital store and the wise assistant will endeavour to get to know the storekeeper personally. He will then become a familiar figure who can supply information readily and make sure that orders are dealt with quickly. Similar advice applies to looking after the equipment. Adequate reserve supplies must be obtained of such items as biopsy valves and spare bulbs and fuses for the light source. A good working relationship should be forged with the suppliers of the unit's equipment as their knowledge and advice can be invaluable. The periodic visits made to most departments by commercial representatives of the fibrescope distribution companies can often provide opportunities to learn more about existing equipment and to keep abreast of new developments in the subject.

Records

The value of an accurate patient list for each endoscopy session and the keeping of an endoscopy book as a record of endoscopies done is extremely important. Add to this, the stock book and the careful filing of all stores requisition notes and instrument repair and it becomes plain that some clerical ability is yet another quality required of a good endoscopy assistant. Once again, in the Third World situation this task will fall on the GI nurse who serves as GI attendant. However, in the ideal situation it is preferable to have a GI clerk who does the following:

1. Makes all the bookings for GI procedures and clinic visits.
2. Ensures the filing of all reports of procedures and medical visits.
3. Carefully indexes all procedures and patient visits so that these are easily retrieved when needed.

Training

Although the vast majority of assistants are trained nurses there is no provision within the nursing profession for a career structure within the endoscopy service. Training for the post of endoscopy assistant comes from two main sources.

1. Established endoscopy assistants. The experienced assistant has a most important role to play in passing on her skills to other staff wishing to establish themselves as competent assistants. This represents the most important source of training.
2. Endoscope distribution companies. In addition there is also some training offered by the instrument companies.

Range of services

In addition to the clinical management of gastrointestinal disease the service should provide the following basic procedures:

1. Upper gastrointestinal endoscopy with biopsy and cytology.
2. Colonoscopy and sigmoidoscopy with biopsy and cytology.
3. Endoscopic retrograde cholangiopancreatography (ERCP) with sphincterectomy and stenting.
4. Injection of oesophageal varices and bleeding peptic ulcers.
5. Small intestinal biopsy.
6. Liver biopsy.
7. Oesophageal dilatation.
8. Peritoneoscopy is also a very important procedure that patients may benefit from in the African context.
9. Motility studies.

Staffing

The gastrointestinal unit must be headed by a gastroenterologist who is usually a physician with special training in gastroenterology. He must be supported by a surgeon with a interest in gastroenterology and other medical staff.

Nursing staff are essential and need to train as gastroenterological nurses and endoscopy assistants. The number required depends on the volume of the service but it is becoming accepted that ideally there should be two assistants in the room during an endoscopy procedure with a third outside in the recovery area supervising arrivals and departures. This level of staffing by competent, well-trained nurse assistants is not always achieved but it needs to be remembered that endoscopy has a small but measurable morbidity and mortality and that it is under conditions of inadequate staffing that the patient is most at risk.

Equipment

This includes gastrointestinal endoscopes together with ancillary equipment. In addition the department will need sigmoidoscopes, proctoscopes and all items of equipment required to provide the services listed. Possession of a dissecting microscope enables biopsy specimens to be inspected and properly orientated before fixation and X-ray viewing boxes are needed to display patient radiographs. Because many gastroenterological procedures require X-ray facilities either access to or even better, possession of X-ray screening equipment is essential.

The present-day cost of obtaining and maintaining the recommended equipment is in the region of US$450 000 and therefore most units need to gather this together over a period of time.

Accommodation

Adequate accommodation for the gastroenterological service should include an endoscopy room and recovery area; a gastrointestinal laboratory where intestinal function tests and biopsies are carried out; an adequate preparation and storage room; toilet facilities; and office accommodation for doctors, nursing staff and secretaries.

The endoscopy room

Planning an endoscopy room is a task of some complexity. The unit is usually run by the physician gastroenterologist who also acts as the senior endoscopist, though less often a gastroenterological surgeon may head the team or very occasionally a radiologist with an interest in endoscopy. When designing an endoscopy room it is suggested that the ideal size should be 5 × 7 m; however, the minimum size is 4 × 6 m. Easy maintenance of equipment and fittings is essential for rapid repair should problems such as electrical or plumbing faults arise. The entrance to the room needs to be double doors sufficiently wide to allow easy passage for a bed-trolley. The room should have a lead-built door and barium plaster if X-ray screening is to be used. The windows should be of frosted glass but capable of being opened. Although darkness is rarely required, the provision of black roller blinds makes this facility possible when needed. For comfort of both patients and staff, air conditioning equipment should be built in, if possible.

The contents of the room must include an endoscopy couch which should be placed at the centre with sufficient clearance at its head for the endoscopy trolley and the nurse assistant. A large sink must be sited near the couch for washing the endoscope insertion tube at the end of each examination and sufficient work-top surface needs to be nearby. Cupboards and drawers can be arranged beneath such surfaces for storage.

An endoscope security cupboard should be attached to a wall of the room in a convenient place. A hand basin separate from the main sink unit is desirable for staff to wash their hands after endoscopic procedures.

The room must have a desk and X-ray viewing boxes. A lamp and telephone should be placed on the desk. Electric points preferably protected by stainless steel covers should be placed around the room at regular intervals but especially at the head and foot of the endoscopy couch. Other items which need to be placed somewhere within the rooms are a drip stand, a waste bin and several stools and chairs. In addition to the endoscopy room itself there is also a need for a recovery area nearby. Once again a purpose designed area with recovery couches in individual cubicles supervised by a nurse/assistant is desirable but not always possible.

Cleaning and disinfection

The proper cleaning and disinfection of endoscopic equipment is of paramount importance in any endoscopy unit. Apart from eliminating the risk of transmission of the HIV virus and other pathogenic organisms, clean, well maintained equipment has a longer life-span and requires less expensive maintenance and repairs.

Salmonella transmission can sometimes lead to fatal septic cholangitis and *Helicobacter pylori* can be transmitted to the uninfected patient and cause gastric inflammation and eventually peptic ulcer disease in some patients. In addition to cleaning the scope itself, the cleanliness of accessories such as forceps, tubing, etc. is also important.

As it is impractical to tailor the degree of disinfection to each patient, any efficiently run endoscopy unit will adopt a policy of universal precautions in terms of disinfection irrespective of the clinical status of the patient or the risk of the procedure. These precautions must fulfil the following: the equipment must be free of pathogens from the last patient which would constitute a risk to the health of the next patient if the equipment were not disinfected. The universal precautions would ensure that patients and staff alike will feel that they are being protected at all times.

It can be seen from the above, that the aim in endoscopy units is not for sterilisation, as this would not be possible, but for, as Cotton states in his book, 'a high level of disinfection' whereby harmful bacterial and viruses will be inactivated. The choice of disinfection is inevitably constrained by the delicate nature of the materials used in the manufacture of endoscopes and their accessories.

The one agent which is used globally in units in both developed and developing countries is glutaraldehyde (2 per cent). It has the properties of being non-corrosive and destroying all bacteria and viruses within a 4-min period. Another important factor in favour of glutaraldehyde is the fact that it is relatively inexpensive when compared with other similar agents. The one drawback is its irritant nature to skin and mucous membranes and hence there is the need to thoroughly wash the instruments after disinfection with the agent and the need for the person performing the disinfection to use some barrier protection e.g. gloves.

Suggested cleaning routine for endoscopes

Ideally in a developed-country situation it is recommended that endoscopes be cleaned using an electronic washing machine. This machine runs off a programme which lasts approximately an hour. The cycle goes through different phases. Firstly the instrument is washed with a soapy detergent and all fat debris, blood and mucus are removed. The second phase involves the injection of a disinfectant to kill off the various viruses and bacteria. In the third phase, the instrument is disinfected using a 2 per cent glutaraldehyde solution. The machine is programmed to run the glutaraldehyde disinfection for approximately 15 min.

In the Third World environment, where funding is a problem, a three bucket system is used to clean endoscope equipment. Three large buckets are used. The first having clean water with a soapy detergent, the second containing the 2 per cent glutaraldehyde solution and the third bucket having clean water. Baby baths may be the most convenient and available containers for use.

When the instrument is removed from a patient it is wiped down with a soft gauze using water from the first bucket. The suction-channel is cleaned using a cleaning brush and aspirating water from the first bucket. The biopsy channel is also cleaned using the same brush. The instrument is then soaked in the bucket of glutaraldehyde for approximately 8 min. The biopsy valves, the air/water valves and the suction valves are removed and also soaked in this bucket.

After 8 min glutaraldehyde is aspirated through the channels and the instrument is wiped down with a gauze. It is then removed from the second bucket and soaked in the clean water. The clean water is aspirated through the different channels. Fresh water is filled into the water bottle and the air/water valve is activated to irrigate the channel thereby removing any glutaraldehyde that may have moved up the channel. Always use a 30 or 50-ml syringe to clean and irrigate the endoscope. Smaller 20-ml syringes do not completely flush the air and water channels.

A new biopsy valve is inserted, the air/water and suction valves are lubricated with a light silicone oil and also reinserted. Lens cleaner is used to polish the distal end. The instrument is now ready to be used for the next patient.

Most instruments have three channels, namely the suction channel, the biopsy channel and air/water channel. It is of paramount importance that all these channels be included in the cleaning and disinfecting process as all of them are potential reservoirs for transmitting infection.

Accessories

Disinfection of accessories is essential. Particular attention should be paid to those which are used parentally – especially if their design makes access for cleaning and disinfecting solutions difficult. For metal and heat-resistant plastic or Teflon accessories there is a clear advantage in using standard steam autoclave procedures for sterilisation. In eye-risk situations in which this full sterilisation is essential, e.g. in variceal sclerotherapy or interventional biliary sclerotherapy, and whenever equipment can be relatively cheaply manufactured, disposable products are increasingly used to avoid time loss, tedium, staff risks and the uncertainty involved in cleaning reusable accessories.

It would be ideal if a purpose-built cleaning area was available for the safe and efficient practice of cleaning the endoscopes and accessories. A double-sink and hand wash basins with ample storage place, good ventilation and extraction facilities would be most suitable.

It is essential that some form of documentary record be kept after any endoscope is cleaned and disinfected. In a unit that does not have too many endoscopes, routine bacteriological test cultures are necessary once a disinfection routine has been established and initially validated. Each instrument should additionally have its own log book to note repair and overall results.

Documentation

Reporting and recording are essential parts of any service. The documents and system should be designed around local needs and limitations, and it is wise to look at a number of ideas from established units, and to incorporate those which fit. The advent of affordable microcomputers – especially easy-to-use systems for endoscopy – transforms the management and record-keeping systems of the past.

Recommended instrumentation

Over the years improvements to the fibreoptic endoscope have been phenomenal. Endoscopes currently being manufactured are completely immersible and the field of view is greater. It is therefore important that when purchases are made that the unit buys wisely. The most widely used endoscopes today are Olympus. The other companies that manufacture fibreoptic endoscopes are Fujinon and Pentax. These companies also manufacture numerous accessories that are compatible with their range of products. The accessories are often interchangeable.

Staff protection

As with all medical procedures, staff protection is an important consideration. Different units have different standards with regards to protective clothing. In a unit, in the developing world where the financial constraints are great, the standards applied must be such that they afford the staff more than adequate protection but on the other hand are not excessive so as to be wasteful and burden an already 'cash-strapped economy'. A plastic apron over the clothing and rubber surgical gloves should be the minimum requirements for routine gastroscopy and sigmoidoscopy. For endoscopic procedures of a more invasive nature where splashing of secretions could be a problem, face and eye protection should be worn.

All surfaces in the endoscopy suite should be kept disinfected and staff should also practise a high degree of personal hygiene.

Conclusion

In the developing world the basic requirement that needs to be fulfilled by a gastrointestinal unit is diagnostic endoscopy (gastroscopy and sigmoidoscopy).

Due to the high turnover of patients and an ever-increasing number of patients with gastrointestinal ailments, it is imperative for any unit to be fully functional that it should be able to make quick and accurate diagnoses, so that both patients and the institution are not over-burdened.

2

Infective Diarrhoea

In the tropics, infective diarrhoeal diseases are among the leading causes of morbidity and mortality in children under the age of 5 years. Breastfeeding confers significant protection against these infections, and diarrhoeal rates are low during the period of exclusive breastfeeding. As weaning occurs, diarrhoeal episodes become more frequent, and it is in these first few critical years of life that diarrhoea exerts its greatest negative effect on child health and survival. In poor, rural areas of the tropics, children under the age of 5 years may experience six to eight episodes of diarrhoea per year, and in poor urban areas these rates may be even higher at ten or more episodes per year. Repeated attacks of diarrhoea lead to a vicious cycle of malnutrition, reduced immunity and further infections of the gastrointestinal tract. The frequency of diarrhoeal episodes and their associated mortality decrease with age. However, adults are not immune from the problem, and food poisoning, gastroenteritis, dysentery and chronic diarrhoea are common causes of illness and admission to hospital in many parts of the tropics. The pathogens responsible for many of the cases of diarrhoea in children and adults are shown in Table 2.1.

The problem of gastrointestinal infection is unrelated to climatic temperature, but rather is the result of crowded conditions in cities or villages where acceptable levels of safe water, domestic and sanitary hygiene are absent. This chapter highlights the important aspects of assessment, diagnosis and management of gastrointestinal infection, and discusses some of the major pathogens in more detail. Gastrointestinal pathogens are discussed according to their most usual clinical presentation.

Assessment of diarrhoeal illness

History

The relevant information which needs to be elicited in the history is summarised in Table 2.2. This helps in determining the possible aetiology of the diarrhoeal episode and to some extent the severity.

10

Table 2.1   Enteric pathogens isolated in children and adults with diarrhoea in the tropics.

	India Inpatient	Bangladesh Largely outpatient	Brazil Rural
Percentage of patients with:			
Rotavirus	8	19	19
Enterotoxigenic *Escherichia coli*	6	20	21
Enteroinvasive *E. coli*	0	—	2
Enteropathogenic *E. coli*	6	—	5
Salmonella	0	1	0
Shigella spp.	2	12	8
Campylobacter	5	14	8
Vibrio cholera O1	30	6	0
Entamoeba histolytica	—	6	2
Giardia intestinalis	—	6	7
Strongyloides stercoralis	—	—	5

Adapted from: Antibiotics in the tropics by S. Enenkel and W. Stille. Chapter on Infections of the Gastrointestinal Tract p 146.

Table 2.2   Clinical assessment of infective diarrhoea: history.

Current illness	Duration of diarrhoea Frequency of bowel movements Stool consistency Presence of visible blood in stool Fever Other symptoms e.g. cough, dysuria
Social/drugs	Friends/relatives affected Residence in institutions Pets Suspect food Antibiotics
Medical history	

Current illness

Duration of illness allows an arbitrary classification of diarrhoea into acute or chronic (longer than 2 weeks). This is useful because, although there is overlap between the two groups, different pathogens need to be considered in each case. A record should be made of the number of bowel movements in 24 h, and the consistency of the motion (faeces, faeculent, fluid or water). Visible blood in the stool indicates colonic ulceration, which in the tropics is commonly due to shigella or *Entamoeba histolytica*. Fever commonly occurs with some intestinal pathogens such as salmonellae and *Shigella*, but it suggests the possibility of systemic infection such as malaria, pneumonia or urinary tract infection; enquiry about cough, chest pain, dysuria, frequency and haematuria should be made.

Social and drug history

It is important to discover whether relatives and friends are similarly affected, or whether the patient comes from a crowded institution such as a prison or military barracks in which other members are afflicted with diarrhoeal illness. Such information suggests a food or water-borne outbreak, and may necessitate appropriate public health measures. Pets may be responsible for disease transmission to humans; *Campylobacter, Salmonella, Shigella* and *Escherichia coli* are commonly present in dogs. Close contact with pets can result in enteritis, and may be one reason for frequent relapses of diarrhoeal illness. The type of foodstuff ingested in the previous 24–48 h may help in identification of the likely cause (see below under food poisoning). A history of antibiotic ingestion in the 4 weeks before gastrointestinal illness suggests infection with *Clostridium difficile* or antibiotic associated diarrhoea. Some antibiotics are more likely to cause this problem than others Table 2.3.

Table 2.3 Antibiotics and *Clostridium difficile* associated diarrhoea.

Association with *C. difficile* diarrhoea	Antibiotics
Common	Ampicillin / amoxycillin Cephalosporins Clindamycin
Uncommon	Tetracycline Sulphonamides Co-trimoxazole Chloramphenicol Erythromycin
Rare	Parenteral aminoglycosides

Medical history

Documentation of past medical or surgical illness is important for two reasons. First, it may provide a clue to aetiology. For example, a person with reduced gastric acidity as a result of gastric surgery or treatment with H_2-receptor antagonists is at increased risk of salmonella and cholera. A patient with a history of herpes zoster and recently treated pulmonary tuberculosis may be immunosuppressed as a result of infection with the human immunodeficiency virus (HIV). Second, it may affect management; for example, a patient with insulin-dependent diabetes mellitus will need close monitoring during a diarrhoeal episode.

Examination

The physical examination should be carried out (1) to assess the degree of fluid deficit and nutritional impairment that has occurred as a result of gastrointestinal illness, and (2) to look for clues to the aetiology of the illness Table 2.4.

In the assessment of hydration status, it is not enough to rely on reduced skin turgor (which may be found in old age and in association with marked weight loss) or dry mucous membranes (a dry tongue may occur with mouth breathing associated with respiratory tract infection). Supine pulse and blood pressure provide a good index of hydration status; however, in young people with moderate dehydration these parameters are often maintained within the normal range, so it is preferable to measure postural changes in pulse and blood pressure. Respiratory rate increases in proportion to the degree of dehydration as a result of attendant acidosis.

Nutritional status can be assessed objectively by measurements of weight, height, mid-upper arm circumference and skinfold thickness. Calculations can be made of mid-arm muscle circumference, and results of these observations give a guide to the amount of fat and protein deficit. Careful clinical examination can reveal specific nutritional deficiencies.

Table 2.4   Clinical assessment: examination.

Fluid deficit	Reduced skin turgor
	Sunken eyes
	Dry mucous membranes
	Pulse and blood pressure (supine and erect)
	Increased respiratory rate
Nutritional state	
General	Fever
	Mental state
	Signs of immunosuppression
	Abdominal mass

Clues to the aetiology of diarrhoea are more often obtained in patients with chronic diarrhoea.

Investigations

Haemoglobin concentration, peripheral white cell count and differential, blood urea and electrolytes are useful in the general assessment of the patient. Specific diagnosis will depend on stool microscopy (with and without concentration techniques) and culture (Table 2.5). DNA probes have now been developed for a number of gut pathogens (viral, bacterial, protozoal and helminthic), but their usage in the developing world will probably remain as a research tool for a long time to come.

Table 2.5   Laboratory investigations: stool microscopy and culture.

Direct microscopy

No special stains required

Protozoa:	Entamoeba histolytica	Helminths:	Strongyloides spp.
	Giardia intestinalis		Fasciolopsis buski
	Balantidium coli		Schistosoma spp.
	Isospora belli		Capillaria philippinensis

Modified Ziehl–Neelsen or acid-fast stain
   Protozoa: Cryptosporidium
                    Isospora belli

Chromotrope-based stain
   Microsporidia

Selective enrichment media before culture
   Alkaline peptone water: vibrios (*Vibrio cholerae, Aeromonas, Plesiomonas*
   Selenite broth: *Salmonellae, Shigella* spp
   Robertson's cooked meat broth: *Clostridium difficile*

Selective culture media
   MacConkey's agar: *Escherichia coli*
   Desoxycholate-citrate-agar (DCA): *Salmonella* spp., *Shigella* spp.
   Xylose-lysine-desoxycholate agar (XLD): *Salmonella* spp., *Shigella* spp.
   Mannitol-lysine-crystal violet brilliant green agar (MLCB): *Salmonella* spp.
   Campylobacter medium: *Campylobacter* spp.
   Thiosulphate-citrate bile salt sucrose agar (TCBS): vibrios
   Cycloserine-cefoxitin blood agar: *Clostridium difficile*

Clinical presentation

Food poisoning

This term refers to a sharp outbreak of gastrointestinal illness affecting two or more people, shortly after sharing a meal. The majority of cases are bacterial in nature Table 2.6, although viral, parasitic and biological toxic causes are also recognised. If the **incubation period is less than 6 h,** the illness is usually caused by ingestion of pre-formed enterotoxin. As there is no bacterial multiplication, constitutional disturbance such as fever is uncommon. These preformed toxins are primarily neurotoxins which act on the emetic centre in the brain. The dominant clinical feature is vomiting, and the illness is usually brief, lasting up to 24 h. However, patients can sometimes be severely ill with abdominal pain, prostration and a high peripheral white cell count.

If the **incubation period is greater than 6 h,** the illness is caused by ingestion of living bacteria in contaminated food, the organisms having to multiply in the gut before causing symptoms. Diarrhoea is more often a feature, and the illness can last a few days. Anthrax involving the small intestine (resulting from poorly cooked meat from infected cattle, sheep or goats) is occasionally responsible for food poisoning. Intestinal anthrax can be severe, and can resemble necrotising enteritis (see below).

Table 2.6   Food poisoning from bacteria or their toxins.

	Principal foods	Dominant clinical features
Incubation period less than 6 h		
Staphylococcus aureus	Meat Poultry Dairy products	Vomiting
Bacillus cereus	Fried rice	Vomiting
Incubation period 6–48 h		
Salmonella spp.	Meat Poultry Dairy products	Diarrhoea Vomiting Abdominal pain
Campylobacter spp.	Poultry	Diarrhoea Abdominal pain
Clostridium perfringens	Cooked meat	Diarrhoea Abdominal pain
Vibrio parahaemolyticus	Sea foods	Diarrhoea Abdominal pain Vomiting

The division of food poisoning into toxin and infective types may be blurred because some organisms cause illness through bacterial multiplication and toxin production in the intestine. For example, type A enteropathic strains of *Clostridium perfringens* multiply in the small intestine, and produce toxins *in vivo* leading to clinical illness. The spores of *C. perfringens* are relatively resistant to heat, and this accounts for infection in meat which appears relatively well cooked. Type C strains of *C. perfringens* may invade the gut mucosa, and through the production of β-toxin can cause necrosis of the full thickness of the intestinal wall – necrotising enteritis. This illness is found in a number of tropical countries, but particularly Papua New Guinea where it commonly follows communal feasting on pigs and is known as pigbel disease. The severity of the illness varies from acute diarrhoea to a severe dysenteric-like illness with extensive necrosis of the small, and to a lesser extent, the large intestine. When peritonitis and signs of intestinal obstruction are present, laparotomy and surgical resection of necrotic intestine may be necessary. Mortality at this stage can be as high as 80 per cent. Specific immunisation with β-toxoid in at-risk population groups has been shown to give significant protection.

Viruses are occasionally implicated in food poisoning outbreaks, particularly rotavirus and Norwalk agent. Gastrointestinal illness with neurological manifestations suggest botulism, shell-fish poisoning and toxic fungi poisoning. *Clostridium botulinum* grows readily in tinned foods which have been badly prepared. An exotoxin, which blocks neuromuscular transmission, is absorbed from the upper small intestine. Symptoms include nausea and vomiting, diplopia, dysphagia, dysphonia, and generalised weakness of the limbs and respiratory muscles. Botulism may be confused with other diseases such as the Guillain–Barré syndrome and myasthenia gravis. In the tropics the mortality rate is high. Certain toxicants in food are well known to cause short-lived diarrhoea usually within an hour of ingestion; a good example is capsicin, the substance which makes chillies hot.

Acute diarrhoea without fever or blood

The main causes of this clinical presentation are preformed toxins from food poisoning (see Table 2.6), viral infections and colonisation of the gut by organisms which make enterotoxins *in situ*.

Rotaviruses (so-called because of a wheel like appearance) were discovered by electron microscopy in 1973. They are a significant cause of infantile gastroenteritis world-wide. In adults, infection also occurs, but is generally mild. It has now been established that adenoviruses are also associated with diarrhoeal disease in infants and children. Other viruses include astrovirus, calicivirus and echovirus.

Enterotoxins alter cellular metabolism so as to promote intestinal secretion without killing the cell. Cholera toxin is the prototype. Figure 2.1 illustrates the mechanism by which this toxin results in massive efflux of water and

CHOLERA ENTEROTOXIN
(One A sub-unit surrounded by five B sub-units)

↓

B sub-units bind irreversibly to
GM-1 monosialoganglioside enteric mucosal receptor

↓

A sub-unit enters enterocyte
irreversibly activates adenylate cyclase

↓

Perpetual increased production of cyclic AMP
for the rest of the life of the enterocyte

↓

Accumulation of cyclic AMP

↓

Net secretion of sodium, chloride and water into
lumen of the small intestine

↓

Colonic absorptive capacity exceeded

↓

Diarrhoea

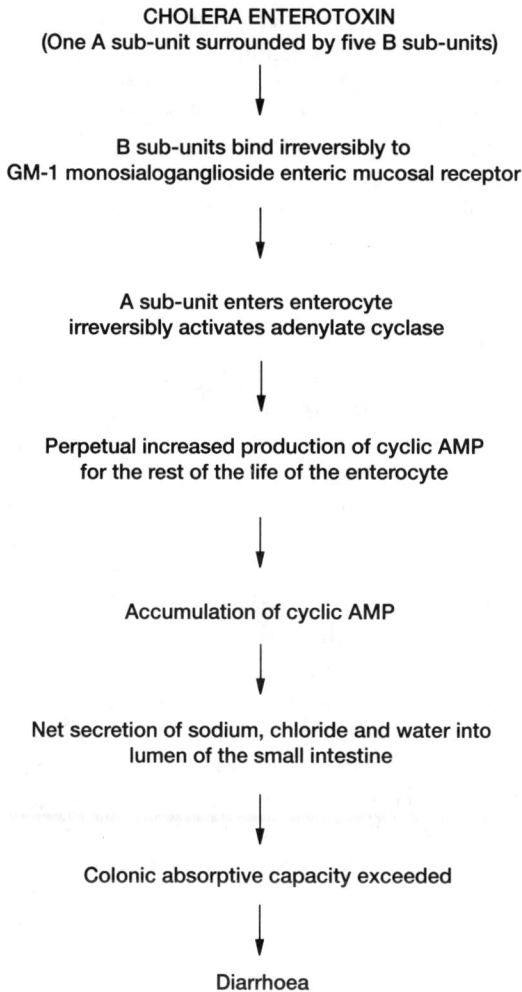

Figure 2.1   Mechanism of action of cholera toxin.

electrolytes into the small intestinal lumen. A number of other bacteria produce enterotoxins, which work either by activating adenylate cyclase or by other mechanisms such as stimulation of guanylate cyclase with production of cyclic GMP. Enteric toxin production is known for several organisms with invasive properties such as *Campylobacter* spp., salmonellae, *Aeromonas*, and *Plesiomonas shigelloides*.

Enterotoxigenic strains of *E. coli* (ETEC)

This is the single most important cause of travellers' diarrhoea and an important cause of infantile gastroenteritis in the tropics. ETEC produce enterotoxins (one heat labile toxin and two heat stable toxins) which cause a non-inflammatory secretory diarrhoea. Clinically, the onset of diarrhoea is sudden, with nausea, vomiting and abdominal colic. Fever is rare. Untreated, the disease is self-limiting, lasting from 1 to 3 days. Clinical recovery is followed by prolonged immunity, for which reason this is mainly a disease of visitors or infants rather than adult residents. **Enteropathogenic *E. coli* (EPEC)** causes a similar, although slightly more severe, disease and is an important cause of diarrhoea in infants and children.

Cholera (see pages 30–36)

Cholera is a bacterial infection of man caused by *Vibrio cholerae*. Up until 1992, all strains of *V. cholerae* isolated from cholera cases possessed O1 antigen. The *V. cholerae* serogroup O1 is divided into classical and El Tor biotypes, and into serotypes Ogawa, Inaba and Hikojima. The classical biotype is largely confined to the Indian subcontinent. The El Tor biotype originated in Indonesia around 1960, subsequently spread to Africa, Europe, Oceania and Latin America, and is responsible for the current seventh pandemic. The gastrointestinal illness produced by the El Tor biotype is indistinguishable from classical cholera, except the former more often gives rise to the carrier state and relatively fewer of those affected develop the 'classical' disease. Non-O1 serotypes have been associated with sporadic cases of gastroenteritis, but not with cholera. However, in 1992 a major shift in isolation rates from O1 serogroup to non-O1 serogroup was noticed in acute diarrhoea cases in the Indian subcontinent. This novel strain (termed *V. cholerae* O139) produces cholera toxin, and causes in sporadic and epidemic form an illness indistinguishable from cholera. The high attack rates among adults demonstrate the ineffectiveness of pre-existing immunity against the previous prevalent strains of El Tor *V. cholerae*. Furthermore, the current parenteral killed whole-cell vaccine and oral vaccines under development, which are derived from *V. cholerae* O1, are likely to be of no benefit in protection. The incubation period in cholera is from a few hours to 5 days. There are no prodromal symptoms (a feature which is important in clinical diagnosis) and the onset is sudden. Mild diarrhoea rapidly gives way to the passage of large volumes of opalescent fluid – the classic 'rice water' stools. Vomiting of fluid occurs, and this is soon followed by clinical signs of severe dehydration associated with painful cramps of limb muscles and abdomen. Collapse from hypovolaemic shock may occur within a few hours, and the untreated patient may be dead within 24 h of onset. In an outbreak, for every case of classical cholera there will be ten or more cases with mild or asymptomatic infections.

Case history 1. Collapse associated with watery diarrhoea and vomiting
An 18-year-old African woman was admitted to hospital in a collapsed and semi-conscious state. According to her relatives, diarrhoea had started **suddenly** the previous day, and for 24 h she had been passing large quantities of 'rice-water' stool

and had been vomiting profusely. During the night she had complained of severe pains in the limbs and abdomen. On examination, she was markedly dehydrated, there was acidotic breathing and the systolic blood pressure was 60 mmHg. Cholera was suspected. A rectal swab was taken into alkaline peptone water, and characteristic colonies of *V. cholerae* were seen on TCBS culture medium the next day. In the meantime, she was rehydrated with intravenous fluids followed by oral rehydration solution and was given doxycycline 300 mg stat. She made an uneventful recovery.

Acute diarrhoea with fever and no blood

The main causes are infections with *Salmonella*, *Campylobacter* and *Shigella* species. The distinction between the three cannot be made clinically, although *Campylobacter* tends to cause more abdominal pain and more prolonged illness than the other two.

A clue to the presence of these invasive bacterial infections is the finding of leucocytes in faecal smears using a methylene blue stain. Other intestinal pathogens may be considered in certain situations: *Clostridium difficile* in association with previous antibiotics; *Plesiomonas shigelloides* and *Vibrio parahaemolyticus* after shell-fish consumption. Patients, and particularly children, should be carefully examined for evidence of systemic infection; infections include pneumonia, urinary tract infection, otitis media and tonsillitis. Other infections such as malaria, typhoid fever and septicaemia may all present with febrile diarrhoea, and blood films for malaria parasites and blood cultures should be taken.

Case history 2. Diarrhoea, abdominal pain and high fever

A 26-year-old African man was admitted to hospital with acute onset of liquid diarrhoea, abdominal pain and shivering. On examination, his temperature was 40.0°C and he had generalised abdominal tenderness. Blood films were negative for malaria parasites. After blood cultures were taken, he was treated for possible toxic salmonella gastroenteritis or typhoid fever with chloramphenicol. The following day he had a cough, and on examination he had evidence of right middle and lower lobe consolidation. Blood cultures grew *Streptococcus pneumoniae*, sensitive to penicillin. His therapy was changed to intravenous benzyl-penicillin. His diarrhoea resolved 24 h after starting benzylpenicillin and he made a full recovery from his pneumococcal pneumonia and bacteraemia.

Salmonella infections

There are more than 1700 different serotypes of *Salmonella* which can be broadly divided into two categories:

1. The serotypes responsible for 'food poisoning'. These are primarily parasites of animals. Only a small number of these serotypes account for human cases e.g. *S. enteritidis*, *S. typhimurium*, *S. virchow* etc.

2. The 'enteric fever' organisms such as *S. typhi* and *S. paratyphi* A, B, and C, which are almost exclusively human pathogens.

Food poisoning *Salmonella* infections are mainly acquired from infected food. A large number of organisms (10^6–10^9) is required to produce disease, which is probably why human to human transmission is rare and why spread is not usually from infected water supplies. Predisposition to infection and more serious illness occur at the extremes of life, in those with lowered immunity and in those with lowered gastric acidity. Salmonellae are invasive, affecting mainly the small intestine, but also occasionally the colon giving rise to bloody diarrhoea.

Blood stream invasion is unusual (less than 5 per cent of cases), but it should be suspected if there is a typhoidal-like illness or metastatic localisation in heart valves, meninges (neonates), joints and bones. In sub-Saharan Africa, *S. typhimurium* is responsible for a large proportion of bacteraemic illness in HIV-positive patients admitted to hospital with a febrile illness, and it is associated with a high mortality. A reactive arthropathy may occur in one or more large joints, especially in genetically predisposed individuals with human lymphocyte antigen (HLA)-B27. After infection, about 5 per cent of patients excrete salmonellae for more than 3 months. This is again more common at the extremes of life and after antibiotic administration. Excretors can act as sources of infection, and it is recommended that food handlers have three negative stool cultures after a proven episode of bacterial diarrhoea.

Enteric fever is endemic throughout the tropics. The source of infection is the faeces or urine of a patient or carrier, and water and food are important vehicles for the spread of infection. After ingestion, the organisms penetrate the intestinal mucosa and travel to the reticuloendothelial tissues. Multiplication occurs followed by bloodstream invasion which marks the onset of the clinical illness. Presentation is often as a pyrexia of unknown origin with very few clinical features. Diarrhoea may occur as the disease progresses. In the third week, about 5 per cent of patients may either develop intestinal haemorrhage (which presents as streaks of blood in the stool or copious melaena) or intestinal perforation. Diagnosis is made by blood culture, although in the second week of illness stool and urine culture may be positive. Serology is of limited value in diagnosis, particularly in a tropical setting.

Campylobacter infections

Campylobacters are found in a wide variety of animal hosts, particularly birds, and most human infections are contracted from infected food. The major enteric pathogen in humans is *C. jejuni*, although *C. coli*, *C. fetus* and *C. laridis* are also human pathogens. The infecting dose is around 10^4 organisms. Campylobacters are invasive and affect both small and large intestine. The acute diarrhoea usually lasts a few days, although symptoms can persist for 1–2 weeks and there may be blood and mucus in the stool. Abdominal pain is a characteristic feature, and it may be severe enough to suggest an acute surgical abdomen. Rarely the pain is a result of acute pancreatitis which can be diagnosed by serum amylase elevation and ultrasonography. Documented bacteraemia is unusual (less than 1 per cent), and chronic disease and carriage are rare. A reactive arthritis is said to affect about 1 per cent of patients. Rare complications include acute cholecystitis and erythema nodosum.

Case history 3. Severe abdominal pain and diarrhoea followed by arthritis
A 32-year-old Indian doctor was hospitalised with a 3-day history of diarrhoea with mucus, fever and severe central abdominal pain. On examination, his abdomen was diffusely tender with guarding; bowel sounds were present. A surgical opinion was requested. The surgical team suggested conservative management with a view to laparotomy if the abdominal signs deteriorated. There was no improvement 48 h after admission, but on that day the laboratory reported that *Campylobacter* spp. had grown in the stool culture. The patient was treated with intravenous followed by oral ciprofloxacin, and within 2 days of starting therapy he was beginning to show marked improvement. He was discharged home with no symptoms after completing 7 days of antibiotics. Two weeks later he was re-admitted with painful swelling of both knees and right ankle, and was diagnosed as having reactive arthropathy. Investigations showed no other cause for the arthropathy, and he was treated with non-steroidal anti-inflammatory drugs. The arthropathy continued for 12 months before it finally resolved.

Yersinia enterocolitica

This organism has emerged as a fairly common human pathogen in many countries in the world. Infection occurs from contaminated food, dairy products or raw pork. The organism invades the intestinal mucosa and multiplies in Peyer's patches.

In adults, an acute ileitis and mesenteric adenitis are common manifestations causing fever, diarrhoea and right lower abdominal pain which can mimic acute appendicitis. Extraintestinal manifestations include reactive arthritis and erythema nodosum.

Septicaemia may occur, usually in immunocompromised individuals. Diagnosis is by isolation of the organism from faeces or by the demonstration of rising agglutination titres in serum.

Clostridium difficile

Toxigenic *C. difficile* is now widely known as a cause of diarrhoea. The clinical features include asymptomatic carriage, mild to moderate diarrhoea, colitis, pseudomembranous colitis and toxic megacolon. The chain of events resulting in illness are disruption of the normal bacterial flora of the colon, colonisation with *C. difficile*, and release of toxins (toxin A and B) that cause mucosal damage and inflammation. Diarrhoea usually occurs during or after antibiotic therapy, but rarely it may occur in individuals who have not received antibiotics. The potential of this organism to spread from patient to patient in hospital, particularly through asymptomatic carriers, has recently become appreciated. Pseudomembranous colitis is the most dramatic presentation of this infection: there are marked systemic symptoms associated with diarrhoea (which can occasionally be bloody) and abdominal tenderness. Sigmoidoscopy reveals characteristic adherent yellow plaques (pseudomembranes), which vary in size from 2 mm to 10 mm, and a hyperaemic non-ulcerated intervening mucosa. The diagnosis of *C. difficile* infection depends on the demonstration of toxins in the stool. A tissue culture assay is the gold standard for toxin identification, although rapid immunoassays for the toxins are now commercially available. A positive stool culture for *C. difficile* is not a useful method of diagnosis, because some strains are non-toxigenic.

Case history 4. Acute bloody diarrhoea after treatment for quinsy
A 24-year-old Australian man was admitted to hospital with a right-sided quinsy. He was treated with intravenous benzyl-penicillin for 4 days, and discharged to take oral amoxicillin at home for 10 days. On the last day of his treatment, he developed fever, abdominal pain and diarrhoea which became mucoid and bloody. He was readmitted to hospital. Sigmoidoscopy revealed a hyperaemic rectal mucosa with a few adherent plaques. Pseudomembranous colitis was suspected. Stool examination showed the toxin of *Clostridium difficile*. He made a rapid recovery with metronidazole 400 mg three times a day for one week.

Acute diarrhoea with blood

Bloody diarrhoea with fever is usually caused by *Shigella*, and less commonly by *Campylobacter* and *Salmonella* spp. Other pathogens to consider are:

1. Enteroinvasive *E. coli* (EIEC) which causes a dysentery syndrome indistinguishable from shigellosis.
2. Enterohaemorrhagic *E. coli* of the serotype O157:H7 which produces a verocytotoxin, and may cause a severe bloody diarrhoea which can be complicated by the haemolytic–uraemic syndrome.
3. *Clostridium difficile*.
4. Acute schistosomiasis with *Schistosoma mansoni* or *Schistosoma japonicum* as part of the spectrum of Katayama fever – a clue to this diagnosis is the presence of an eosinophilia in an area where schistosomiasis is endemic.

   Bloody diarrhoea without fever is usually caused by invasive *Entamoeba histolytica*. A rare cause is colonic ulceration due to *Balantidium coli*, humans generally being infected from pigs.
   In small children who eat dirt, or in mentally subnormal patients in institutions, massive infection with *Trichuris trichiura* can cause bloody diarrhoea.

Shigella infections

Bacillary dysentery is caused by one of four species: *S. dysenteriae, S. sonnei, S. flexneri* and *S. boydii. S. sonnei* is the predominant species in industrialised countries, while in the tropics *S. dysenteriae* and *S. flexneri* are the predominant pathogens. The organism is most commonly transmitted by person to person contact, although bacterial contamination of food and water can result in point source outbreaks. There is also good evidence that houseflies can act as mechanical vectors of infection. Whatever the route, the spread is faecal-oral; as few as 10–100 organisms of the most virulent species, *S. dysenteriae* type 1, are sufficient to cause clinical dysentery in an otherwise healthy adult. Following a major epidemic of bacillary dysentery in Mexico and Central America in 1970 due to *S. dysenteriae* type 1, there have been many epidemics in Asia and Africa. The manifestations of the disease are due to invasion and ulceration of the colonic mucosa.

The incubation period is 2–4 days. The illness usually starts with fever followed by watery diarrhoea, then bloody diarrhoea and dysentery. The classic dysentery stool is composed only of a small amount of blood and mucus. In severe cases, stool frequency can be up to 100 times a day associated with abdominal cramps and tenesmus. Severe abdominal pain and tenderness can mimic acute appendicitis. Complications, both intestinal and systemic, are frequent. Toxic megacolon is a serious life-threatening condition, with a high mortality rate if perforation of the dilated gut occurs. A protein-losing enteropathy may occur which can lead to generalised oedema and ascites. Systemic complications include: meningism and convulsions in babies and children; Reiter's syndrome in those who are HLA-B27 positive; haemolytic-uraemic syndrome (mainly in children) or thrombotic thrombocytopaenic purpura (mainly in adults). Shigellae are excreted in the stools for a few weeks after illness, but chronic carriage is rare.

Amoebic dysentery

Amoebiasis is widespread throughout the tropics, and is caused by the protozoon *Entamoeba histolytica*. Amoebiasis is discussed in detail on pp 42–56. Infection is acquired through cysts ingested either from person-to-person contact or from infected food and water. The cysts are digested in the gut to release several small amoebic trophozoites. The main clinical differences between amoebic and bacillary dysentery are shown in Table 2.7. Amoeboma, stricture, perforation and haemorrhage may all complicate intestinal amoebiasis. Liver abscess may present acutely with fever, pain and tenderness in the right hypochondrium, or the presentation can be more insidious as a pyrexia of unknown origin.

The diagnosis of amoebic dysentery depends on finding haematophagous trophozoites (i.e. amoebae with ingested red cells in their cytoplasm) either in fresh stool specimens or rectal mucosal scrapes. In diarrhoea due to another cause, amoebic trophozoites may be found in the stools of a patient who was previously passing cysts, but these trophozoites do not contain red cells and are

Table 2.7 Amoebic and bacillary dysentery – clinical differences.

	Amoebic	Bacillary
Community	Sporadic	May be epidemic
Onset	Gradual	Acute
Prodromata	None	Common
Fever	None	Common
Prostration	None	Common
Vomiting	None	Common
Abdominal cramps	Mild	May be severe
Tenesmus	Uncommon	Common
Diarrhoea	Bloody	Bloody
	Faeculent	Watery

not invasive. Other methods of diagnosis include rectal biopsy and amoebic serology (the immunofluorescent antibody test IFAT is the commonest).

Case history 5. Bloody diarrhoea after travel to India
A 40-year-old British woman developed gradual onset of bloody diarrhoea after a 4-week holiday in India. Stool microscopy and culture performed by her general practitioner were reported as normal. She was seen in the outpatient department where on sigmoidoscopy she had several ulcers visible in the rectum. Rectal mucosal scrapes were performed, and the material was placed on a slide and at once examined in the microbiology laboratory; motile haematophagous trophozoites of *Entamoeba histolytica* were seen under the microscope. The woman made a good recovery with metronidazole 800 mg three times a day for 7 days.

Chronic diarrhoea

In patients with chronic diarrhoea, the usual infectious causes to be considered include tuberculosis of the small bowel, prolonged infestation of the gut by parasites such as *Giardia* and *Strongyloides*, and enteropathic AIDS. However, many of the infectious agents which have already been discussed have the potential to cause persistent diarrhoea. Mechanisms include: (1) interference with bowel absorption either as a result of damage to the mucosal brush border (disaccharidase deficiency) or the mucosa, or (2) continued increased secretion from the bowel because of bacterial toxins, inflammatory products, inflammatory reaction due to invasive pathogens or activation of the enteric nervous system. Pathogens implicated in chronic diarrhoea include *Escherichia coli*, salmonellae, *Shigella*, *Campylobacter*, *Aeromonas*, *Yersinia enterocolitica*, *Clostridium difficile*, rotavirus and *E. histolytica*.

Chronic bloody diarrhoea in the tropics may be due to *S. mansoni* or

S. japonicum (through large bowel granulomatous polyps) and amoebiasis.

Chronic diarrhoea in HIV-infected patients is discussed on pp 26 and 75–82.

Tuberculosis (pages 85–102)

Chronic diarrhoea, wasting and fever in the tropics used to be highly suggestive of tuberculosis, although enteropathic AIDS is now a much more common cause of this presentation. Ileocaecal tuberculosis is the predominant problem, and is either a sequel to disseminated tuberculosis or follows ulceration of the ileum from ingestion of infected sputum. Tuberculosis is suggested by productive cough, an abdominal mass in the right iliac fossa and ascites with or without palpable mesenteric lymph glands. Diagnosis may be difficult and requires radiology (barium follow-through or enema) and/or laparotomy. Acid fast bacilli are rarely found in the stool.

Giardiasis

Giardiasis is an infection of the small intestine with the flagellate protozoon *Giardia intestinalis*. Infection is acquired through ingesting cysts, usually via contaminated water. Cysts form trophozoites in the proximal small intestine, and these multiply by binary fission. Encystation occurs in the ileum and colon, and cysts are excreted in the faeces. The mechanism by which disease occurs is unclear, but there is often mucosal damage, an inflammatory infiltrate and associated small bowel bacterial overgrowth. Most patients are asymptomatic carriers. In a proportion of infected patients, acute small bowel diarrhoea results after an incubation period of 2 weeks, and in 20–30 per cent of these patients chronic diarrhoea and weight loss can ensue. Stools are typically pale, offensive, bulky and are accompanied by much flatus. Abdominal distension is common. Cysts are intermittently excreted, and detection by stool microscopy is therefore erratic. Trophozoites may be detected by duodenal aspiration or by using the 'hairy string' test, but often when no parasites are detected and the diagnosis strongly suspected, a therapeutic trial with metronidazole is warranted.

Strongyloidiasis

Infection with *Strongyloides stercoralis* occurs throughout the tropics, but especially in South-East Asia, West Africa and the Caribbean. *S. fulleborni* is found in Papua New Guinea and Central Africa, and may be associated with severe malabsorption and weight loss. Infection with the strongyloides nematode is usually caused by larval penetration of intact skin. Following a complex life cycle, the larvae reach the proximal small intestine where they live in the mucosa and crypts. Autoinfection can occur by larvae penetrating the perianal skin or bowel wall, and in this way infection can persist for more than 40 years. In the early stages of infection there may be an itchy eruption at the site of larval penetration, cough and wheeze due to larvae passing through the lungs, and upper abdominal pain and diarrhoea. Established strongyloidiasis is associated with the characteristic skin eruption of 'larva currens' and chronic intermittent diarrhoea. In immunosuppressed patients, a 'hyperinfection syndrome' can result whereby enormous numbers of larvae invade the body causing severe diarrhoea, paralytic ileus, Gram-negative septicaemia, serous effusions, meningitis and often death.

Diagnosis of strongyloidiasis by stool microscopy is difficult (because of intermittent excretion of larvae), and the most useful diagnostic test is the 'hairy string' test. Eosinophilia is a useful clue; in the hyperinfection syndrome peripheral eosinophils are not seen.

Case history 6. Chronic intermittent diarrhoea and skin eruptions

A 65-year-old man who had been a Far East Prisoner of War in Malaysia during the Second World War was seen in the outpatient clinic with a complaint of intermittent diarrhoea for 20 years. He also complained of an itchy, erythematous skin rash which appeared every 3 or 4 months in localised areas of his chest and abdomen; the rash lasted 1–2 weeks and then disappeared. He had a peripheral blood eosinophilia of 950 cells/mm³. Several stool specimens for microscopy were reported to be negative for ova, cysts and parasites. A 'hairy string' test was carried out, and the juice which was obtained from the upper small intestine was found to contain larvae of *Strongyloides stercoralis*. He was treated with albendazole 400 mg twice daily for 5 days. His skin rash never returned, but he continued to have intermittent diarrhoea which was finally explained on the basis of an irritable bowel syndrome.

Other parasites

Capillaria philippinensis is associated with diarrhoea and malabsorption in the Philippines and Thailand, and is acquired through ingestion of raw fish. *Fasciolopsis buski* is a trematode found in South-East Asia: man is infected by swallowing the infected metacercariae when eating water chestnuts and water caltrops. Both parasitic infections are diagnosed by finding eggs in the stool.

Chronic diarrhoea in HIV-infected patients

Chronic diarrhoea with weight loss ('slim disease') is a common clinical manifestation of HIV-infection in the tropics. In fact, diarrhoea for longer than 30 days is one of the major criteria of the World Health Organization for the diagnosis of AIDS in Africa. Published studies from Africa focusing on 'slim patients' have found that *Cryptosporidium* occurs in about 30 per cent and *Isospora belli* in 10–15 per cent of patients. Less than 5 per cent of patients respectively have *Giardia intestinalis*, *Strongyloides stercoralis*, and *Entamoeba histolytica*. Bacterial infections with salmonellae, *Shigella*, *Campylobacter* and mycobacteria are very uncommon. No aetiological agent is identified in

40–50 per cent of patients. There are various explanations for seemingly pathogen negative diarrhoea in HIV-positive patients (Table 2.8); the extent to which these are important in the tropics is unknown.

The commonest mode of presentation is with large volume, secretory diarrhoea associated with small bowel cramping, clinical signs of dehydration and evidence of malabsorption. *Cryptosporidium, Isospora belli* and *Microsporidium* are the likely pathogens in this setting.

The diagnosis of specific infections in HIV infected patients is discussed on pp 73–82 (see Chapter 5 and Table 2.9).

Miscellaneous presentations

These mainly include helminthic enteropathies which are summarised in Table 2.10. Diagnosis is largely by finding typical ova in the stool.

General management of diarrhoea

Rehydration

This is the essential component in the treatment of acute diarrhoeal disease. During the past decade, oral rehydration therapy (ORT) has become the mainstay of treatment for mild to moderate dehydration; intravenous fluids being reserved for severe dehydration and in cases where ORT has failed. WHO oral rehydration solution (ORS) (which is made up to one litre) consists of glucose 20 g, sodium chloride 3.5 g, sodium bicarbonate 2.5 g and potassium chloride 1.5 g. Substitution of glucose by other carbohydrates is sometimes more acceptable and cheaper; for example, ORS with rice powder at 30 g/l is just as good as standard ORS. If ORS is not available, then homemade sugar–salt solutions (4 heaped teaspoons of sugar to one level teaspoon of salt in 1 litre of water) can be used instead. In adults, ORS should be taken

Table 2.8 Causes of 'seemingly pathogen negative' diarrhoea in HIV-positive patients with chronic diarrhoea.

Inadequate number of stool samples for microscopy:
    Cryptosporidium; Isospora belli

Microsporidia

Viruses

Other mechanisms – small bowel overgrowth
                 – autonomic dysfunction
                 – disaccharidase deficiency
                 – HIV infection itself

Table 2.9 Therapeutic agents which have been tried in HIV-positive patients with Cryptosporidium.

Ineffective treatments

Antiparasitic drugs: – chloroquine

                                   – quinine

                                   – pyrimethamine

                                   – co-trimoxazole

Macrolide antibiotics: – spiramycin

Diclazuril (vetinerary compound)

Treatments which may be effective, but not yet proven

Macrolide antibiotics: – azithromycin

Paromomycin (non-absorbable aminoglycoside)

Octreotide (synthetic analogue of somatostatin)

Oral hyperimmune bovine colostrum

Table 2.10 Helminthic enteropathies.

Helminth	Clinical features
Ascaris lumbricoides	Visible worms Obstruction in small bowel, biliary tree, pancreatic duct
Hookworm	Iron-deficient anaemia
Whip worm (*Trichuris trichiura*)	Heavy infections only: bloody diarrhoea; rectal prolapse
Enterobius vermicularis	Perianal pruritus
Angiostrongylus costaricensis	Right iliac fossa mass (confined to central and South America)
Taenia saginata (beef tapeworm)	White motile proglottides in stool
Taenia solium (pork tapeworm)	White motile proglottides in stool Cysticercosis
Hymenolepis nana (dwarf tapeworm)	Mild gastrointestinal upset
Diphyllobothrium latum (fish tapeworm)	Vitamin B_{12} deficient anaemia

at the rate of 500–1000 ml/h until rehydration has been achieved. Maintenance therapy with ORS at 500–750 ml/h should be taken until diarrhoea ceases. It is important that both doctor and patient realise that ORT does not stop diarrhoea, and that continuation of diarrhoea does not imply failure of therapy. Intravenous fluids are best given as physiological solutions with potassium supplements.

Antibiotics

In the majority of cases of acute diarrhoea, antibiotics are not indicated because they do not influence the clinical course of the illness, the patient is exposed to possible side effects, the cost of treatment is increased and drug resistance is encouraged. Moreover, in *Salmonella* infections faecal carriage and excretion may be prolonged. However, there are certain situations where antibiotic treatment is indicated. Patients with diarrhoea who have a high fever and systemic toxicity, dysenteric disease and travellers' diarrhoea warrant empirical therapy Table 2.11. Antibiotics are also useful for milder forms of amoebiasis, *Campylobacter*, *Cholera*, giardiasis and a variety of other laboratory-defined enteropathogens Table 2.11. The treatments of helminthic enteropathies are summarised in Table 2.12.

Other measures

Antimotility and anti-emetic agents are generally not recommended in acute diarrhoea because they can interfere with the excretion of pathogens and toxins from the intestine. However, in immunosuppressed patients with chronic diarrhoea due to non-treatable pathogens such as *Cryptosporidium*, drugs such as kaolin, diphenoxylate, codeine, loperamide and morphine may have a useful antidiarrhoeal effect. Micronutrient supplements such as vitamin A and zinc may have a role in reducing duration of diarrhoea, particularly in malnourished children.

Prevention

Diarrhoeal disease can be largely prevented by education, a safe water supply and proper disposal of excreta and rubbish. Epidemiological research has demonstrated the reduction in gastrointestinal infection which may result from hygiene behaviour modifications such as washing of hands, washing of food and utensils, and the disposal of children's stools. It is now recognised that the quantity of water used by people is at least as important as the quality of that water in relation to diarrhoeal disease control. Fly control measures and limiting the access of flies to human faeces by 'VIP' (ventilated improved pit) latrines have reduced the transmission of shigellosis in communities at risk. Diarrhoeal disease burden could also be substantially reduced by the introduc-

Table 2.11 Antibiotic therapy for gastrointestinal infections.

Indication	Antibiotic	Dose (adults)	Duration (days)
Febrile, toxic	Chloramphenicol	500 mg q.d.s.	10–14 diarrhoea
	Co-trimoxazole	2 tabs b.d.	10–14
	Ciprofloxacin	500 mg b.d.	10–14
Febrile dysentery (includes shigellosis)	Co-trimoxazole	2 tabs b.d.	7
	Nalidixic acid	1 g q.d.s.	7
	Ciprofloxacin	500 mg b.d.	7
Traveller's diarrhoea (ETEC)	Co-trimoxazole	2 tabs b.d.	3
	Ciprofloxacin	500 mg b.d.	1–3
Campylobacter	Erythromycin	500 mg q.d.s.	5–7
	Ciprofloxacin	500 mg b.d.	5–7
Cholera	Tetracycline	500 mg q.d.s.	5
	Doxycycline	300 mg once	1
Clostridium difficile colitis	Metronidazole	400 mg t.d.s.	7
	Vancomycin	125 mg q.d.s.	7
Giardiasis	Metronidazole	400 mg t.d.s.	7
	Metronidazole	2 g daily	3
	Tinidazole	2 g once	1
Amoebiasis	Metronidazole	800 mg t.d.s.	7
Isosporiasis	Co-trimoxazole	2 tabs q.d.s.	10
Microsporidiosis	Metronidazole	400 mg t.d.s.	14
	Albendazole	400 mg b.d.	28
Balantidium coli	Tetracycline	500 mg q.d.s.	10

b.d. = twice a day; t.d.s. = three times a day; q.d.s. = four times a day
Co-trimoxazole tablets = 80 mg trimethoprim plus 400 mg sulphamethoxazole

tion of enteric vaccines. Oral vaccines against typhoid fever (Ty21a) and cholera (using killed whole vibrios alone or in combination with purified B subunit) give approximately 60 per cent protection against their target diseases in rural communities. Several vaccine candidates against enterotoxigenic *E. coli*, enteropathogenic *E. coli*, *Shigella* and rotavirus are in preparation. These will not completely prevent an infection from becoming established, but used together with existing or upgraded public health measures the disease burden and childhood mortality from diarrhoeal pathogens could be significantly reduced.

Table 2.12 Treatment of helminthic enteropathies.

Helminth	Therapy: dose and duration (adults)
Ascaris lumbricoides	Piperazine hydrate 75 mg/kg daily 2 days
Hookworm	Pyrantel pamoate 10 mg/kg once Bephenium hydroxynaphthoate 5 g once Mebendazole 100 mg b.d. 3 days Levamisole 2.5 mg/kg once Albendazole 400 mg once
Trichuris trichiura	Mebendazole 100 mg b.d. 3 days Levamisole 2.5 mg/kg Albendazole 400 mg once
Enterobius vermicularis	Mebendazole 100 mg once and repeated after 2 weeks Albendazole 400 mg once
Strongyloides stercoralis	Albendazole 400 mg b.d. 3–5 days Thiabendazole 25 mg/kg b.d. 3 days
Capillaria	Thiabendazole 25 mg/kg b.d. 30 days Mebendazole 200 mg b.d. 20 days
Taenia saginata *Taenia solium* *Hymenolepis nana* *Diphyllobothrium latum*	Niclosamide 1 g taken twice 1 h apart Praziquantel 25 mg/kg once
Schistosoma mansoni *Schistosoma japonicum* *Fasciolopsis buski*	Praziquantel 40 mg/kg once Praziquantel 60 mg/kg once Praziquantel 15 mg/kg once

b.d. = twice a day

Further reading

Alam AN, Alam NH, Ahmed T, Sack DA. Randomised double blind trial of single dose doxycycline for treating cholera in adults. BMJ 1990;300:1619–21.

Bell DR. Lecture notes in tropical medicine. Oxford: Blackwell Scientific Publications, 1990.

Char S, Farthing MJG. DNA probes for diagnosis of intestinal infection. GUT 1991;32:1–3.

Cohen D, Green M, Block C *et al*. Reduction of transmission of shigellosis by control of houseflies (*Musca domestica*). Lancet 1991;337:993–7.

Cook GC. Tropical gastroenterology. Oxford: Oxford University Press, 1980.

Curry A, Canning EU. Human microsporidiosis. J Infect 1993;27:229–36.

Dallabetta GA, Miotti PG. Chronic diarrhoea in AIDS patients in the tropics: a review. Trop Doct 1992;22:3–9.

DuPont HL, Ericsson CD. Prevention and treatment of traveller's diarrhoea. N Engl J Med 1993;328:1821–7.

Enenkel S, Stille W. Antibiotics in the tropics. Berlin: Springer-Verlag, 1988.

Gorbach SL. Bacterial diarrhoea and its treatment. In Infection today. A Lancet Review, 1988:31–42.

Grohmann GS, Glass RI, Pereira HG *et al.* Enteric viruses and diarrhoea in HIV-infected patients. N Engl J Med 1993;329:14–20.

Guerrant RL. Baillière's Clin Trop Med Com Dis 1988. Diarrhoeal diseases.

Hibbs RG. Diarrhoeal disease: current concepts and future challenges. Trans R Soc Trop Med Hyg 1993;87 (Suppl 3):1–53.

Kelly CP, Pothoulakis C, LaMont JT. *Clostridium difficile* colitis. N Engl J Med 1994; 330:257–62.

Mandal BK. Epidemic cholera due to a novel strain of *V. cholerae* non-O1 – the beginning of a new epidemic? J Infect 1993;27:115–17.

Pape JW, Verdier R, Johnson WD. Treatment and prophylaxis of *Isospora belli* in patients with the acquired immunodeficiency syndrome. N Engl J Med 1989; 320:1044–7.

Petersen C. Cryptosporidiosis in patients infected with the human immunodeficiency virus. Clin Infect Dis 1992;15:903–9.

3

Specific Infections Causing Diarrhoea

Cholera

Cholera is a bacterial infection of man caused by *Vibrio cholerae* (of classical or El Tor biotypes) which characteristically causes severe diarrhoea, and death (in those severely affected) from water and electrolyte depletion. Spread is directly from person to person by the faecal–oral route, or indirectly by infected food or water. The disease spreads easily and is endemic in areas of the world where environmental sanitation and personal hygiene are low. Man is the only reservoir of infection. The El Tor biotype has now largely displaced classical cholera as the major pathogen of public health importance.

Clinical presentation

The incubation period usually lasts 1–5 days. This is followed by an acute onset of diarrhoea. After the colon has been evacuated of faecal material, profuse painless, watering diarrhoea follows. Typically the stools are watery, white and flecked with mucus and this has been referred to as 'rice-water stool'. In 80 per cent of cases, vomiting follows soon after the diarrhoea. Fever is unusual except in children and is short-lived. The temperature is usually subnormal when the patient is first seen. The illness is self-limiting and diarrhoea ceases in a week if the patient survives.

Changes in fluid and electrolytes

Dehydration is caused by the profuse diarrhoea, compounded by the inability to retain fluids by mouth. Collapse with hypovolaemic shock may occur within a few hours of the onset, and the untreated patient may die within 24 h.

Cramps of the muscles of the limbs and abdomen are a typical feature of

33

severe cases. They are painful and result from reduction in the concentration of calcium and chloride ions.

The specific toxin 'choleragen' produced by the multiplying vibrios in the small intestine causes a breakdown of the functional barrier between the intestinal epithelium and the blood. The result is an outpouring of protein-free fluid with an electrolyte composition similar to that of plasma although the potassium (average 13 mmol/l) and bicarbonate average 44 mmol/l) concentrations are both higher than in the plasma. The values both refer to adults. In children the potassium loss is twice as great. In children the loss of water is relatively more than the loss of electrolytes resulting in hypertonic dehydration.

Diagnosis

Clinical diagnosis is only possible in classical cases with profuse, painless diarrhoea, rice-water stools, gross dehydration and muscle cramps. Very rarely do other infections produce this picture. A definite diagnosis can only be made by isolating the organism.

Direct diagnosis by microscopy

In severe cases the watery stool contains cholera vibrios in almost pure culture. They can be recognised with a high degree of confidence by darkfield examination of a wet preparation. Identification can be confirmed by adding specific antiserum which immobilises the vibrios immediately. In milder cases and asymptomatic cases microscopic identification is much more difficult. Fluorescence microscopy, using a fluoroscein-conjugated specific anti-cholera serum is more sensitive than darkfield microscopy but less widely available.

Direct diagnosis by culture

Various media are used for primary isolation, among the best being TCBS (thiosulphate-citrate-bile-salts-sucrose) agar. Small numbers of vibrios can only be detected using an enriched liquid medium such as alkaline peptone water. The specimen is best taken by a sterile rubber catheter inserted into the anus or by a rectal swab. Specimens taken in the field can be transported to the laboratory in sealed plastic bags or after inoculation into a holding medium.

Indirect diagnosis

After recovery from an attack of cholera, various antibodies appear in the serum. Provided cholera vaccine has not been given previously this may allow a retrospective diagnosis to be made by serological tests. This has no clinical importance and is only of use in epidemiological studies.

Management

Initial rehydration and resuscitation

Rehydration is the mainstay of cholera treatment. In severe cases with hypovolaemic shock, the restoration of blood volume is a matter of extreme urgency and this can only be achieved by rapid intravenous infusion. A central line is usually necessary since the peripheral veins are collapsed in such patients.

Fluid in the initial stages is run in as quickly as possible: an initial rate of 4 l/h for the first few litres is the norm in adults. The best guide to success is the return of a palpable arterial pulse. As soon as the systolic blood pressure reaches 90 mmHg, renal function usually returns.

Choice of rehydration fluid

Patients usually have a metabolic acidosis due to bicarbonate loss, a deficiency of potassium and a loss of water greater than of salts. A slightly hypotonic alkaline fluid enriched with potassium is the most suitable physiological choice. The single fluid that meets all these needs and is suitable for both adults and children is Ringer lactate solution, BP. This contains sodium 131 mmol/l, potassium 5 mmol/l, calcium 2 mmol/l, lactate 27 mmol/l and chloride 11 mmol/l. It is suitable for both the initial rehydration and maintenance therapy.

Maintenance rehydration

When the patient has been resuscitated, careful charting of fluid intake and output must be done. The uncontrollable watery diarrhoea will often continue for several days. To measure this accurately it is best for the patient to be nursed on a special 'cholera cot', a frame bed covered in rubber sheeting with a hole in the middle, to allow the fluid escaping from the anus to be funnelled into a calibrated collecting bucket below. The urine output must also be charted accurately. The period of maintenance parenteral fluid can be shortened by tetracycline administration and early resumption of oral rehydration with sugar–electrolyte solution.

Oral rehydration with glucose–electrolyte solution

This should be given frequently, but in small amounts. The following solution is suitable for oral rehydration of adults and children.

In 1 litre of sterile water:-

dextrose (glucose)	20 g
sodium chloride	3.5 g
sodium bicarbonate	2.5 g
potassium chloride	1.5 g

If glucose is not available, sucrose can be used instead but the dose should be increased to 40 g, as it generates only half its weight of glucose on hydrolysis. Various pre-packaged commercial preparations are available in sachets and have obvious advantages.

The dosage of the oral rehydration solution depends on the severity of the diarrhoea. In severe continuing diarrhoea the dose should be 15 ml/kg per hour, in frequent divided doses. In mild to moderate cases a dose of 5–10 ml/kg per hour is recommended.

Tetracycline

Tetracycline is given to cholera patients as soon as vomiting stops. The normal adult dose is 500 mg 6 hourly for 3 days. This shortens the duration of the diarrhoea and the stools should be free of vibrios within 24–48 h, in contrast to 7 days in untreated cases. Furazolidone 400 mg daily for 3 days is equally effective.

Prevention

This depends on improving standards of environmental sanitation. The treatment of carriers and known contacts is relatively unimportant. Cholera vaccine has no significant part to play in controlling the disease. Vaccination gives perhaps 50 per cent immunity for up to 6 months but the disease is not of reduced severity when it develops in vaccinated individuals. Administration of the cholera vaccine is no longer recommended for travellers to endemic areas.

Typhoid and paratyphoid fevers (enteric fevers)

Enteric fevers are caused by *Salmonella typhi* and *S. paratyphi*: A, B and C. They are characterised by a systemic septicaemic illness. Typhoid and paratyphoid organisms are commonest where standards of personal and environmental hygiene are low. The causal organisms are all Gram-negative bacilli with flagellae. They possess somatic (O) and flagellar (H) antigens. *S. typhi* and *S. paratyphi* C sometimes possess a surface (Vi) antigen that coats the O antigen and potentially protects it from antibody attack.

Patients with typhoid and paratyphoid fever are encountered in all parts of the world, but are now found mainly in those countries of the developing world where sanitary conditions are poor.

Although there is little reliable information on the incidence, morbidity and mortality of enteric fever in the countries of the developing world, reports from Central and South America, Sub-Saharan and North Africa, the Middle East, the Indian subcontinent and Southeast Asia indicate that typhoid is still a major problem.

Pathogenesis of typhoid fever

Infection is transmitted in water (*S. typhi*) and food, and is largely dose-related. All these organisms can multiply in suitable foods maintained at a favourable temperature, and so greatly enhance the efficiency of human food-handlers in transmitting the infection. The most important reservoirs of infection are asymptomatic human carriers.

After ingestion, the organisms attach to the small intestinal mucosa, penetrate it, and are transported by the lymphatics to the mesenteric lymph glands. There they multiply and enter the blood stream via the thoracic duct. The main location of bacilli is inside the macrophages. From this bacteraemia, which corresponds to the end of the incubation period, the organisms are carried to the bone marrow, spleen, liver and gall bladder.

Following this there is a secondary invasion of the bowel via the infected bile. Organisms multiply in macrophages, and the pathological changes are greatest where macrophages are present in large numbers such as in the intestinal lymph follicles. The largest of these are Peyer's patches in the ileum.

At this time there is a strong inflammatory response with infiltration by inflammatory cells (macrophages and lymphocytes) and the Peyer's patches become hyperplastic. If the inflammation does not resolve, necrosis occurs within 7–10 days and the patches ulcerate. Involvement of the blood vessels may lead to bleeding, and if the whole of the bowel is involved, perforation follows.

The natural course of the disease is variable. In a 'classical' case fever subsides at the end of the third week and repair processes begin. In some cases, however, fever may continue for weeks while in others the course is brief and unspectacular. Death most commonly occurs from perforation, haemorrhage or toxaemia and rarely from complications such as meningitis.

Much of the pathology in various organs of the body is due to the obvious local inflammatory response to the bacilli, as in the gut. But serious disease of the brain, lung, and kidneys is not usually accompanied by typhoid nodule formation. It has been speculated that the cause is some unidentified toxin. *S. typhi* endotoxin does not seem to be the cause.

Clinical presentation

The incubation period is 2 weeks but can vary from 1 to 3 weeks. The most common symptoms are fever and headache. The untreated illness normally lasts 3 weeks but could last longer. The fever is of the remittent type. Patients with typhoid often feel unwell with malaise, anorexia and generalised aches. The following symptoms also commonly occur: abdominal pain/discomfort, constipation, diarrhoea and cough. In Papua New Guinea the diarrhoea is often accompanied by blood, and neurological manifestations such as deafness or cerebellar ataxia may occur.

The physical signs depend on both the severity of illness and the length of time the patient has been ill. In the early stages the patient looks relatively well and is mentally alert. In contrast, a patient who has been ill for 2 weeks often has serious toxaemia, is mentally stuporous and gravely dehydrated. The pulse rate is relatively slow compared with the fever and may not reach 100 even when the temperature is 40°C. The commonest signs are: fever, a disproportionately slow pulse, hepatomegaly, splenomegaly (often tender), mental changes, signs of bronchitis, rose spots, meningism and deafness.

Complications

Complications may develop as the illness progresses and may follow a clinically mild attack. So the clinician must remember that patients with typhoid may present with the complication itself rather than symptoms of typhoid fever. These patients are often difficult diagnostic problems and a high index of suspicion is required.

Practice point
• *Typhoid patients may present with a complication rather than the disease itself.*

1. **Perforation** This typically occurs in the third week. Patients with toxaemia show few signs of peritonitis, except for abdominal distension, increasing toxaemia and a rising pulse. Surgery gives a better chance of survival than conservative management (pp 377–379).
2. **Haemorrhage** also tends to occur in the third week. There may be massive bleeding or repeated small bleeds. Surgery is seldom needed provided blood transfusion is available.
3. **Haemolytic anaemia** is common in patients with G6PD deficiency and typhoid depresses G6PD levels in normal as well as in deficient patients.
4. **Typhoid lobar pneumonia** is a rare complication occurring in the second and third week of the illness. Rusty sputum is not produced.
5. **Meningitis** may be the only obvious manifestation of typhoid, when it resembles other causes of bacterial meningitis.

6. **Renal disease** may present as renal failure or an acute nephrotic syndrome, and is probably an immune-complex nephritis. Recovery after successful chemotherapy is usual.
7. **Typhoid abscess** is a late complication that can occur almost anywhere, especially in the spleen, liver, brain and skeletal system.
8. **Skeletal complications** include suppurative arthritis and osteomyelitis. Either may have a delayed onset. Pyomyositis can also occur.
9. **Other complications or sequelae** include suppurative parotitis, myocarditis, acute cholecystitis, deep venous thrombosis and the Guillain–Barré syndrome.

Diagnosis

Culture

Culture of the organism is the mainstay of diagnosis. Unfortunately some hospitals in the developing countries may not have this facility.

Blood culture is the most useful investigation in the first week, but may also be positive later. Marrow culture is more likely to be positive (95 per cent *versus* 43 per cent) even after chemotherapy has been started.

Stool culture often becomes positive in the second week or earlier if the patient has diarrhoea. More recently a string capsule used to sample duodenal contents has been shown to have higher positive rate than blood culture (86 per cent *versus* 42 per cent).

Urine culture becomes positive in about 25 per cent of cases after the second week, but its main use is in the detection of urinary carriers.

Other materials, such as aspirates from rose spots, cerebrospinal fluid or pus from abscesses may also yield positive culture results.

Serodiagnosis

The most widely used test is the Widal test which measures agglutinating antibodies to the somatic 'O' and flagellar 'H' antigens. The test is usually non-specific because numerous non-typhoid salmonellae share 'O' and 'H' antigens with *S. typhi*. In addition a significant number of culture-positive patients develop no rise in titre and in those where there is a rise, the titres often rise before the clinical onset making it difficult to demonstrate the 'diagnostic' four-fold rise between the initial and subsequent specimens.

So the Widal test has many pitfalls but if the test is interpreted intelligently, a significant number of patients will be correctly diagnosed by the Widal test when other methods have failed.

Other laboratory findings

The white blood count is usually normal but leucopenia may occur. Leucocytosis can also occur particularly if complications are present. A relative lymphocytosis is common.

Biochemical tests normally show minor changes, such as slight elevation of transaminases and bilirubin.

Management

General care

Good nursing care is essential for patients who are often critically ill and mentally unco-operative when first admitted. Good supportive care including the maintenance of fluid and electrolyte balance is essential. However the mainstay of specific treatment is antimicrobial chemotherapy and management of complications.

Antibiotic therapy

Chloramphenicol used to be the drug of choice, but in recent years resistance has become a major problem. For example, in Bangkok almost half of all strains are chloramphenicol-resistant and significant numbers are also resistant to ampicillin and co-trimaxole.

Chloramphenicol

A prolonged course must be given to prevent relapse; a total of 14 days, or 12 days after fever has subsided. The dose is 1 g 6-hourly to 0.5 g 4-hourly until the patient is afebrile, followed by 500 mg 6-hourly for 10–12 days. It commonly takes 48 h before the fever shows a response and 5 days or more before the patient becomes completely afebrile.

Amoxycillin

This drug is much more expensive than chloramphenicol, but is equally effective if given in high doses. It must be given for chloramphenicol resistance in a dose 500 mg to 1 g 6-hourly for 14–21 days. Ampicillin is not as effective as chloramphenicol.

Co-trimoxazole

The dose is 2 tablets 8-hourly until afebrile, then 2 tablets 12-hourly for 10 days. The clinical response is at least as rapid as with chloramphenicol.

Ciprofloxacin

Ciprofloxacin is being used in some developed countries but is expensive. The dose is 750 mg b.d. for 10–14 days. It may be effective in shorter courses but this has not been proved.

Steroids

One small study has shown high dose dexamethasone (3 mg/kg) to be beneficial but moderate doses of hydrocortisone are not. The use of steroids is one of personal preference but perforation has proved to be a problem so steroids should be avoided in the third week of illness.

Carrier state

This commonly occurs for some months into the convalescence period and when it terminates spontaneously such patients are called convalescent carriers. They are an obvious source of infection to others during those months but an even more important source are chronic carriers (1–3 per cent of cases) in which a persisting focus of infection smoulders on in the gallbladder (faecal carriers) or urinary tract (urinary carriers).

Treatment of chronic carriers

Co-trimoxazole 2 tablets twice daily for 3 months is the most cost-effective treatment. Ampicillin and amoxycillin in high dosage for the same length of time combined with probenecid, may also be effective. Faecal carriers with gallstones or cholecystitis only respond to chemotherapy temporarily and cholecystectomy is indicated to terminate the carrier state.

Typhoid vaccine

The old TAB vaccine contained paratyphoid organisms also but was never proved to provide worthwhile immunity to the paratyphoids, and often produced severe reactions. A monovalent vaccine using killed *S. typhi* organisms is now most widely used.

The first dose is 0.5 ml subcutaneously and this gives protection for 6 months. If long-term (3 year) protection is needed, a booster dose of 0.1 ml intradermally is given 1 month later. These two doses constitute the 'primary course'. Immunity can be maintained by repeating booster closes every 3 years. Immunity begins to develop 10 days after the first dose. The degree of protection given by the vaccine is 90 per cent.

Paratyphoid fever

Paratyphoid A and B

These usually infect via contaminated foods in which the organisms have multiplied. Diarrhoea and vomiting may precede septicaemia. Many mild cases occur. Treatment is as for typhoid.

Paratyphoid C

This produces septicaemia without involvement of the gut and abscess formation is common. Treatment is as for typhoid.

Amoebiasis

Entamoeba histolytica, an enteric pathogen, is the causative agent of amoebiasis. This protozoan is the third leading parasitic cause of morbidity and mortality in the developing world. Approximately 10 per cent of the world's population is infected by the parasite. Disease usually manifests as colitis or liver abscess and is largely confined to infected individuals either living in or with a history of travel to subtropical or tropical areas.

Life cycle

Trophozoites of *E. histolytica* range in size from 10 to 50 μm and are uninucleate. Cysts are the infective stage of the parasite; these are 12–17 μm in size and have between one and four nuclei. After ingestion the cysts excyst in the small intestine to release trophozoites which infect the colon. Trophozoites do not play any role in disease transmission because they cannot survive outside the body due to their sensitivity to changes in temperature and humidity and furthermore once ingested are destroyed by gastric acidity. Mature cysts may survive for up to 2 months in water and cool, damp conditions.

Epidemiology

Transmission of cysts occurs via the faecal–oral route. Cysts can survive for about 10 min on the surface of hands and even longer under fingernails. Infected material can readily be transmitted from one person to another when personal hygiene is not observed. In such situations intrafamilial spread results in the clustering of infection; higher infection rates are also seen in mental institutions. The ingestion of faecally contaminated water or vegetables is also implicated in parasite transmission. Absence of proper sanitation facilities, in part due to cultural rejection of latrines, results in contamination of water supplies after heavy rains. Use of human waste as agricultural fertiliser may also facilitate transmission.

In developing countries, which are tropical or subtropical, the damper conditions favour cyst survival. This together with poverty, overcrowding, poor sanitation and hygiene result in higher prevalence of infection, reaching 50 per cent in some areas of Mexico and India. Low prevalence of infection is observed in developed countries; here, infection tends to be more common in the lower socioeconomic groups, immigrants from developing countries and male homosexuals.

There is now abundant evidence indicating the existence of pathogenic and non-pathogenic strains of *E. histolytica*. These strains were initially distinguished by characteristic isoenzymes. More recently, pathogenic strains have been shown to be resistant to lysis by human complement and can be further characterised from non-pathogens by unique monoclonal antibodies and distinct differences in genomic and ribosomal DNA sequences. Pathogenic *E. histolytica* is always associated with invasive disease or seropositive asymptomatic carriers. Non-pathogenic strains exist as commensals even in patients with severe immunosuppression of the acquired immunodeficiency syndrome. It is now accepted that previous observations of *in vitro* conversion of a non-pathogenic strain to a pathogenic one was due to incomplete cloning of the amoeba used.

Pathogenesis and pathology

Adherence of *E. histolytica* to colonic mucins is mediated by a lectin-like adherence molecule on the surface of the parasite. This adhesion also facilitates attachment of the amoeba to colonic epithelium, leukocytes and other cells. Contact with target cell results in lysis of the host cell. Lysed leukocytes release proteolytic enzymes that contribute to tissue damage. In addition, proteolytic enzymes are also released by *E. histolytica* which further damages tissue. The parasite also has enterotoxigenic properties which may be causally related to the diarrhoeal symptoms of colonic disease.

There is now evidence that after tissue invasion the trophozoites invade blood vessels causing a vasculitis with subsequent thrombosis and infarction. This leads to the sharply demarcated lesions seen in transmural colitis. Involvement of the vasa brevis causes an irregular patch of necrosis; triangular ischaemia is due to vas longum thrombosis and kissing ulcers have been described with longum trunk ischaemia. Affected areas become occluded by omental wraps which prevent gross peritoneal soiling. Subsequent healing is effected by neovascularisation and re-epithelialisation. This process is invariably associated with stenosis of the affected segment.

Amoebae reach the liver via the portal vein. The 'liver abscess' is in fact an area of liquefactive necrosis caused by a combination of contact mediated lysis of hepatocytes, proteolytic enzymes released by amoebae and leukocytes and infarction due to thrombosis of portal vein radicles.

It is not yet known to what extent immunological responses protect against reinfection. Reports from Mexico indicate that recurrence of amoebic liver abscess is rare. An Indian study showed that subjects with anti-amoebic antibodies have a lower incidence of intestinal colonisation with *E. histolytica*. Ninety-six per cent of patients with invasive amoebiasis have an antibody response to the galactose-inhibitable lectin described above. Gerbils immunised with this lectin were successfully protected from developing liver abscess after intrahepatic challenge. Cell mediated immunity may play a role in preventing reinfection. In patients with invasive amoebiasis, T-lymphocytes become sensitised to amoebic antigen; these lymphocytes exhibit cytotoxic activity and are capable of producing γ-interferon upon antigen challenge. Exacerbation of disease with concurrent corticosteroid therapy also indicates a role for protective immunity in limiting disease progression.

Clinical manifestations and complications

Intestinal disease

Carriage of non-pathogenic *E. histolytica* strains does not result in clinical disease. Mild diarrhoea in such patients can usually be attributed to other intestinal pathogens. Mucosal invasion by pathogenic strains presents as dysentery which is of gradual onset. These patients may also complain of abdominal pain and tenesmus and only a third of them will have fever. Less commonly, patients may have an intermittent mucoid diarrhoea (non-dysenteric colitis), abdominal pain, flatulence and weight loss.

Transmural disease presents acutely with signs of bacterial peritonitis occurring secondary to bowel perforation. Patients usually have a profuse bloody diarrhoea and toxaemia and are hypotensive and febrile. Some patients develop a slow leak from the site of perforation; this tends to become walled off by omental wraps resulting in an abdominal mass. Toxic megacolon and intestinal haemorrhage are less common presentations of transmural colitis.

Perianal disease may result from direct extension of mucosal disease to the skin or from a fistulous tract. The lesions are either ulcerative or condylomatous and manifest as pain or bleeding.

Extra-intestinal disease

The commonest presentation is with liver abscess. Pain is the principal symptom and is usually of a pleuritic nature. The discomfort is frequently in the right upper quadrant of the abdomen or right lower chest. Epigastric pain occurs with involvement of the left lobe. Pain is occasionally referred to the shoulder tip when the abscess encroaches on to the diaphragm. Anorexia, weight loss, fever and cough are all common symptoms. Concomitant dysentery occurs in only 10 per cent of cases. Patients are usually febrile and have a tender hepatomegaly; jaundice is infrequent. When the abscess is located high up against the diaphragm there may be no apparent hepatomegaly; chest signs including an impaired percussion note, decreased breath sounds, crackles and a pleural rub may be present. Point tenderness over a palpable hepatomegaly and intercostal tenderness are useful clinical signs.

Extension of an abscess into the pleural space may be preceded by a sympathetic effusion. Rarely, direct extension into the lungs could result in a lung abscess or bronchohepatic fistula. Left lobe abscesses may rupture into the pericardium and manifest as retrosternal pain or cardiac tamponade. Rupture into the abdominal cavity produces peritonitis or a walled off abscess. Secondary bacterial infection is a serious complication which only occurs subsequent to percutaneous aspiration of an initially sterile abscess.

Diagnosis

Dysentery due to intestinal amoebiasis is difficult to differentiate from bacillary dysentery. Ulcers can be identified in 80 per cent of patients by sigmoidoscopic examination. Demonstration of haematophagus trophozoites in freshly voided stools or rectal scrape is central to confirming the diagnosis. Leukocytes are scanty and Charcot–Leyden crystals may be identified on stool microscopy. Examination of wet mount stool specimens is most helpful. Alternatively, smears may be fixed in Schaudinn's solution or polyvinyl alcohol and stained with either iron-haematoxylin, trichrome or Sargeaunt's solution for later examination.

Amoebic liver abscess must be differentiated from pyogenic liver abscess and other causes of tender hepatomegaly such as primary or secondary neoplasms and subphrenic abscess as well as gallbladder disease, pseudocyst, hepatobiliary ascariasis and hydatid cyst. Ultrasound scan demonstrates a hypoechoic lesion with an irregular margin (Figures 3.1a, b, c); the hepatic defect persists for a variable period after successful treatment. Gas within a pyogenic abscess shows up as bright echoes on ultrasound (Figure 3.4) and hepatic tumours are hyperechoic (Figure 3.5). Radioisotope scan demonstrates a space occupying lesion and does not differentiate hepatic amoebiasis from other liver lesions. Anaemia (normocytic, normochromic), mild to moderate leukocytosis, hypoalbuminaemia and mildly elevated transaminases and alkaline phosphatase are also present.

The amoebic 'pus' is bacteriologically sterile with scanty leukocytes; *E. histolytica* may occasionally be identified.

Anti-amoebic antibodies can be detected in up to 98 per cent of patients with invasive disease. A number of serological tests are available; however none of them can presently identify active disease since antibodies persist for years after clinical cure. A negative test is of value in excluding disease.

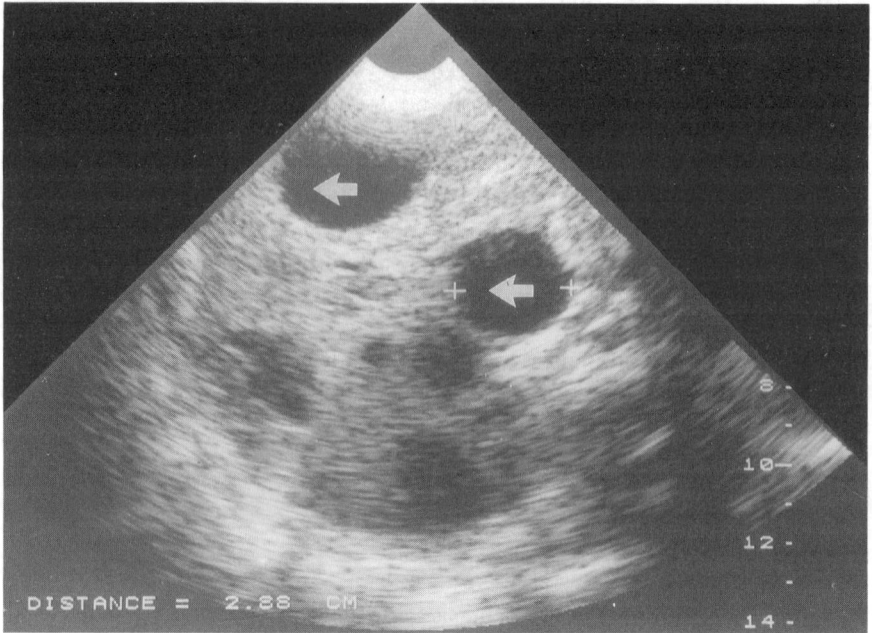

(a) Multiple abscesses – arrows indicate hypoechoic lesions.

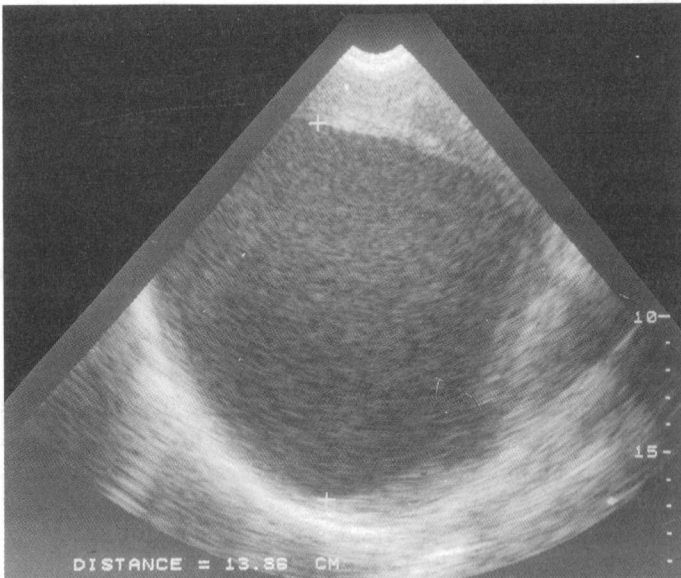

(b) Large abscess with slightly less dense echoes than surrounding liver tissue.

Figure 3.1   Ultrasound features of amoebic liver abscess.

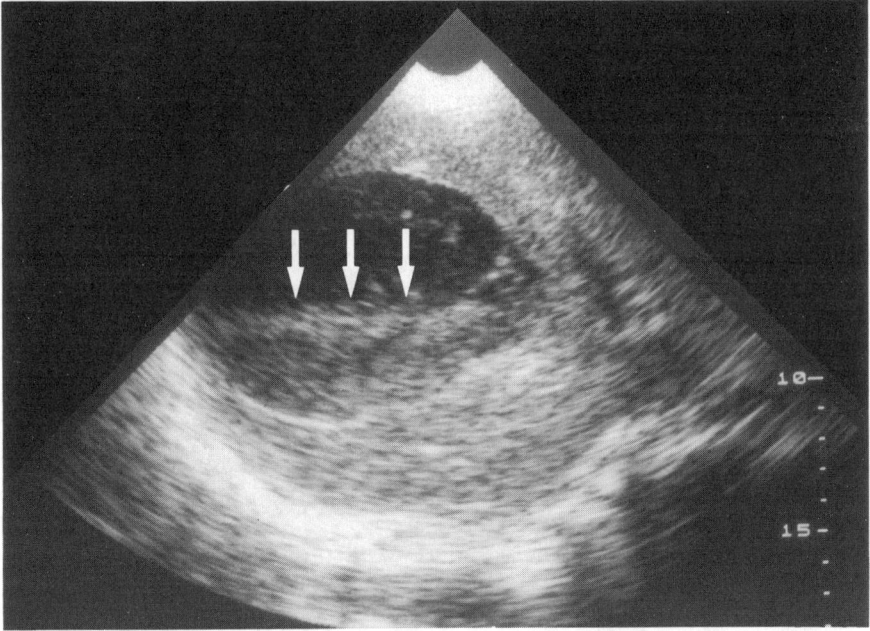

(c) Large abscess – the debris within has gravitated resulting in an echo level (arrows).

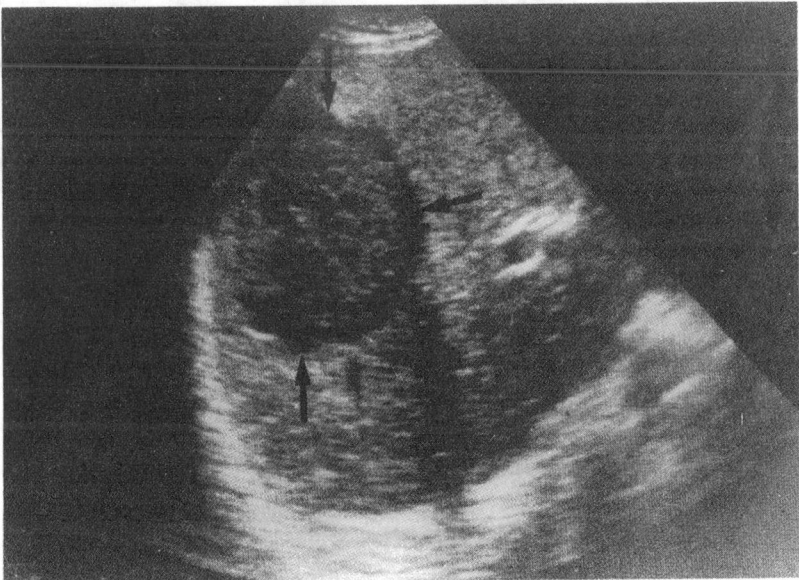

(d) Large abscess – early lesion showing a hypodense area ('halo') circumscribing the abscess.

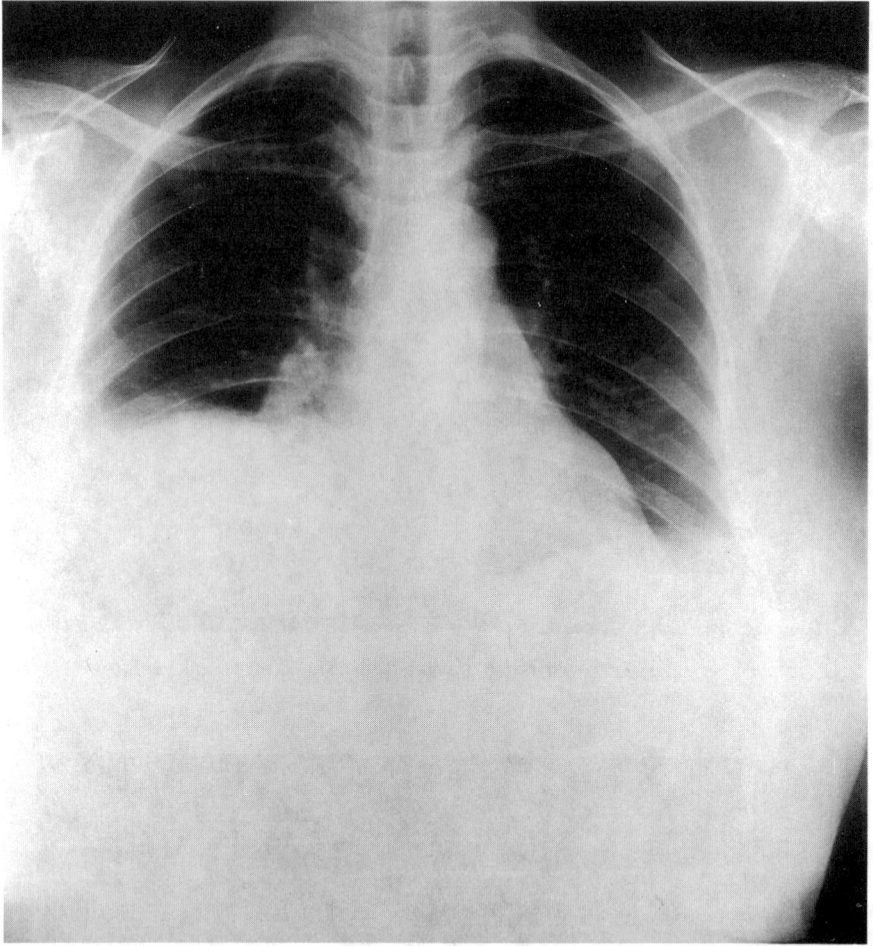

(a) Chest X-ray showing elevated right diaphragm. There is blunting of right costophrenic angle indicating a pleural effusion.

Figure 3.2   Pleural complications of amoebic liver abscess.

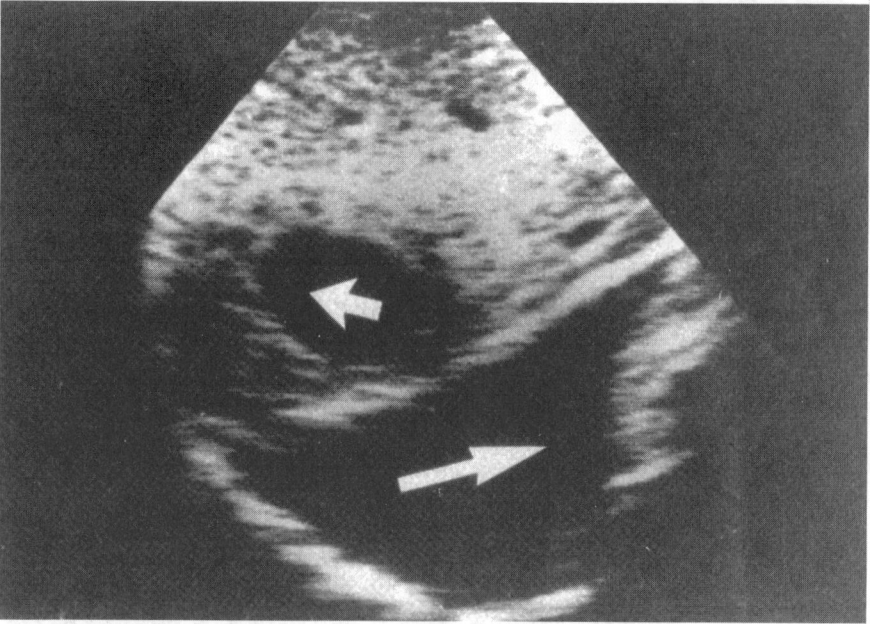

(b) Same patient – ultrasound showing hypoechoic abscess close to diaphragm (small arrow) and pleural effusion (large arrow). Note the diaphragm is intact.

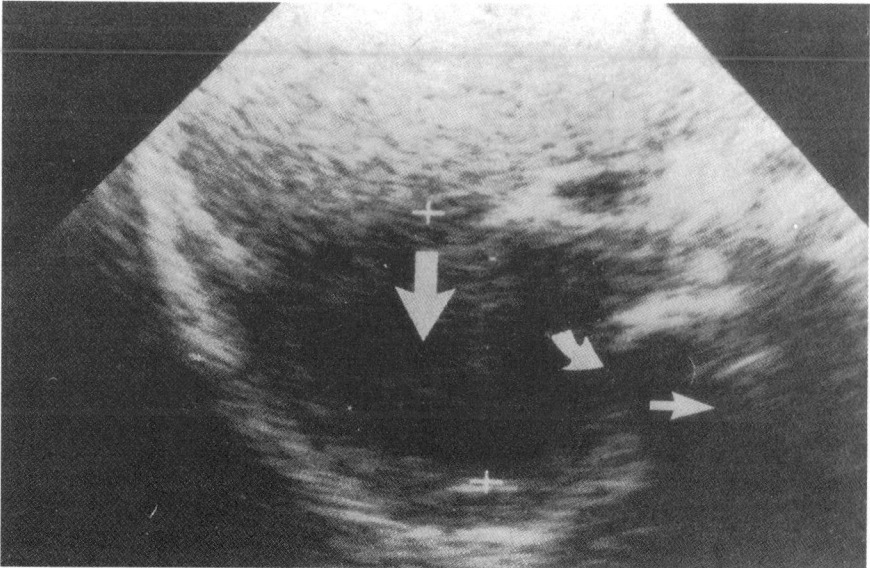

(c) Same patient – ultrasound showing hypoechoic lesion (large arrow) adjacent to diaphragm and pleural effusion (small arrow). Note the defect in the diaphragm (curved arrow).

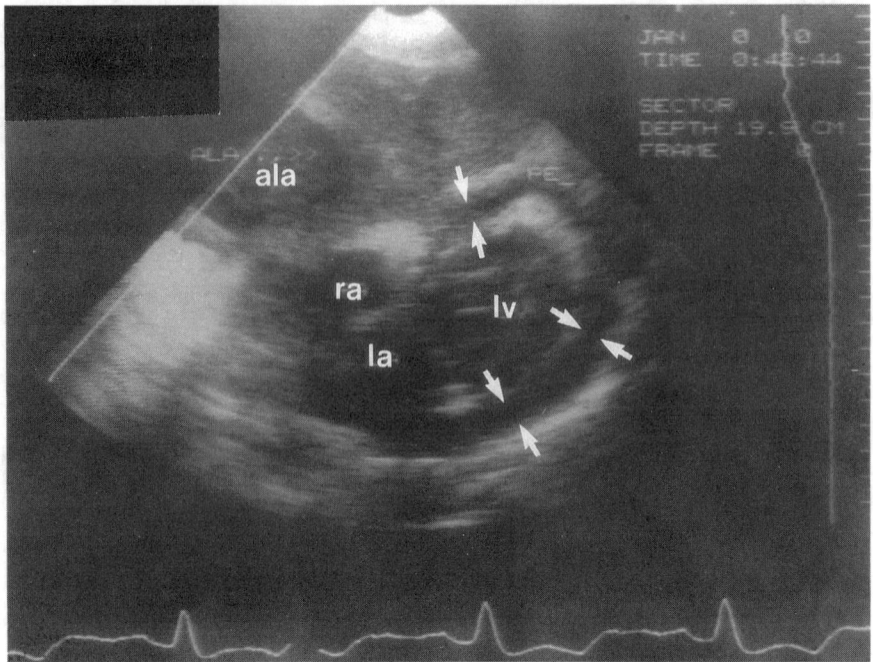

Figure 3.3   Amoebic pericarditis. Echocardiogram showing liver abscess (ala), right atrium (ra), left atrium (la), left ventricle (lv) and pericardial effusion (arrows).

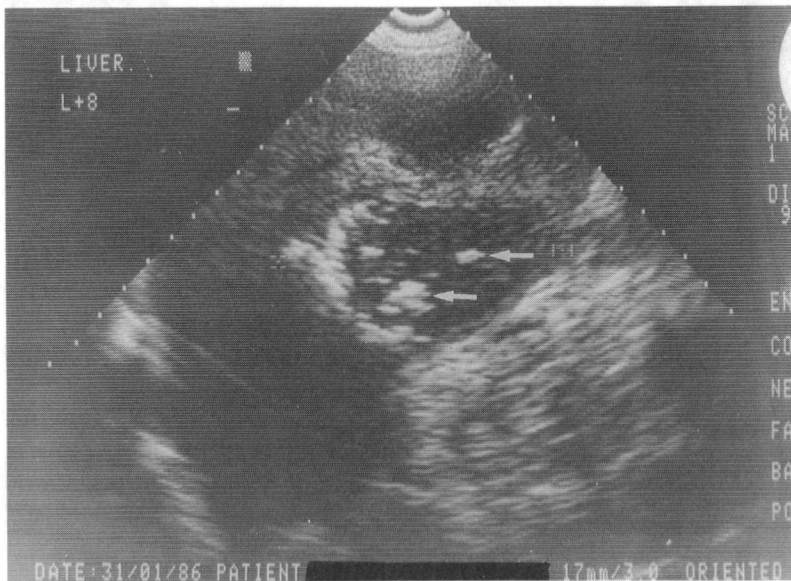

Figure 3.4   Pyogenic liver abscess. Ultrasound. Dense echoes (arrows) within abscess cavity indicates presence of air.

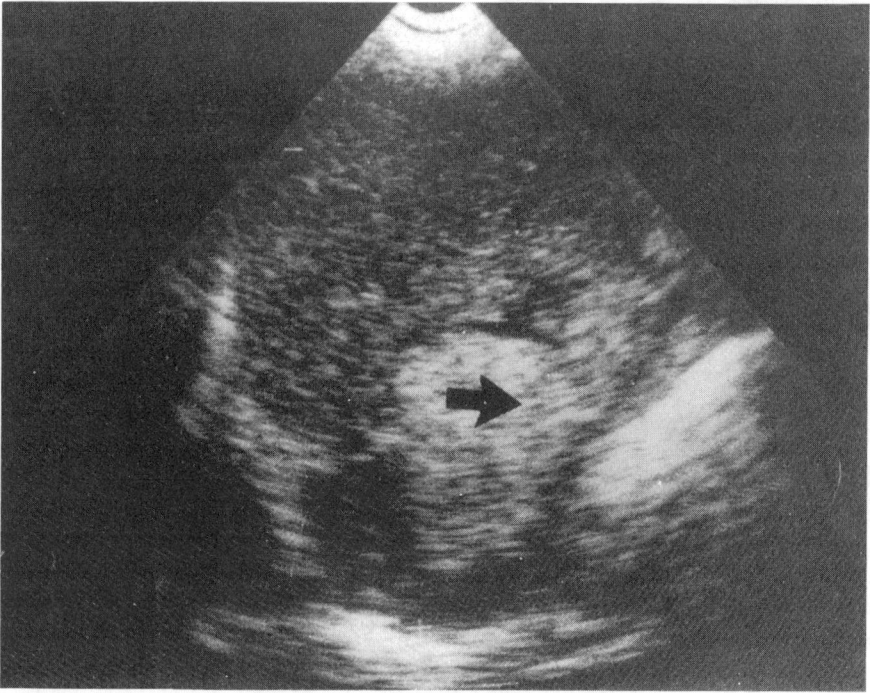

Figure 3.5 Hepatoma. Ultrasound. The lesion appears dense (arrow).

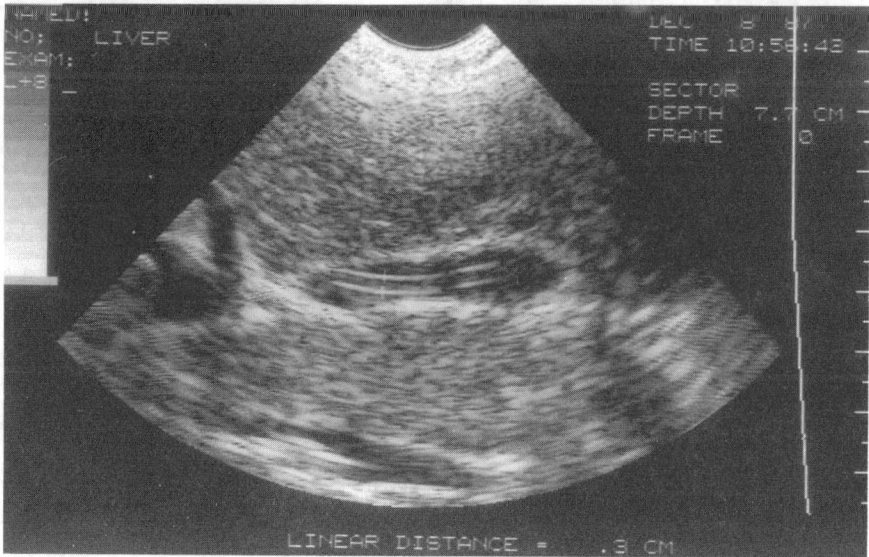

Figure 3.6 Hepatobiliary ascariasis. Ultrasound. Linear shadows indicating presence of worm within intrahepatic bile duct.

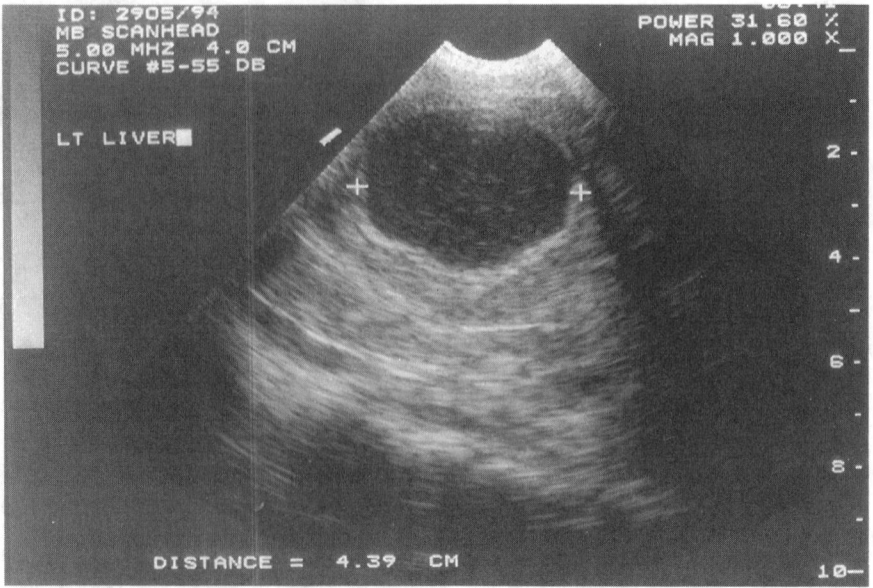

(a) Ultrasound showing hypoechoic lesion indistinguishable from amoebic liver abscess.

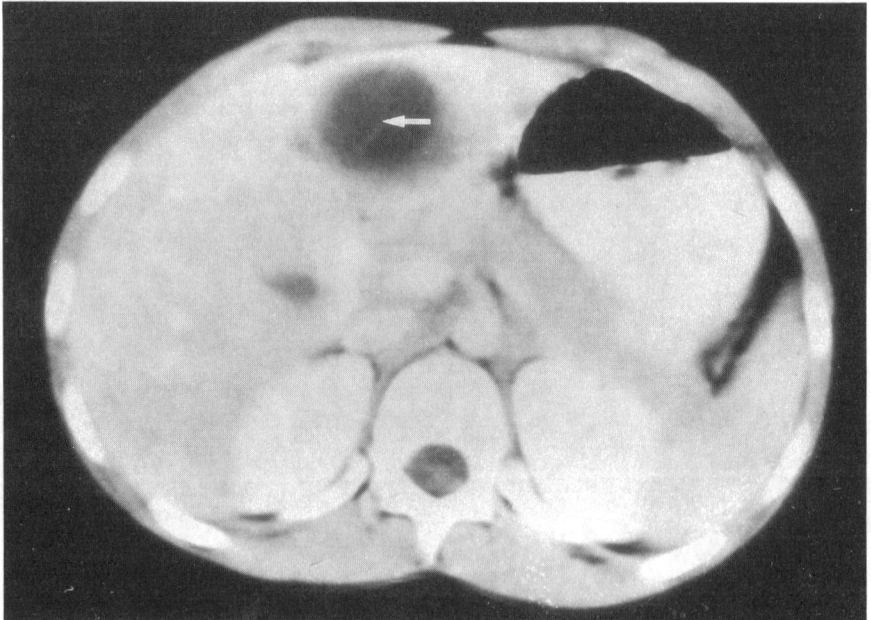

(b) CT scan of lesion above showing septae (arrow) within cyst.

Figure 3.7   Hepatic hydatid cyst.

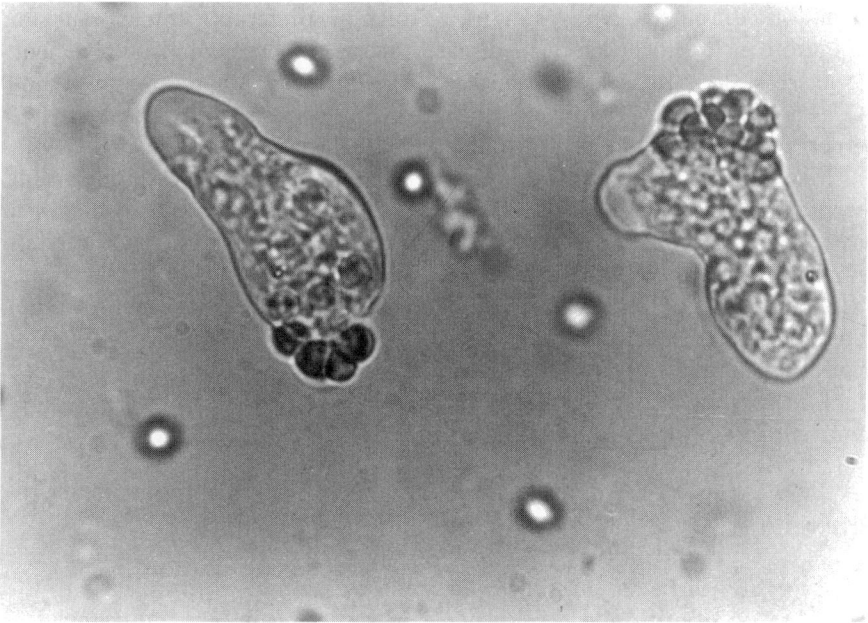

Figure 3.8 Colonic amoebiasis. Photomicrograph of haematophagus trophozoites at higher magnification.

Treatment

General supportive measures include rehydration, pain relief and the correction of anaemia. Mucosal intestinal disease responds well to the nitroimidazoles (metronidazole or tinidazole; 2–2.4 g daily for 5 days in adults and 35–50 mg/kg daily in 3 divided doses for 10 days in children). Ingestion of alcohol should be avoided especially with metronidazole. Transmural colonic amoebiasis should be managed in hospital. Concomitant bacterial peritonitis necessitates the use of broad-spectrum antibiotics in addition to specific antiamoebic treatment. Mortality has been significantly reduced by isolating the affected bowel segment with a colostomy; the omental wraps should not be disturbed as any attempt to do so will cause new perforations. The colostomy is closed after 4–6 weeks; a gentle barium enema will confirm closure of perforation; if leakage is present the perforation can be closed at the same time as the colostomy.

Liver abscess responds well to metronidazole or tinidazole (2–2.4 g daily for 1–5 days in adults and 34–50 mg/kg daily in 3 divided doses for 10 days in children). A third of patients continue to be asymptomatically colonised after treatment. Percutaneous aspiration relieves symptoms and may be diagnostic but carries the risk of introducing nosocomial infection if aseptic procedures are not observed. The needle is inserted at the point of maximal tenderness or, if facilities are available, aseptic aspiration under direct visualisation by ultrasound or computed tomography (CT) scan is preferable. Indications for aspiration include: (1) left lobe disease to prevent pericardial involvement, (2) abscess close to a serosal surface, (3) poor response to treatment and (4) negative serology. Amoebic empyema and pericarditis respond well to percutaneous drainage plus specific antiamoebic therapy.

Asymptomatic intestinal colonisation may be eradicated with diloxanide furoate (500 mg t.d.s. for 10 days) or paromomycin (30 mg/kg body mass per day in 3 divided doses for 5–10 days). However, treatment of such carriers remains controversial. Most carriers are infected with non-pathogenic strains and do not require treatment. There is no simple means of identifying pathogenic *E. histolytica* infection; a positive serological test is supportive. In most developing countries, where serological tests are too costly and access to good stool microscopy remains a problem, it may be prudent not to treat asymptomatic carriers.

Prevention

The provision of better housing to improve overcrowding, coupled with the ready availability of good quality water in sufficient amounts and improvement of sanitary disposal facilities are the only means of decreasing parasite transmission. A vaccine designed to boost local gut immunity may facilitate the spontaneous clearance of cysts, however, this still remains a distant possibility.

Case history 1

On admission a 31-year-old black male complained of right upper quadrant abdominal pain and fever of 6 weeks' duration. He was pyrexic (38.8°C) and slightly pale. A 6-cm tender hepatomegaly was palpable. Chest radiograph demonstrated elevation of the right hemidiaphragm and an ultrasound scan showed multiple hypoechioc lesions in the liver (Figure 3.1a). The patient was slightly anaemic (10 g/dl) with a leukocytosis of 14.2×10^9/l. Hypoalbuminaemia and mildly elevated alkaline phosphatase and transaminases were also present. Amoebic serology was positive and the patient responded well to metronidazole.

Case history 2

A 25-year-old black male presented with complaints of right upper quadrant abdominal pain, poor appetite and malaise of 3 weeks' duration. The patient was febrile (38.4°C), had mild pallor and a 10-cm hepatomegaly with point tenderness in the midclavicular line just below the right costal margin. There was no preceding history of dysentery. His blood count showed an anaemia of 8.2 g/dl and leukocytosis of 13.3×10^9/l. The patient had hypoalbuminaemia (28 g/dl), mildly elevated alkaline phosphatase and transaminases. The chest X-ray was normal and ultrasound examination of the liver revealed a large (14 cm) hypodense lesion in the liver consistent with a liver abscess (Figure 3.1b). The amoebic serology (agar-gel diffusion test) was positive. Sonar guided aspiration of the abscess yielded 1.4 litres of sterile greenish pus. The patient responded well to metronidazole 2 g daily for 5 days.

Case history 3

A 34-year-old black female patient presented to hospital with a 3 week history of pleuritic pain in the right lower chest, fever, poor appetite and malaise. She was febrile (39.3°C), had signs consistent with a right pleural effusion as well as a 2-cm hepatomegaly. Intercostal tenderness was present in the right chest laterally. Chest X-ray (Figure 3.2a) revealed marked elevation of the right hemidiaphragm and blunting of the costophrenic angle on that side. Ultrasound scan showed a hypoechoic lesion in the liver and a low density lesion in the right chest consistent with a pleural effusion (Figure 3.2b); percutaneous aspiration of the latter yielded clear exudative fluid. The patient was treated with metronidazole 2 g daily. Fever and chest pain persisted and on the third hospital day she became tachypnoeic. Ultrasound scan confirmed the previous findings; additionally a defect could be seen in the diaphragm (Figure 3.2c). Percutaneous needle aspiration of both liver lesion and pleural effusion produced reddish brown fluid ('anchovy sauce') which was bacteriologically sterile. A diagnosis of amoebic empyema was made and treatment with metronidazole continued. The patient then made an uneventful recovery.

Case history 4

A black male aged 45 years presented to hospital with dyspnoea and retrosternal chest pain of 8 days' duration. He admitted to having epigastric pain and fever for the past 2 months. The patient was febrile and had a tachycardia of 124 beats/min with pulsus paradoxus. An elevated jugular venous pressure, tender hepatomegaly and pericardial rub confirmed the diagnosis of pericarditis. This was verified by an echocardiogram (Figure 3.3) which showed a pericardial effusion as well as a hypoechoic defect in the liver. Amoebic liver abscess with rupture into the pericardium was diagnosed. Percutaneous aspiration of the pericardium yielded typical amoebic pus. The patient responded well to metronidazole. There was no evidence of pericardial constriction upon recovery.

Case history 5

A 25-year-old black male, complained of pyrexia, malaise, weight loss (2.5 kg), and pain in the right upper quadrant of the abdomen for one month. He was febrile (39.8°C) and a tender hepatomegaly was present; chest X-ray showed an elevated right diaphragm. The patient had a leukocytosis of $19.8 \times 10^9/l$ (78 per cent neutrophils) and anaemia of 7.2 g/dl. Blood cultures were done and the patient was initially treated with metronidazole (800 mg t.i.d. orally). Ultrasound examination revealed a hypoechoic hepatic lesion with dense echoes within it (Figure 3.4). The liver abscess was aspirated percutaneously. Microscopic examination of the pus showed numerous leukocytes and Gram-positive cocci. Treatment was changed to soluble penicillin (one million units q.d.s. intravenously) and the patient referred for open surgical drainage of the abscess. Culture of both pus and liver aspirate grew *Streptococcus milleri*. The patient made an uneventful recovery.

Case history 6

A 13-year-old black female presented with a one week history of right upper quadrant abdominal pain and fever. She had jaundice, fever and tender hepatomegaly. X-ray of the chest showed an elevated right diaphragm. The patient was initially treated with metronidazole. Ultrasound examination of the abdomen revealed linear shadows in a dilated intrahepatic bile duct (Figure 3.6). Stool microscopy confirmed infection with *Ascaris lumbricoides*. Blood cultures were negative. Metronidazole was stopped; the patient responded well to conservative management with a single dose of albendazole (400 mg orally); the adult worms spontaneously migrated back into the duodenum.

Case history 7
A 9-year-old boy was referred to hospital for investigation of hepatomegaly. There was no history of fever or weight loss. Chest radiograph was normal. Ultrasound examination demonstrated a hypoechoic lesion in the liver (Figure 3.7a). Amoebic serology was negative. CT scan of the abdomen confirmed a hypodense hepatic lesion; however septae were identified within the lesion (Figure 3.7b). A diagnosis of hepatic hydatid was entertained and the patient referred for surgical excision.

Case history 8
A black male aged 28 complained of severe abdominal pain for 3 days and profuse vomiting of 1 day duration. He admitted to having diarrhoea for about 3 weeks. He was toxic with a temperature of 39.4°C and hypotensive (90/60 mmHg). There were signs of peritonitis. Sigmoidoscopy demonstrated small ulcers in the rectum; microscopy of a rectal scrape showed numerous haematophagus trophozoites of *E. histolytica* (Figure 3.8) and biopsy confirmed an amoebic ulcer. Erect abdominal radiograph demonstrated dilated transverse colon but there was no air in the mid-transverse colon. Amoebic colitis with transmural disease and bowel perforation with peritonitis were diagnosed. The patient was stabilised and intravenous antibiotics (ampicillin and metronidazole) commenced. The following day the patient was taken to theatre. Apart from peritonitis, disease involving the entire transverse colon was discovered. A colostomy was performed; the diseased bowel was irrigated and left intact. Before closing the colostomy at 6 weeks a barium enema was performed which showed no stricture and the perforation had healed.

Further reading

Cholera

Anon. Status of new cholera vaccines. Bull Pan Am Health Organ 1991;25:278–80.
Anon. Cholera prevention and control; environmental health measures. Epidemiol Bull 1991;12:13–14.
Barua D, Burrows W, (editors) Cholera. Philadelphia: WB Saunders, 1974.
Behrens RH. Diarrhoeal disease: current concepts and future challenges. The impact of oral rehydration and other therapies on the management of acute diarrhoea. Trans R Soc Trop Med Hyg 1993;87(Suppl 3):35–8.
Carpenter CCJ. Cholera and other enterotoxin-related diarrhoeal illnesses. J Infect Dis 1972;126:551–64.
Dupont HL. Diarrhoea disease: current concepts and future challenges. Antimicrobial therapy and prophylaxis. Trans R Soc Trop Med Hyg 1993;87(Suppl 3):31–4.

Lindenbram J, Greenough WB, Islam MR. Antibiotic therapy of cholera. Bull World Health Organ 1967;36:871–83.

Pierce NF, Greenough WB, Carpenter CCJ. *Vibrio cholerae* enterotoxin and its mode of action. Bacteriol Rev. 1971;35:1–13.

Simeant S. Cholera 1991. Viel ennemi, *nouveau visage*. World Health Stat Q 1992; 45:208–19.

Typhoid and paratyphoid

Benevant L *et al.* (1984). Diagnosis of typhoid fever using a string capsule device. Trans R Soc Trop Med Hyg 1984;78:404–6.

Cornwell J *et al.* Multiple presentations of salmonella infection. NZ Med J 1992; 105:131–2.

Guerra – Caceres JG *et al.* Diagnostic value of bone marrow culture in typhoid fever. Trans R Soc Trop Med Hyg 1979;73:680–3.

Hoffman SI *et al.* Reduction of mortality in chloramphenicol treated severe typhoid fever by high-dose dexamethasone. N Engl J Med 1984;310:82–8.

Huckstep R. Typhoid fever and other salmonella infections. Edinburgh: Churchill Livingstone, 1962.

Islam N. A new look at typhoid. Trop Doct 1992;22:84–5.

Wahdan MH *et al.* A controlled field trial of live oral typhoid vaccine ty 21a. Bull World Health Organ 1980;58:467–74.

Welch TP, Martin NC. Surgical treatment of typhoid perforation. Lancet 1975;i:1078.

Amoebiasis

Adams EB, MacLeod IN. Invasive amoebiasis. I. Amoebic dysentery and its complications. Medicine (Baltimore) 1977;56:315–23.

Adams EB, MacLeod IN. Invasive amoebiasis. II. Amoebic liver abscess and its complications. Medicine (Baltimore) 1977;56:325–34.

Ravdin JI, editor. Amoebiasis: human infection by *Entamoeba histolytica*. New York: John Wiley.

Ravdin JI, Petri WA. *Entamoeba histolytica* (amoebiasis). In: Mandell, Douglas, Bennet editors. Principles and Practice of Infectious Diseases. New York: Churchill Livingstone, 1990.

Wilmot AJ. Clinical amoebiasis. Oxford: Blackwell Scientific Publications, 1962.

4

Diarrhoea in Children

Diarrhoea is one of the commonest symptoms in children; there can be many causes, from simple, self-limited conditions requiring little active intervention to serious and life-threatening diseases requiring emergency treatment. Many episodes of diarrhoea in children are due to gastrointestinal infections; these are particularly important in tropical, developing countries where they cause the deaths of more than 3 million under-fives annually.

Definitions

It is important to agree on definitions of **diarrhoea** and its various forms (see below). 'Diarrhoea' depends to a large extent on parents' perceptions about what are normal stools in infants and young children. There is a wide range of normality; Italian infants had a median number of 2.7 stools daily in the first year of life while in children over 6 years old a single daily stool was the norm. The following definitions are generally accepted:

diarrhoea: the passage of abnormally loose or fluid stools more frequently than normal – the passage of 3 or more loose stools daily after 12 months of age is usually considered abnormal

acute diarrhoea: the symptom has had a rapid onset (i.e. within 24 h or less), often with an illness starting in the preceding 48 or 72 h

chronic (or persistent) diarrhoea: the stools have been abnormally loose for 14 days or more, irrespective of whether they are watery, mucoid, bloody, pasty, or abnormally bulky; this form of diarrhoea can have begun with an acute illness or had a slow, insidious onset

dysentery: diarrhoeal illness in which abnormally loose or fluid stools are mixed with blood and mucus

intractable diarrhoea: episodes of chronic or persistent diarrhoea, not usually with an identifiable cause, that do not respond to usual, standard treatment regimes and which may require special interventions, such as parenteral nutrition.

58

From a public health perspective, it is important to know whether parents (particularly mothers) perceive their infants' faeces to be a potentially important source of gastrointestinal infections or diarrhoeal illnesses. A study in an urban setting in Papua New Guinea found that children whose mothers did not perceive babies' faeces to be important in causing diarrhoeal illness were more than seven times more likely to develop diarrhoea than those whose mothers recognised the relationships; the risk from contaminated food was also almost 7:1 compared with children of mothers who recognised the link. Work in Cali, Colombia, has also found mother's perception of malnutrition, knowledge about diarrhoea and her age, birthplace and other factors to be predictive of diarrhoea in young children.

This chapter classifies childhood diarrhoea into:

1. infectious, and
2. non-infectious causes.

Because of the importance of infectious causes of diarrhoea in tropical countries, these will be discussed first.

Infectious diarrhoea

Transmission and epidemiology

Some of the factors involved in transmission of diarrhoea-causing micro-organisms are shown in Table 4.1. Many episodes of childhood gastrointestinal infections (often called 'gastroenteritis') are transmitted by the faecal–oral route and so are facilitated by contact with infectious agents (e.g. bacteria, viruses, parasites) via fingers or lips or by means of inanimate objects such as feeding utensils or items of clothing (called fomites) that have become contaminated by infected faecal material.

Clearly, these routes of transmission are encouraged by inadequate personal and community living conditions, inadequate hygiene, overcrowding and

Table 4.1   Some routes of diarrhoea transmission.

Direct

Faeces – Human, animal

Fingers – Particularly infants, toddlers, young children, foodhandlers

Fomites – Objects such as feeding bottles, eating utensils, mothers' clothing, bedding materials

Indirect

Food – Contaminated in the food chain, in preparation, distribution, sale, or in the household

Fluids – Contaminated at source or during delivery, storage or *via* utensils

Insect vectors – Such as flies

Infected animals – e.g. dogs, cattle

Air-borne droplets – e.g. for rotavirus (?)

behaviour that permits the spread of faecally contaminated material through families and communities. Likewise, interruption of transmission depends on improved personal and domestic hygiene and breaking routes of transmission or sources of contamination whether they are inside or outside the household. Aspects of the household environment in a poor, rural agricultural area of Egypt that were associated with diarrhoea in children under 3 years of age included house structure, water usage, toilet and bathing area, animal management, the food preparation area, hygiene, and wastewater management; protection of infants from flies during napping appeared to be protective. Some co-factors that predispose to infectious diarrhoea are summarised in Table 4.2.

In many parts of industrialised countries, these factors have improved significantly over recent decades so that infectious childhood diarrhoea is now less prevalent and serious; however, even in the United States this is still a serious problem and diarrhoeal illnesses cause at least 500 deaths in the 1-month to 4-years age group annually. In tropical, developing countries childhood diarrhoea is a much more serious community problem and is a major cause of deaths in infants and young children as well as being a prominent contributor to high levels of ill-health, hospitalisation and morbidity. The main infectious agents that cause these illnesses are bacteria, viruses and parasites. Some of the agents most frequently isolated from young patients with diarrhoea are shown in Table 4.3.

Diagnosis

One of the great difficulties and frustrations in managing children with diarrhoea in developing countries is that adequate laboratory services and facilities to make a microbiological diagnosis are often lacking; furthermore, results

Table 4.2 Some co-factors that predispose to infectious diarrhoea.

Unhygienic, overcrowded living conditions
Inadequate facilities and/or services for sewage disposal
Living in close contact with domestic and farm animals
Contaminated food and water; infected foodhandlers and vendors
Unsafe personal and domestic hygiene practices (e.g. faeces disposal, food handling, hand washing, food and drink storage)
High-risk feeding and weaning practices (e.g. use of feeding bottles)
Undernutrition, including low birthweight
Impaired immune function, including AIDS and malnutrition
Gatherings of incompletely toilet-trained young children (e.g. at daycare or preschool centres) increased risk of cross-contamination and spread into the community
Travel (infants, children and adults) from low-risk to high-risk areas

---

Table 4.3 Commonest enteric pathogens isolated from young children with diarrhoea in some recent studies.

Locations	Pathogens	Authors
Korea	rotavirus, enterotoxigenic *Escherichia coli* (ETEC), *Clostridium difficile*, enteroadherent *E. coli*, (EAEC), enteropathogenic *E. coli* (EPEC)	Kim *et al.* (1989)
Bangladesh	ETEC, *Shigella*, *Campylobacter*, *Ascaris*, *Trichuris*, *Giardia*	Stanton *et al.* (1989)
Egypt	ETEC, *Campylobacter*, *Shigella*	Mikhail *et al.* (1989)
Somalia	rotavirus, ETEC, *Shigella*, *Aeromonas*, *Campylobacter*, *Vibrio cholerae* non-O1	Casalino *et al.* (1988)
Australia (Aborigines)	*Salmonella*, *Shigella*, ETEC, *Campylobacter*, *Cryptosporidium*, *Giardia*	Gracey *et al.* (1992)
China	rotavirus, *Campylobacter jejuni*	Ming *et al.* (1991)
Pakistan	ETEC, rotavirus EPEC, *Campylobacter*	Khalil *et al.* (1993)
Multicentre study in China, India, Mexico, Myanmar and Pakistan	ETEC, rotavirus, *Shigella*	Huilan *et al.* (1991)

may take so long that clinical management decisions must be made without a laboratory diagnosis. However, microbiological methods have improved greatly in recent years so that this situation is slowly improving; Mahmud and others showed that 'it is possible to establish a well functioning and reliable micro-biological laboratory in a setting with restricted trained personnel and material resources in a developing country' and urged for improved laboratory resources in developing countries. In a prospective study in Lahore, Pakistan (with international collaboration), enteric pathogens were isolated in 73.4 per cent of patients; bacteria in 53.5 per cent and viruses in 19.9 per cent. An enteric pathogen was isolated from more than two-thirds of patients with diarrhoea in a multicentre study involving five hospitals in China, India, Mexico, Myanmar and Pakistan; however, pathogens were isolated from 30 per cent of their control subjects. This emphasises the difficulties in attributing an episode of diarrhoea in any patient to a particular pathogen simply because it has been isolated. In the tropics, particularly in areas where hygiene is poor, multiple infections and simultaneous bacterial (or viral, or both) and parasitic infections are common.

There are some general clinical features that might help suggest the occurrence of a bacterial on viral gastrointestinal infection, including:

Bacterial gastroenteritis
- commoner in the tropics
- quick onset with high fever
- vomiting not usually prominent
- ill, toxic appearance
- stools may be bloody

Viral gastroenteritis
- commoner in temperate and cooler climates
- often occurs in outbreaks or epidemics that may be seasonal
- low-grade fever
- vomiting common, sometimes profuse
- large-volume, watery stools
- rapid dehydration

Management

Oral rehydration therapy (ORT) has become established in recent years as the mainstay of management for most infants and children with diarrhoeal dehydration. The initial step is assessment of the severity of dehydration (Table 4.4). This is often difficult due to associated malnutrition, acidosis and viraemia or bacteraemia. Signs of dehydration can be present with loss of as little as 3 per cent extracellular fluid; some of the widely accepted signs of dehydration,

Table 4.4 Some indicators of dehydration (from Gracey, 1993).

Mild dehydration (4–5% body weight loss)	• Dry mucous membranes • Decreased skin turgour • Irritability, anorexia • Mild oliguria
Moderate dehydration (8–10% weight loss)	• All of the above, exaggerated • Sunken frontanelle (if it is still open) • Sunken eyes • Rapid pulse • Restlessness, lethargy and/or irritability • Oliguria • Pinched skin returns slowly
Severe dehydration (more than 10% weight loss)	• All of the above, but worse • Lethargy, floppiness or unconscious • Drinks poorly, if at all • Peripheral circulatory failure • Thready, weak pulse and hypotension (these are all **very serious signs** indicating a poor prognosis unless treated promptly and appropriately)

such as dry mouth, low urine output and sunken frontanelle, are not necessarily reliable predictors of dehydration.

The World Health Organization (WHO) has developed a simple, practical scheme to help assess dehydration (Table 4.5). This categorises children with diarrhoea as having 'no dehydration', 'some dehydration' or 'severe dehydration'; these patients then enter Treatment Plan A, Plan B or Plan C.

Plan A is used to teach the mother to continue to treat the child's current episode of diarrhoea at home and to give early treatment for future episodes of diarrhoea. Treatment at home can include oral rehydration solution (ORS), food-based fluids (such as soup, rice water, and yoghurt drinks) and plain water – as much as the child will take:

Age	Amount of ORS after each loose stool	Amount of ORS for use at home
Up to 2 years	50–100 ml	500 ml/day
2 to 10 years	100–200 ml	1 litre/day
10 years or more	as much as wanted	2 litres

The child should be given plenty of food to prevent malnutrition, breastfeeding should be continued or if the child is not breast-fed the usual milk should be continued. For children 6 months or older or already on solid food cereals, starchy foods, pulses, vegetables, and meat or fish should be given; fresh fruit juice or mashed banana should be given for extra potassium and frequent, small meals should be encouraged. Extra food will be needed for at least 2 weeks.

Plan B attempts to rehydrate the patient orally while the mother is encouraged to continue breastfeeding; the approximate amount of ORS solution to be given in the first 4 hours is shown in Table 4.6. The patient's age should be used with these guidelines only when the weight is not known; if the infant is breast-fed this should be continued and if the patient wants more ORS than shown in the Table, more should be given. Infants under 6 months who are not breast-fed should be given an extra 100–200 ml of clean water during this early rehydration phase. Infants or children managed by this 'Plan B' should be carefully supervised and their continued treatment depends on whether their hydration status is corrected or worsens. If they become more dehydrated or for patients who are initially in the category of 'severe dehydration' (Tables 4.4 and 4.5), more active and urgent management is needed.

Plan C requires intravenous fluids; treatment regimes tend to differ from place to place and depending on the availability of intravenous solutions and adequately trained staff and supervision. If the patient can drink, give ORS orally while the drip is being set up. The WHO guidelines suggest 100 ml/kg of Ringer's lactate solution or, if that is not available, normal saline as follows:

Table 4.5 World Health Organization guidelines for assessment of dehydration (WHO, 1992).

	No dehydration	Some dehydration	Severe dehydration
Clinical observations			
1. General condition	Well, alert	*Restless irritable*	*Lethargic or unconscious floppy*
2. Eyes	Normal	Sunken	Very sunken and dry
3. Tears	Present	Absent	Absent
4. Mouth and tongue	Moist	Dry	Very dry
5. Thirst	Drinks normally, not thirsty	*Thirsty, drinks eagerly*	*Drinks poorly; or unable to drink*
6. Skin test pinch	Goes back quickly	*Goes back slowly*	*Goes back very slowly*
Decide	The patient has **no signs** of dehydration	If two or more signs including at least one marked (*sign*) there is **some** dehydration	If two or more signs, including at least one marked (*sign*) there is **severe** dehydration
Action (see text)	Treatment Plan A	weigh the patient, if possible, and use Plan B	weigh the patient and use Treatment Plan C **URGENTLY**

Table 4.6 World Health Organization guidelines to treat dehydration: Approximate amount of ORS solution to be given in the first 4 hours (WHO, 1992).

Patient's age	Less than 4 months	4–11 months	12–23 months	2–4 years	5–14 years	15 years or older
Weight	< 5 kg	5–7.9 kg	8–10.9 kg	11–15.9 kg	16–29.9 kg	30 kg or more
Volume of ORS	200–400 ml	400–600 ml	600–800 ml	800–1200 ml	1200–2200 ml	2200–4000 ml

Intravenous Ringer's lactate or saline

Age	Initially give 30 ml/kg in	Then give 70 mg/kg in
Under 12 months	1 h*	5 h
Older	30 min*	2.5 h

*repeat once if the pulse is still very weak

For patients with peripheral circulatory failure and shock, plasma expanders (e.g. 5 per cent normal serum albumin) may be required in the initial phase of rehydration. After acute fluid losses have been replaced, maintenance needs can be calculated from normal body weight and surface area; an approximate guide is to give 10 ml/kg per hour intravenously plus oral fluids, as tolerated. Patients who are rehydrated intravenously need close supervision and their continued management (e.g. with Plan A, B or C) should be determined by their progress every few hours, initially. If there are difficulties in establishing intravenous rehydration, nasogastric intubation and ORT can help, particularly if the mother can encourage her child to drink. The type of fluid to be given intravenously should be determined by the type of dehydration (i.e. isotonic, hyponatraemic or hypernatraemic with or without acidosis) which is obviously facilitated by access to biochemical investigations such as electrolytes, $P\mathrm{co}_2$ and pH.

Dietary management

Dietary management of diarrhoeal illnesses is extremely important, particularly in the tropics where the nutritional status of infants and young children is often marginal and can be severely compromised by infections, especially by gastrointestinal infections which are often accompanied by anorexia, vomiting and excessive gastrointestinal losses. There are some important basic principles:

1. breastfeeding should be continued during diarrhoea and other fluids should be given to replace faecal losses of water and electrolytes,
2. in children who are on other milks, these can be reintroduced when rehydration is achieved; low-lactose or lactose-free milks can be given if lactose intolerance occurs, e.g. due to damage to the small intestinal mucosa,
3. food-based ORT (e.g. based on rice powder) can be used to help reduce stool fluid losses,
4. after 4–6 months all children should be given soft or semi-solid food that should be mashed, pureed or otherwise prepared for them and given at least six times daily. Food should **not** be withheld or restricted until the diarrhoea stops,
5. extra food should be given after the diarrhoea has stopped, for at least 2 weeks.

Drugs

Antibiotics have very little role in the management of acute infectious diarrhoea in children yet they are often used indiscriminately in the tropics; in Indonesia, for example, nearly 60 per cent of children with illnesses including diarrhoea were given prescriptions for four or more drugs and almost 90 per cent of children under 5 years were given an antibiotic, yet oral antibiotics were usually given in sufficient amounts for only 2 days; in Pakistan 75 per cent of children with diarrhoea were given antibiotics, maximally to those in upper middle classes. There are several reasons why antibiotics should not generally be used in childhood gastroenteritis including the fact that some episodes (e.g. those caused by viruses) would not be affected; many enteric bacteria are already antibiotic-resistant; indiscriminate usage of antibiotics facilitates the development of plasmid-transmitted drug resistance; and antibiotic treatment can prolong the carrier state with some micro-organisms, such as *Salmonella*. Furthermore, antibiotics are expensive and have significant side-effects. WHO sanctions the use of antibiotics only for dysentery and for suspected cholera cases with severe dehydration. For shigellosis, oral therapy for 5 days with the antibiotic recommended in your area is suggested; this might be trimethoprim–sulphamethoxazole (co-trimoxazole), ampicillin, nalidixic acid, norfloxacin, or ciprofloxacin; enteroinvasive *Escherichia coli* (EIEC) can be treated as for shigellosis. Antibiotics are also indicated for the treatment of bacterial infections that can produce bacteraemia, such as typhoid fever, for which chloramphenicol, ampicillin or ciprofloxacin can be used.

Antiparasitic drugs should be used for amoebiasis only after antibiotic treatment of bloody diarrhoea for *Shigella* has failed or there is microscopic evidence of trophozoites of *Entamoeba histolytica* containing erythrocytes seen in the faeces. It is problematical to know when to treat patients with cysts or trophozoites of *Giardia intestinalis (G. lamblia)* identified by microscopy in stool specimens or upper intestinal aspirates because in localities where giardiasis is common, asymptomatic carriage is not unusual; WHO recommends treatment in such patients when diarrhoea has lasted at least 14 days. All children with strongyloidiasis should be treated in an attempt to eradicate the infection to prevent autoinfection. The drug of choice is thiabendazole but it is not always effective and recurrent courses may be required.

Anti-diarrhoeal drugs (such as opiates) and anti-emetics should never be used in infants or children. They are not efficacious and can be dangerous.

It is important to make clinical judgements about the use of antibiotics in children with diarrhoea based on other considerations, such as the presence or suspicion of another serious bacterial infection, e.g. pneumonia, meningitis or otitis media. The likelihood of malaria should also be dealt with appropriately in areas where falciparum malaria is endemic and other endemic diseases, such as tuberculosis, should also be considered.

Table 4.7 Possible risk factors for persistent diarrhoea in infants and young children (WHO, 1988).

Host factors	• Young age, particularly under 12 months • Malnutrition • Impaired cell-mediated immunity
Previous infections	• Recent acute diarrhoea • Previous persistent diarrhoea
Feeding practices	• Recent introduction to animal milk
Microbial isolates during acute phase	• Enteroadherent *Escherichia coli* (EAEC) • Enteropathogenic *E. coli* (EPEC) • *Shigella* • Multiple pathogens
Drugs used during acute phase	• Antiparasitic drugs • Antimicrobials

Persistent diarrhoea

Persistent diarrhoea after acute gastroenteritis is a very important problem in children in tropical countries, particularly in poorer communities where hygiene is poor and undernutrition is prevalent. Sugar intolerance is a common cause which can easily be recognised at the bedside or in the clinic on consulting rooms by use of the Clinitest method for reducing substances in the stools. Allergy to food proteins, particularly to milk and soy protein, may also cause prolonged diarrhoea. In many children, multiple factors, including bacterial overgrowth in the upper intestinal lumen and, perhaps, degradation of intraluminal bile salts and increased faecal bile acid excretion may be involved. WHO has defined persistent diarrhoea to mean three or more liquid stools per day for 14 days or more and, excluding known causes of chronic or recurrent diarrhoea such as tropical sprue, coeliac disease, hereditary disorders and the contaminated small bowel syndrome, has linked this with a number of risk factors (Table 4.7). Between 3 and 20 per cent of acute diarrhoeal episodes in children under 5 years of age become persistent.

Malnourished children are more prone to gastrointestinal infections and patients with acquired immune deficiency syndrome (AIDS) are particularly prone to intestinal infections with unusual micro-organisms such as *Isospora*, *Mycobacterium avium intracellulare*, *Cryptosporidium* and cytomegalovirus; see also Chapter 5.

Non-infectious diarrhoea

Despite the continuing importance of infectious causes of diarrhoea in children in developing countries, the clinician must be alert to the possibility of other underlying causes for diarrhoeal illnesses, particularly for episodes that do not respond to rehydration and nutritional treatment as outlined above or for illnesses that recur or become refractory to treatment. Some clinical clues to examples of underlying diseases associated with diarrhoea are shown in Table 4.8. Investigation of such a formidable list of possibilities will usually require referral to a specialist centre for opinion from a consultant with appropriate experience and where specialised investigative techniques are available. Conditions once thought to be very rare or non-existent in many developing countries must be considered; cystic fibrosis (CF), for example, has now been well documented in patients in South India.

Professor Charlotte Anderson lists 77 main causes of persisting diarrhoea in children, which can be categorised into smaller sub-sets of disorders that are listed in Table 4.9. This shows the complexities that can be involved in investigation of persistent diarrhoea and emphasises the need for expert advice and assistance in this process whenever possible. This can help prevent the use of inappropriate and expensive investigations that are not risk-free, particularly in small children, for example intestinal biopsy in the hands of occasional operators.

Table 4.8 Some clinical clues to underlying diseases associated with diarrhoea.

Clinical feature	Underlying disease
In infants and young children	
Diarrhoea from birth	Congenital defects in digestion or absorption (e.g. glucose–galactose malabsorption)
Diarrhoea after weaning	Bulky stools: coeliac disease
	Watery stools: sucrase–isomaltase deficiency
Chronic cough with pale, greasy stools ± family history	Cystic fibrosis
After gastrointestinal surgery	Secondary sugar intolerance
Older children	
Chronic cough, pale bulky stools, ravenous appetite	Cystic fibrosis (CF)
Chronic diarrhoea, growth failure	Coeliac disease
Severe weight loss	Inflammatory bowel disease (IBD), malabsorption (see Table 4.9), TB, malignancy
With liver disease	IBD, Wilson's disease, CF, malignancy with secondaries
With eosinophilia	Intestinal parasitosis
Frequent infections	AIDS, other immunodeficiency disorders (see Chapter 5)
With unusual parasites	AIDS
Arthritis	IBD, Whipple's disease, infection with *Yersinia*
Response to antibiotics	Intestinal bacterial overgrowth (e.g. postoperative), tropical sprue
Lymphadenopathy	Lymphoma, AIDS

Table 4.9 Classification of causes of persisting childhood diarrhoea, with or without malabsorption (from Anderson, 1993).

Pathophysiology	Clinical condition
The mucosa	
Morphological:	
• Non-specific	Malnutrition ± chronic infections, infestations, coeliac disease, allergy to food proteins
• Specific (very rare)	Immune deficiencies, intestinal lymphangiectasia, Whipple's disease
Functional:	Specific defects in intestinal digestion (e.g. glucose–galactose malabsorption) or transport (e.g. sugars, amino acids, chloride, zinc, vitamins, lipoproteins)
	Non-specific abnormalities associated with mucosal damage
The lumen	Exocrine pancreatic insufficiency (including cystic fibrosis); altered enterohepatic bile salt circulation; bile salt deconjugation (e.g. intestinal bacterial overgrowth); impaired ileal reabsorption of bile salts (e.g. in tuberculosis, post-surgical); altered bacterial flora in upper small intestine
Abnormal small intestinal anatomy	Surgical resection; intermittent malrotation; anatomical abnormalities (and severe chronic constipation and congenital pseudo-obstruction syndrome) associated with bacterial overgrowth
Miscellaneous	Toddler diarrhoea or irritable colon syndrome; endocrine diseases; inflammatory bowel disease; other forms of colitis

Appendix

A basic, simple formula for oral rehydration salts (ORS) is:

Ingredient	Amount
Sodium chloride	3.5 g
Sodium bicarbonate (Sodium hydrogen carbonate)	2.5 g
Potassium chloride	1.5 g
Glucose	20 g
Clean drinking water	1 litre

The formula for oral rehydration salts (ORS) recommended by WHO and UNICEF is given in the following table:

Ingredient	Grams/litre
Sodium chloride	3.5
Trisodium citrate, dihydrate	2.9
Potassium chloride	1.5
Glucose*	20
Clean drinking water	2.0

*can be replaced by glucose monohydrate 22 g or sucrose 40 g.

When dissolved as instructed, those mixtures provide the following components:

Molar concentrations of components of ORS solutions

Component	mmol/litre of water	
	ORS – Bicarbonate	ORS – Citrate
Sodium	90	90
Potassium	20	20
Chloride	80	80
Citrate	–	10
Bicarbonate	30	–
Glucose	111	111

There are numerous brands of ORS packets that are now available commercially and that should approximately match the formulations given above and their components in those oral rehydration solutions.

A very simple rice-based ORS can be made by adding 50 g of rice to 3.5 g of sodium chloride, 2.5 g of sodium bicarbonate and 1.5 g of potassium chloride dissolved in water. The rice should be ground and made into paste with water then boiled in one litre of water for 5–7 min before the salts are added to complete the mixture.

Further reading

Anderson CM. The child with persistently abnormal stools. In: Gracey M, Burke V, editors. Pediatric Gastroenterology and Hepatology, 3rd ed. Boston: Blackwell Scientific Publications, 1993:373–9.

Bern C, Martines J, de Zoysa I, Glass RI. The magnitude of the global problem of diarrhoeal disease: a ten-year update. Bull World Health Organ 1992;70:705–14.

Bertrand WE, Walmus BF. Maternal knowledge, attitudes and practice as predictors of diarrhoeal disease in young children. Int J Epidemiol 1983;12:205–10.

Bukenya GB, Kaser R, Nwokolo N. The relationship of mothers' perception of babies faeces and other factors to childhood diarrhoea in an urban settlement in Papua New Guinea. Ann Trop Paediatr 1990;10:185–9.

Casalino M, Yusuf MW, Nicoletti M, *et al.* A two-year study of enteric infections associated with diarrhoeal diseases in children in urban Somalia. Trans R Soc Trop Med and Hyg 1988;82:637–41.

Deivanayagam CN, Venugopalan K, Mallikesan S, Madhavan K, Mathukumaraswamy N. A clinical profile of cystic fibrosis in South India. Lung India 1990;VIII:167–72.

Fontana M, Bianchi C, Cataldo F, *et al.* Bowel frequency in healthy children. Acta Paediatr Scand 1989;78:682–4.

Gazzard B. AIDS: an overview. Baillière's Clin Gastroenterol 1990;4:259–89.

Gracey M. Treatment of acute diarrhoea in different settings. In: Gracey M, Burke V, editors. Pediatric Gastroenterology and Hepatology. 3rd ed. Boston: Blackwell Scientific Publications, 1993:301–17.

Gracey M. Environmental hygiene, undernutrition, and diarrhoea. In: Gracey M, Burke V, editors. Pediatric Gastroenterology and Hepatology. 3rd ed. Boston: Blackwell Scientific Publications, 1993:332–50.

Gracey M, Sullivan H, Burke V, *et al.* Intestinal pathogens and parasites in Australian Aboriginal children from birth to two years of age. Trans R Soc Trop Med Hyg 1992;86:222–3.

Griffiths JK, Gorbach SL. Other bacterial diarrhoeas. In: Gracey M, Bouchier IAD, editors. Infectious diarrhoea, Baillière's Clin Gastroenterol 1993;7:263–305.

Grove DI. Parasitic intestinal infections. In: Gracey M, Burke V, editors. Pediatric Gastroenterology and Hepatology. 3rd ed. Boston: Blackwell Scientific Publications, 1993:318–31.

Ho M-S, Glass RI, Pinksy PR, *et al.* Diarrheal deaths in American children. Are they preventable? JAMA 1988;260:3281–5.

Huilan S, Zhen LG, Mathan MM, *et al.* Etiology of acute diarrhoea among children in developing countries: A multicentre study in five countries. Bull World Health Organ 1991;69:549–55.

Khalil K, Lindblom G-B, Mazhar K, Khan SR, Kajiser B. Early child health in Lahore, Pakistan: VIII. Microbiology, Acta Paediatr 1993;390 (Suppl):87–94.

Kim K-H, Shu I-S, Kim JM, Kim CW, Cho Y-J. Etiology of childhood diarrhoea in Korea. J Clin Microbiol 1989;27:1192–6.

Mahmud A, Jalil F, Karlberg J, Lindblad BS. Early child health in Lahore, Pakistan: VII. Diarrhoea. Acta Paediatr 1993;390 (Suppl):79–85.

Mikhail IA, Hyams KC, Podgore JK, *et al.* Microbiologic and clinical study of acute diarrhoea in children in Aswan, Egypt. Scand J Infect Dis 1989;21:59–65.

Ming ZF, Xi ZD, Dong CS, *et al.* Diarrhoeal disease in children less than one year of age at a children's hospital in Guangzhou, People's Republic of China. Trans R Soc Trop Med Hyg 1991;85:667–9.

Pickering LK. Therapy for acute infectious diarrhoea in children. Pediatrics 1991;118:5118–28.

Stanton B, Silimperi DR, Khatun K, *et al.* Parasitic, bacterial and viral pathogens isolated from diarrhoeal and routine stool specimens of urban Bangladeshi children. J Trop Med Hyg 1989;92:46–55.

WHO. Persistent diarrhoea in children in developing countries: Memorandum from a WHO meeting. Bull World Health Organ 1988;66:709–17.

WHO. Seventh Programme Report, 1988–1989. Programme for Control of Diarrhoeal Diseases. WHO/CDD 190.34. Geneva: World Health Organization, 1990.

WHO. Management of the patient with diarrhoea. Programme for Control of Diarrhoeal Diseases. Geneva: World Health Organization, 1992.

Wright CE, El Alamy M, DuPont HL, *et al*. The role of home environment in infant diarrhoea in rural Egypt. Am J Epidemiol 1991;134:887–94.

WHO. A manual for the treatment of diarrhoea. Programme for the Control of Diarrhoeal Diseases, WHO/CDD/SER/80.2 Rev. 2 1990, Geneva: World Health Organization, 1990.

5

HIV infection in the Gastrointestinal Tract

The gastrointestinal tract is the largest lymphoid organ in the body so it is not surprising that the human immunodeficency virus (HIV), a virus that specifically attacks the immune system, affects the gut in many patients. In the early days of the AIDS epidemic in North America, diarrhoea was a commonly reported symptom. In some cases a specific pathogen was identified, in others usually non-pathogenic organisms were blamed but, in many cases, no cause for the diarrhoea was found. Early reports of AIDS in Africa also noted that chronic diarrhoea and weight loss were common clinical manifestations; so much so that local people in Uganda coined the phrase 'slim disease' to describe this new problem.

Diarrhoea, both acute and chronic, are the commonest problems associated with HIV. About half of the patients presenting with HIV in Zambia had diarrhoea as a major symptom. Many cases of diarrhoea related to HIV are due to infection. It must be remembered that the prevalence of potential gastrointestinal pathogens varies from region to region, so that the findings in one part of the tropics may differ from the findings in other parts. Although infection is common, tumours may also affect the gut. However, many patients with HIV may have diarrhoea with no obvious cause. In addition, HIV may be associated with symptoms other than diarrhoea.

This chapter will outline the spectrum of problems that HIV may cause in different parts of the GI tract. Much of the information comes from data gathered in North America, Europe and Africa. It is to be expected that more, and sometimes different, data will be reported from Latin America and Asia as the HIV epidemic increases in these areas. Although we know a lot about the clinical manifestations of HIV, there is still much that is not known and we are only just beginning to understand the basics of the pathophysiology of HIV-related diseases.

Oropharynx

Inspection of the teeth and oral cavity in people with HIV infection frequently reveals abnormalities. Some of these may be incidental findings but others may be the cause of symptoms or have prognostic significance. An early sign that the immune system is damaged by HIV is the development of oropharyngeal candida, or thrush. Although this has many appearances, it often looks like whitish-yellow milk curds stuck on to the oral mucosa. The underlying mucosa is often slightly inflamed and red compared with the unaffected tissue. The plaques of candida are easily removed with a spatula and, when Gram-stained and examined microscopically, have the typical appearance of *Candida* species with budding yeasts and hyphae. Candida may cause atrophic glossitis. Extensive candidiasis may lead to oral ulcers and discomfort or may impair taste and appetite.

Oral candidiasis is usually easy to treat. In the early stages it may respond to topical antifungal agents such as nystatin suspension, clotrimazole troches or amphotericin B lozenges. Later, oral systemic antifungals are required, such as ketoconazole, fluconazole or itraconazole. Continuous prolonged use of these imidazole antifungals may lead to the development of resistant *Candida*. This can be a difficult problem, particularly in end stage HIV disease, and may require intravenous amphotericin B therapy.

Hairy oral leukoplakia was recognised to be a feature of HIV disease early in the epidemic and appears to be associated with more rapid disease progression. This lesion, which superficially may resemble candida, usually appears as a poorly demarcated, slightly raised and corrugated white plaque on the side of the tongue. It may also appear on the buccal mucosa. Unlike candida, it cannot be scraped off.

Most lesions are asymptomatic. Epstein–Barr virus has been found in the lesions of oral hairy leukoplakia but the significance of this finding is unclear. High dose acyclovir may sometimes cause the lesions to regress.

Aphthous ulceration is more common in HIV disease than in seronegative individuals. The ulcers are painful and may become quite large. Sometimes symptoms are severe enough to warrant steroid therapy, either locally or systemically.

Periodontal disease is seen frequently in the setting of HIV. Suppurative gingivitis may cause halitosis or may lead to more serious sequelae, such as necrosis and mandibular osteomyelitis.

Purplish plaques or raised areas in the palate are indicative of Kaposi's sarcoma. When these are present there are usually further Kaposi's sarcoma plaques in the stomach and elsewhere in the gastrointestinal tract.

Oesophagus

Oesophageal candidiasis is an AIDS-defining infection that is a common and expected continuation of severe oral candidiasis. The patients presents with a painful dysphagia of fairly gradual onset. Such patients, if endoscoped, will usually be found to have a carpet of candida throughout the length of the oesophagus in association with a marked ulcerative oesophagitis. Anyone who has oral candida and dysphagia in the context of HIV infection should be treated for oesophageal candidiasis and only needs to be endoscoped if symptoms do not improve on antifungal therapy. Topical antifungals are not useful, so the more expensive systemic drugs are required. The condition commonly relapses in the absence of antifungals.

Less common causes of infective oesophagitis are cytomegalovirus (CMV) and herpes simplex virus (HSV). Both are rare but may mimic disease due to candida with painful dysphagia. Oral candida is absent, the oesophagus is ulcerated and friable on endoscopy and viral inclusions will be seen in histological sections of mucosal biopsies. Specific antiviral therapy with ganciclovir and acyclovir respectively will usually bring about improvement but, as both are expensive, histological proof of viral infection should be sought.

Rarely, the oesophagus may be the site of painful, solitary ulcers. The cause of these ulcers is not known but in many instances they respond to high dose oral prednisolone. Thalidomide has also been shown to be helpful.

Practice point
• *Patients presenting with the triad of weight loss, oral candida and painful dysphagia can be assumed to have oesophageal candida and treated empirically with systemic antifungals. Endoscopy is only required if the symptoms do not settle within a couple of weeks. The presence of oral or oesophageal candida should lead to consideration of HIV testing.*

Case history 1
A 30-year-old man presented to a clinic in Kampala complaining of weight loss and retrosternal pain when swallowing. Examination revealed generalised lymphadenopathy and oral candidiasis. Upper gastrointestinal endoscopy revealed an ulcerative oesophagitis with plaques of candida along the length of the oesophagus. Oral nystatin suspension helped to clear his oral candida but his retrosternal discomfort only abated after he was switched to ketoconazole.

Stomach

This organ is relatively spared in patients with HIV. It should be noted, however, that in moderately to severely advanced disease, many patients are achlorhydric and this may affect the absorption of some drugs, such as ketoconazole. The stomach may be the site of HIV-related tumours. Both Kaposi's sarcoma and non-Hodgkin's lymphoma may present in the stomach with nausea, pain, bleeding etc. Kaposi's in the stomach, as in other sites in the gut, may rarely present with protein-losing enteropathy.

Small bowel

HIV may affect the small intestine along any or all of its length, often with serious consequences. The most common problem is diarrhoea, which is usually chronic and intermittent. Infective causes include protozoa, bacteria and viruses.

Infections

Protozoa

The most common parasite to affect the small bowel in HIV disease is *Cryptosporidium parvum*, a coccidian parasite that invades enterocytes. This organism can affect many species and is transmitted to man via food or water. Human to human transmission has also been described. Immunocompetent people may have only mild symptoms but those with HIV may have severe, watery diarrhoea resembling cholera. This can lead to profound dehydration and marked weight loss. The diarrhoea is often accompanied by cramping abdominal pain and sometimes by nausea and vomiting. Some patients may develop an ascending cholangitis and acalculus cholecystitis due to *Cryptosporidium*, with severe pain and abnormal liver function tests. Diagnosis is relatively easy. The *Cryptosporidium* oocysts are round, about 4–5 μm in diameter and stain red with a modified acid-fast stain, such as Kinyoun's. The parasite may also be seen adhering to villi on histological sections of small bowel mucosa. The main problem with cryptosporidiosis is that no specific therapy is available. A large number of drugs have been tried and success has been claimed for some initially. However, because the symptoms can be intermittent, drug trials need to be placebo-controlled to show a real benefit and to date no drug has been shown to be useful. Therefore, the most important aspects of therapy are rehydration and correction of electrolyte imbalance, which may have to be with intravenous fluids if nausea and vomiting are severe, and anti-diarrhoeal drugs, such as loperamide or codeine phosphate. The oocysts of *Cryptosporidium* are very hardy and resistant to many common disinfectants, so care must be taken to prevent nosocomial transmission of this parasite. (See also Table 2.9 p 28)

Case history 2
A 24-year-old Zambian woman had already had two admissions to hospital for diarrhoea in the past 6 months. On this occasion, she gave a week's history of watery diarrhoea, opening her bowels 10 to 12 times daily. In addition, she had severe nausea and had been unable to eat or drink for the past 24 hours. On examination she was dehydrated with a systolic blood pressure of 90 mmHg and had oral candida. She was treated initially with IV saline with added potassium. Her initial blood results showed a plasma potassium of 2.3 mmol/l and a plasma urea of 25 mmol/l. Stool cultures were negative but showed cysts of *Cryptosporidium* on microscopy. She required 10 litres of IV fluids over the first 36 hours. Her symptoms slowly resolved over the next week and she was discharged with a supply of Imodium (loperamide hydrochloride).

Isospora belli, another coccidian parasite, can produce symptoms very similar to those due to *Cryptosporidium*. The diarrhoea is usually less dramatic and abdominal pain is less of a feature. The parasite can also be found by careful examination of the stool using a modified acid-fast stain and appears as an elliptical oocyst 20–30 μm by 10–15 μm. As for cryptosporidiosis, stool concentration methods in the laboratory may increase in the diagnostic yield if few oocysts are shed in the faeces. Unlike cryptosporidiosis, there is reasonable evidence to support the use of co-trimoxazole in the treatment of diarrhoea due to *Isospora belli*. High doses (2 tablets [each tablet contains 80 mg trimethoprim and 400 mg sulphamethoxazole] four times daily) are required for 2 to 3 weeks. Many clinicians put patients on 2 tablets daily of co-trimoxazole to prevent recurrences.

Recently, a new group of human pathogens has been described in association with the HIV pandemic. Microsporidia are parasites of a wide variety of animals, including insects. The main species found in patients with HIV are *Enterocytozoon bienusi* and *Encephalitozoon cuniculi*. The main symptoms due to microsporidiosis are chronic diarrhoea and weight loss. Abdominal pain does not seem to be a feature. These parasites can become disseminated and may cause eye infections, meningoencephalitis and infection of the renal tract. Diagnosis is difficult because the spores are only about 2 μm in diameter. Species diagnosis can only be made using electron microscopy but spores are visible with light microscopy in histological sections. In experienced hands, touch preparations of bowel biopsies and stool smears can be appropriately stained and microsporidial spores identified. Because of these diagnostic difficulties, the prevalence of microsporidial infection in HIV positive people is not known. Improvements in diagnosis will undoubtedly lead to more cases being identified. Although there is no established therapy for microsporidiosis, anecdotal reports suggest albendazole may have a role. This needs further evaluation.

Although *Giardia intestinalis* and cysts of *Entamoeba histolytica* are found more commonly in homosexual men than in heterosexual men in Europe and North America, there is no evidence that they cause particular problems in HIV disease. In the tropics, where these two enteric protozoa are more prevalent, they have not been identified in association with HIV with or without diarrhoea.

Bacteria

Bacteria may cause diarrhoea in a variety of ways but there is little evidence that the common causes of bacterial gastroenteritis are more common or worse in those with HIV. It is clear, however, that non-typhoidal salmonella infections are much more likely to result in bacteraemia and increase the risk of death in those with HIV compared with HIV negative individuals.

Autonomic neuropathy may occur in some patients with HIV and lead to intestinal stasis. This predisposes to bacterial overgrowth and sometimes to malabsorption and diarrhoea. Although rare, this may respond to treatment with broad-spectrum antibiotics, such as tetracycline or erythromycin.

Mycobacteria

Mycobacterial infections are much more common in HIV infection than in the general population, particularly in the tropics. There is a clear link between HIV and *Mycobacterium tuberculosis* in Africa, South America and, increasingly, in North America. Although most cases are pulmonary tuberculosis (TB), extrapulmonary TB is also an increasing problem and sometimes affects the abdomen. Primary TB peritonitis may occur, presenting either as ascites or as a 'doughy' abdomen, but TB may affect the gastrointestinal tract itself. This may present with weight loss, abdominal discomfort, malabsorption or as an acute abdomen. Tuberculosis does not account for the syndrome of 'slim' disease, however. Disease due to *M. tuberculosis* should be treated with standard anti-tuberculous chemotherapy according to national guidelines. Patients with HIV appear to respond to therapy as well as those without HIV but there is evidence from Africa that the recrudescence or re-infection rate is higher with HIV, at least with pulmonary TB. In addition, HIV infected patients with TB to have a decreased survival compared with HIV negative TB patients, probably because they succumb to other HIV-related infections.

A different mycobacterium causes most of the problems in Europe and North America but is rarely identified in the tropics. *Mycobacterium avium-intracellulare* complex (MAI) is a common environmental organism that can cause clinical infection in HIV positive patients with severe immunosuppression. The bacillus probably has the gut as its portal of entry, being ingested with food or water. Clinical symptoms usually result from dissemination of MAI but diarrhoea is a common association. Infected patients usually have high fevers, often with rigors, and usually have accelerated weight loss. The diagnosis should be suspected if acid-fast bacilli are seen on stool microscopy. MAI may be cultured from stool, lymph nodes, bone marrow, blood and urine. Because symptoms due to MAI are seen only in late disease, with very low CD4 lymphocyte numbers, it is not seen in tropical countries where very few patients survive with such marked immunodeficiency. Treatment of MAI is difficult as the organisms are frequently resistant to first-line anti-TB drugs. A common anti-MAI regimen used in Europe is a combination of rifabutin, ethambutol, clarithromycin and ciprofloxacin. There are no good clinical trials on which to base decisions about therapy, the regimens in common use are expensive and not all patients get symptomatic relief.

Practice point

- *'Slim disease' is not due to mycobacterial infection and therefore should not be treated as tuberculosis. This will lead to wastage of expensive anti-tuberculous drugs and may promote the development of antibiotic resistance. Atypical mycobacterial (MAI) infection is exceedingly rare in the tropics.*

Viruses

There are few viruses, other than HIV itself, which are known to cause specific problems in the small bowel of patients with HIV. Cytomegalovirus can cause small bowel ulceration which may lead to bleeding or even to perforation.

It should be noted that people with HIV cannot readily clear live poliovirus from the gut. They should, therefore, be immunised with the parenteral killed vaccine (Salk type).

Helminths

Despite the wide distribution of a large number of species of worms in the tropics and subtropics, helminth infections have not emerged as a significant problem in HIV infected people. Although there have been anxieties about the hyperinfection syndrome with *Strongyloides stercoralis* in immunocompromised HIV positive patients, experience has shown that this syndrome does not occur in the HIV setting.

Tumours

Lymphoma

Better prevention and treatment of the common infections associated with HIV has resulted in prolonged survival of HIV positive patients. One consequence of this has been an increased incidence of non-Hodgkin's lymphoma. Lymphoma may present at a variety of sites, including the small bowel. Symptoms related to small bowel lymphoma include abdominal pain, diarrhoea and bleeding associated with the tumour in the bowel and weight loss, malaise and fever as systemic symptoms of the lymphoma. The mass may be diagnosed by ultrasound, barium studies, sometimes by CT scan or at laparotomy. Tissue is required to make a definitive diagnosis, however. Treatment is often disappointing, largely because other HIV-related problems intervene, but is based around conventional chemotherapy, sometimes in association with surgical resection. Bowel lymphoma in association with HIV appears to be rare in tropical countries, probably because lymphoma is usually a feature of late disease.

Case history 3
A British haemophiliac was found to be HIV positive in 1985. Five years later he was admitted with *Pneumocystis carinii* pneumonia (PCP) and recovered uneventfully. Over the next year he remained fairly well but his CD4 lymphocyte count fell to around 0.01×10^9/l. He subsequently complained of increasingly severe abdominal pain and became mildly anaemic. He had two episodes of rectal bleeding and one of melaena. Colonoscopy revealed a mass in the terminal ileum which turned out, on biopsy, to be a poorly differentiated non-Hodgkin's lymphoma. He declined surgery and died a month later.

Kaposi's sarcoma

This may involve the small bowel and is often asymptomatic. However, bleeding can occur and, rarely, may be involved in intussusception. Chemotherapy and surgery both have a role in symptomatic small bowel Kaposi's.

Small bowel diarrhoea of uncertain cause (HIV enteropathy)

Up to 50 per cent of HIV-associated diarrhoea do not have an infective cause established. Affected patients tend to have chronic secretory diarrhoea, i.e. there are no pus cells or red blood cells in the stool. There is a relatively high stool frequency and volume. In general, there are no clinical clues that separate this sort of diarrhoea from infective causes and, in fact, the two may co-exist. There are a variety of possible explanations for HIV enteropathy, none of which is mutually exclusive.

Some people with HIV develop an autonomic neuropathy. In a manner analogous to that seen with diabetic neuropathy, this may sometimes result in diarrhoea. Nocturnal diarrhoea may be particularly troublesome. Histological studies of small bowel biopsies from patients with HIV enteropathy have shown loss of small never fibres, likely to be autonomic nerves, compared with normal controls.

In some patients with HIV, small bowel biopsies show partial villous atrophy, the degree of which correlates with severity of symptoms in some studies. It is conceivable that villous atrophy will result in malabsorption and lead to the diarrhoea and weight loss that characterises slim disease. However, it is unusual to be able to document malabsorption in most patients using standard techniques such as xylose absorption, red blood cells indices, vitamin levels, faecal fat estimates etc. Some studies have shown vitamin B_{12} malabsorption or abnormal xylose absorption tests in some patients but in the majority these tests are normal. In addition, there is no evidence to suggest that pancreatic function is seriously impaired in these patients so maldigestion is not the cause.

There is good evidence that the small bowel mucosa becomes excessively 'leaky' with HIV enteropathy with the net result that water and electrolytes flow into the gut lumen and overwhelm the absorptive capacity of the bowel. The mechanism by which this occurs is completely unclear but may involve either direct damage to enterocytes by HIV or a disturbance of local cytokine regulation.

Any or all of the above explanations for HIV enteropathy may be true. However, until the real mechanisms are known, treatment can only be symptomatic.

Practice point

* *Chronic diarrhoea and weight loss are common with HIV in the tropics. Most patients will not have a treatable cause. Attention should be focused on*

symptom relief with IV fluids and simple anti-diarrhoeal medication. Investigation should be kept to a minimum but ought to include at least two stool examinations using a modified acid-fast stain to exclude Isospora belli, *which will often respond to co-trimoxazole.*

Large bowel

Compared with the involvement of the small intestine, disorders of the large bowel are rarely a problem in HIV disease. In homosexual men in North America and Europe, CMV may affect the large bowel. CMV colitis is characterised by diarrhoea, usually with blood, in association with abdominal pain. Sigmoidoscopy may reveal a frankly haemorrhagic colitis or may show discrete ulceration. The diagnosis is made on histological grounds on the basis of typical CMV inclusions or immunocytochemistry. The disease often responds to intravenous ganciclovir or foscarnet but may relapse. Generally, CMV colitis is a feature of late stage disease and is rarely seen in the tropics.

Case history 4
Initially diagnosed as HIV positive 3 months before when he presented with nodules of Kaposi's sarcoma on his right thigh, a 36-year-old man from Tanzania was admitted with a cough, haemoptysis and an abnormal chest X-ray. He was started on treatment for tuberculosis but sputum microscopy was negative. Soon after admission he began to have rectal bleeding. Sigmoidoscopy revealed Kaposi's lesions in the rectal mucosa. Over the next few weeks his chest worsened and he died in respiratory failure. Post mortem revealed extensive Kaposi's sarcoma in his lungs and large bowel.

Case history 5
A 40-year-old bisexual man from Brazil presented to the gastroenterology clinic with diarrhoea and weight loss of a few weeks duration. He was thin and weighed 60 kg. He had tenderness and some guarding in the left iliac fossa. His stools were positive for occult blood and sigmoidoscopy revealed a friable rectal mucosa with some contact bleeding. A provisional diagnosis of ulcerative colitis was made but histological examination of a rectal biopsy showed characteristic inclusions of cytomegalovirus (CMV). After appropriate counselling, he was tested for HIV and found to be positive. His symptoms slowly settled after 2 weeks of IV ganciclovir therapy.

Patients with HIV are more likely to harbour sexually transmitted diseases than seronegative individuals and some of these infections may cause rectal or perineal problems. Herpes simplex infections may become chronic and lead to rectal and perineal discomfort and discharge. Homosexual men are more likely to have rectal symptoms but women can be similarly affected. Lymphogranuloma venerum (LGV), due to certain serotypes of *Chlamydia trachomatis*, and granuloma inguinale, caused by *Calymmatobacterium granulomatis*, may be more aggressive in the setting of HIV infection and both may cause rectal disease. LGV can cause a proctitis, fistula *in ano* or even rectal stricture. In very rare instances, granuloma inguinale can cause sufficient scarring to cause anal stricture.

Ischiorectal abscesses appear to be more common in HIV infection but can be incised and drained in the usual way (see Chapter 23). There is anecdotal data to suggest that surgical wounds are slower to heal in HIV positive patients, however.

Conclusions

It can be seen that HIV and its complications often affect the gastrointestinal tract and can cause problems at any site from the teeth to the anus. Some of these problems are simple to diagnose with the minimum of resources and can often be dealt with using available drugs or procedures. It should be remembered that infecting pathogens may vary from place to place, so local knowledge and experience is often more useful than the medical literature. Even with adequate treatment, some infections, such as oesophageal candidiasis, may recur when treatment stops. Local experience and resources will dictate whether chemoprophylaxis or intermittent therapy for relapses are used.

Unfortunately, the most common clinical problem in the tropics is chronic diarrhoea and wasting (slim disease in Africa) and this is poorly understood at present. Although sometimes due to treatable infections, such as *Isospora belli*, most cases are of unknown aetiology and can only be treated symptomatically. This is an area that needs further research. In the meantime, prevention is vitally important to try to reduce the chances of new HIV infections.

Drugs for HIV-related gastrointestinal diseases

Anti-diarrhoeal agents

Codeine phosphate (generic) 30–60 mg 4–6 hourly when required for diarrhoea.
Lomotil (diphenoxylate hydrochloride 2.5 mg with atropine sulphate 25 μg); 4 tablets initially, followed by 2 tablets every 6 h when required.
Imodium (loperamide 2 mg) 2 capsules initially, followed by 1 capsule after every loose stool up to 5 times a day.

Antifungals for oral and oesophageal candida

Nystatin suspension (100 000 units per ml) 1 ml 6-hourly for oral candida.
Canesten (clotrimazole) 100 mg vaginal tablets, can be used orally for candida.
Nizoral (ketoconazole) 200 mg daily, may need to double for oesophageal disease.
Diflucan (fluconazole) 50–100 mg daily, may need to increase dose.
Sporanox (itraconazole) 100–200 mg daily.
Fungizone (amphotericin B) IV infusion; 1 mg/kg daily for severe candidiasis.

Antiparasitic drugs

Albendazole; 400 mg daily for microsporidiosis.
Septrin (co-trimoxazole); each tablet contains 80 mg trimethoprim and 400 mg
sulphamethoxazole; dose for *Isospora belli* infections: 2 tablets 6-hourly.

Anti-cytomegalovirus drugs

Cymevene (Ganciclovir) for IV infusion; 5 mg/kg 12-hourly for 14–21 days for CMV
colitis; rarely need maintenance.
Foscavir (foscarnet) for IV infusion; 200 mg/kg per 24 h continuous infusion;
14–21 days for CMV colitis.

N.B. Both of the above are very expensive and rarely required in the tropics.

Anti-herpes simplex drugs

Zovirax (acyclovir) 200–400 mg 5 times daily for oesophageal or perianal disease; oral
hairy leukoplakia may respond to 800 mg 5 times daily.

Anti-tuberculous drugs

Rifabutin 300 mg daily for non-tuberculous mycobacterial disease including *Myco-
bacterium avium-intracellulare*. Expensive.
Ciprofloxacin 250–750 mg b.d.
Ethambutol 25 mg/kg initially then 15 mg/kg daily.
Clarithromycin 250–500 mg b.d. for 7–14 days.

Further reading

Anon. HIV-associated enteropathy. Lancet 1989;ii:777–8.
Cello JP. Gastrointestinal manifestations of HIV infection. In: Sande MA, Volberding
PA editors. The Medical Management of AIDS. Philadelphia: WB Saunders Com-
pany, 1988:141–52.
Colebunders R, Lusakumuni K, Nelson AM, *et al*. Persistent diarrhoea in Zairian AIDS
patients: an endoscopic and histological study. Gut 1988;29:1687–91.
Conlon CP, Pinching AJ, Perera CU, Moody A, Luo NP, Lucas SB. HIV-related
enteropathy in Zambia: A clinical, microbiological and histological study. Am J Trop
Med Hyg 1990;42:83–8.
DeHovitz JA, Pape JW, Boncy M, Johnson WD Jnr. Clinical manifestations and therapy
of *Isospora belli* infection in patients with the acquired immunodeficiency syndrome.
N Engl J Med 1986;315:87–90.

Smith PD, Quinn TC, Strober W, Janoff EN, Masur H. Gastrointestinal infections in AIDS. Ann Intern Med 1992;116:63–77.

Van Gool T, Hollister WS, Schattenkerk JE *et al*. Diagnosis of *Enterocytozoon bieneusi* microsporidiosis in AIDS patients by recovery of spores form faeces. Lancet 1990;336:697–8.

6

Abdominal Tuberculosis

Tuberculosis is a disease caused by *Mycobacterium tuberculosis*. Abdominal tuberculosis is the term used to describe this disease in the intra-abdominal organs of the digestive system, their peritoneal covering and the draining lymph nodes. Thus, it includes tuberculosis of stomach, small intestine, large intestine, hepatobiliary system, spleen, pancreas, peritoneum and the lymph nodes. Tuberculosis of the genitourinary system, adrenals and vascular system is not included in this term.

There are three major clinical subtypes of abdominal tuberculosis.

1. intestinal tuberculosis and tubercular involvement of other organs of the digestive system;
2. peritoneal tuberculosis;
3. intra-abdominal glandular tuberculosis (synonym: tabes mesenterica).

Intestinal tuberculosis is the commonest form of abdominal tuberculosis. The other structures affected are, in order of frequency, the peritoneum, abdominal lymph nodes and other abdominal organs.

Epidemiology

Abdominal tuberculosis was frequent before chemotherapy for pulmonary tuberculosis was introduced. Publications before 1940 reported 6–90 per cent abdominal involvement in patients with pulmonary tuberculosis. This high incidence has declined wherever pulmonary tuberculosis has been controlled. Unfortunately, control programmes for tuberculosis have not been very successful in many developing countries. In India the incidence remains high and recent studies have reported abdominal tuberculosis in 0.8 per cent of admissions, 7 per cent of small bowel obstruction and 6 per cent of intestinal perforation. In another Indian study, 44 per cent of exudative ascites and 8 per cent of all ascites in a tertiary care hospital were due to tuberculosis. Similar reports from Iraq and South Africa indicate that abdominal tuberculosis is still a common problem in other developing countries.

The disease has a higher prevalence in low socioeconomic groups in the

85

age group 20 years to 40 years. Females suffer more than the males. The emergence of drug resistant mycobacteria and association of tuberculosis with human immunodeficiency virus (HIV) infection has changed the epidemiology of this disease during the last decade.

Pathogenesis

The organism

Mycobacterium tuberculosis (bovine strain) acquired through ingested milk was the main infecting agent before pasteurisation. After pasteurisation, the incidence of bovine tuberculosis declined and currently the human strain is the principle cause of the abdominal tuberculosis.

Routes of entry

The possible routes of infection of *M. tuberculosis* include direct invasion by the ingested organisms, haematogenous seeding, transport through bile and direct extension from adjacent diseased organs or tissue.

Ingestion of bacilli

Tuberculosis bacilli may be ingested through swallowing infected sputum in patients with pulmonary tuberculosis, or contaminated foodstuffs, particularly in developing countries where sharing of food from a common source is widespread. After being ingested the acid-fast bacilli reach the ileum where they spread to the submucosa and mesenteric lymph nodes through the lymphatics.

Hematogenous spread

Silent bacteraemia may occur in miliary tuberculosis, or during the primary phase of pulmonary tuberculosis, thus enabling bacilli to become seeded in the abdominal organs. However clinical and experimental evidence do not support this hypothesis.

Transportation through bile

Sequestration of bacilli by the liver with biliary excretion is a potential but unproven route of infection.

Extension from contiguous organs

Direct extension from infected organs and tissues such as the female genital tract may occur. However invasion of the bowel does not arise from involvement of the peritoneum but intestinal tuberculosis may spread to the peritoneum through the draining lymph nodes which may then ulcerate to involve the peritoneum.

Pathogenic process

The tuberculosis bacillus reaches a tissue such as the intestinal mucosa and passes through the lymphatics to the submucosa, and lymph nodes, or reaches the peritoneum through the bloodstream. It is the engulfed by tissue macrophages for antigen processing. When its determinant antigen is presented to cytotoxic T lymphocytes, cytokines – particularly α-interferon – are released which activate macrophages to secrete other cytokines such as tumour necrosis factor (TNF), interleukin-1 (IL-1) and other cytotoxic enzymes which, in trying to destroy the bacillus, damage the surrounding tissue resulting in caseation necrosis. The constitutional symptoms in tuberculosis are due to the liberated cytokines and the local symptoms depend upon the organ involved. The cytokines also cause endothelial changes to adjacent vascular structures resulting in endarteritis and intravascular microthrombi. When this active inflammatory process heals the ensuing fibrosis may result in contraction and stenosis.

This process may continue over a long period of time. Depending upon the time of presentation, one may encounter ulceroconstrictive and ulcerohypertrophic types of intestinal tuberculosis. However, in the lymph node and on the peritoneal surface, caseation surrounded by participating lymphocytes and histiocytes (the classical tubercle) is commonly found. Three factors seem to determine the severity of a lesion:

1. virulence of the organism,
2. concentration of the innoculum, and
3. competence of the cell mediated immunity (CMI).

When the CMI is compromised, the bacillus, through proteolytic and lysosomal enzymes, causes extensive damage as seen in tubercular ulcerative enteritis associated with open cavitary tuberculosis in the prechemotherapeutic era and in patients with HIV infection.

Pathology

Gross appearance

Intestinal tuberculosis

Intestinal tubercular lesions can be categorised into ulceroconstrictive and ulcerohypertrophic types depending upon the gross morphological appearance.

Ulceroconstrictive type (Figure 6.1)

Endarteritis causes mucosal ulceration surrounded by an inflammatory reaction which initiates collagen formation, particularly during the process of healing, and results in circumferential strictures in the bowel lumen. The mucosal surface may show single and multiple ulcers with skip areas. The ulcers are characteristically circumferential and transverse and do not usually penetrate the muscularis propria. The margins of the ulcers are nodular and shaggy. The draining mesenteric lymph nodes are enlarged, firm and its cut surface may show caseation. During the acute phase the lumen of the bowel may be narrow due to an element of spasm.

Ulcerohypertrophic type (Figure 6.2)

This type of lesion usually occurs in the ileoacecal region of the caecum and colon. Such lesions show an intense fibroblastic reaction in the submucosa and subserosa. The mesenteric lymph nodes and bowel wall are invariably thickened. The mucosal surface may show a exophytic mass lesion indistinguishable from a neoplasm. Such lesions are probably associated with fewer bacilli with increased CMI, whereas the ulceroconstrictive lesions are associated with higher numbers and greater virulence.

Peritoneal tuberculosis

Depending upon the laparosopic appearance, three types of peritoneal morphology have been described in patients with peritoneal tuberculosis.

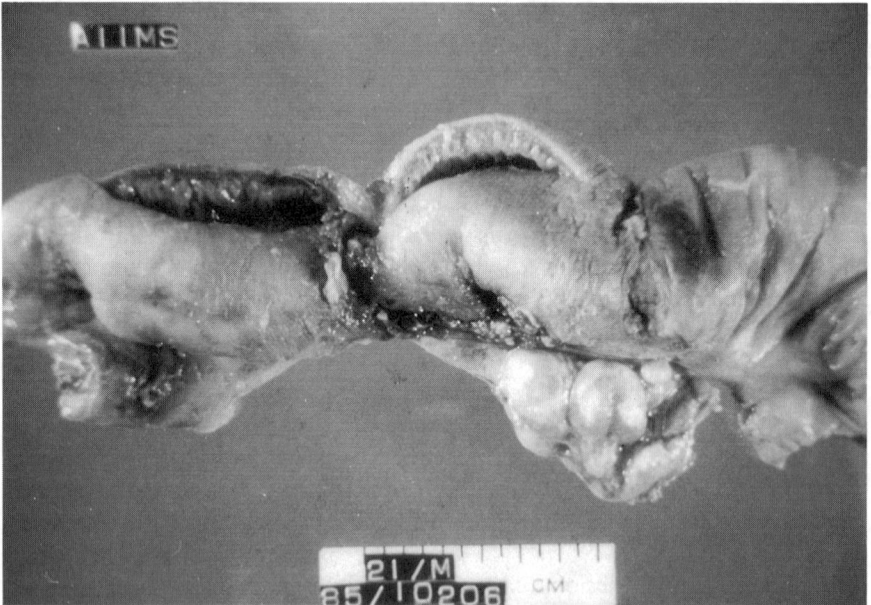

Figure 6.1 Ulceroconstrictive lesion of the intestine.

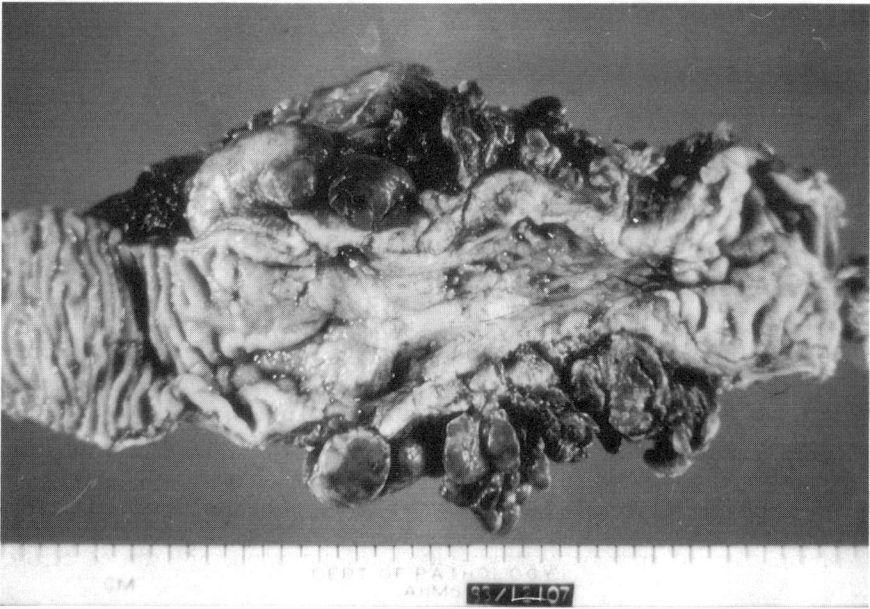

Figure 6.2 Ulcerohypertrophic lesion of the intestine.

Thickened peritoneum with tubercule

Tubercules are present in two-thirds of patients with peritoneal disease. Ascites is invariable. Laparoscopy shows:

- Yellowish white nodules of uniform size (4–5 cm) on the parietal and visceral peritoneum as well as on the bowel wall and omentum.
- Parietal peritoneum that has lost its lustre and looks thickened. The vascular pattern of the peritoneum is lost.
- Multiple adhesions between the parietal peritoneum and other abdominal organs like liver and intestines are present.
- Ascites, which is always present.

Thickened peritoneum without tubercle (20 per cent)

There are no nodules but the other findings described above are present including ascites.

Fibroadhesive type

These patients have grossly thickened peritoneum to which omentum and bowel loops are invariably adherent, resulting in a mass, often palpable in the upper abdomen. Ascites and nodules are rarely seen. Previous laparotomy may result in the patient presenting with intestinal fistula because of the difficult adhesions.

Glandular tuberculosis

Mesenteric and less frequently retroperitoneal lymph nodes are almost always involved in intestinal tuberculosis. When peritoneal tuberculosis occurs secondary to glandular tuberculosis, then simultaneous involvement of both is encountered. However, in children, isolated glandular tuberculosis is observed in about 20–25 per cent of cases.

Histology

The diagnostic feature in all types of tubercular lesion is the caseating granuloma (Figure 6.3). It cannot always be demonstrated, particularly in intestinal disease. In developing countries where tuberculosis is endemic, demonstration of non-caseating granulomas is also diagnostic of tuberculosis. Unfortunately, only 40–50 per cent of the intestinal tubercular lesions may show a granuloma. The reasons for the absence or non-detection of a granuloma include:

1. previous antitubercular therapy which has been empirically started before histology is available;
2. the draining lymph nodes may contain the granuloma even when the intestinal lesions do not;
3. a granuloma may be located in the submucosal layer so that endoscopic biopsy, which is often limited to the mucosa, may miss a submucosal

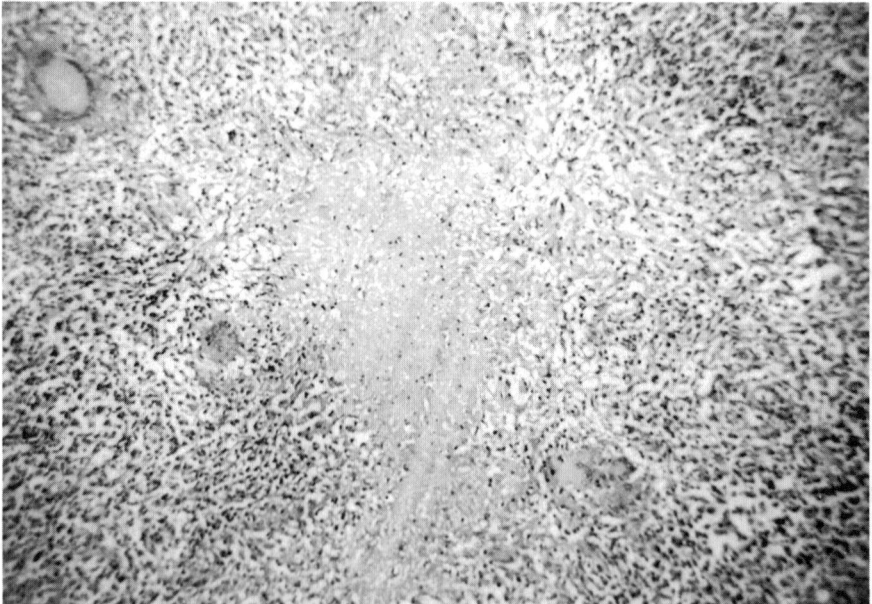

Figure 6.3 Granuloma showing a typical Langhans' giant cell.

granuloma and the characteristic lesion may only be obtained by surgical biopsy of the whole wall.

Demonstration of acid fast bacilli (AFB) is also rare. However bacteriological culture of the tissue homogenate grows AFB on specific media in about 40 per cent of cases. Thus combining histology and bacteriological culture a definite diagnosis can be achieved in 60–70 per cent of patients.

In contrast to intestinal tuberculosis, a characteristic granulomatous lesion in peritoneal tissue is documented in about 80 per cent of patients. However, the laparoscopic appearance of the peritoneum has been reported to be reliable in 95 per cent if cases with peritoneal tuberculosis. In glandular disease demonstration of a granuloma is almost always possible unless the patient had received prior antituberculosis therapy.

Clinical features

The clinical manifestations depend on the site of involvement. The small intestine is most often affected with peritoneal and lymph node spread in a third of intestinal cases. The ileocaecal region is affected in 50–60 per cent of cases. Other sites affected in decreasing order of frequency, are the ileum, caecum, ascending colon, jejunum, appendix, transverse and descending colon, rectum, duodenum, stomach and oesophagus. Colonic tuberculosis is usually segmental.

Primary and secondary abdominal tuberculosis have the same clinical features except for the association of pulmonary tuberculosis in the latter. The symptoms and signs of abdominal tuberculosis are not specific and can be broadly grouped into two categories:

1. Constitutional symptoms like fever, weight loss, anorexia and lethargy, which occur if the disease is active and are the result of cytokines liberated during the ongoing necro-inflammatory process. Such features are encountered in about one-third of all patients with abdominal tuberculosis.
2. Symptoms and signs due to the specific organ involved – these are discussed below.

Intestinal tuberculosis

Intestinal tuberculosis usually presents with one of the following features:

1. **Subacute intestinal obstruction** due to intestinal luminal narrowing which is the most frequent form of presentation in patients with intestinal tuberculosis; there is a characteristic history of pain in periumbilical region associated with increased borborygmi, often accompanied by abdominal distension, constipation and vomiting. In some tropical countries 12–60 per cent of those with intestinal tuberculosis present with obstruction and

39–60 per cent of intestinal obstruction is due to abdominal tuberculosis (only 5 per cent in non-endemic areas). The cause of obstruction may be due to strictures, adhesions, lymph nodes or extrinsic compression by a mass. Strictures are the commonest cause and in India a study of 300 patients with intestinal tuberculosis found 119 (39.7 per cent) had at least one stricture. The ileum was most frequently affected in 81 (68 per cent), the jejunum in 15 per cent and both in 17 per cent. Multiple strictures were encountered in 60 per cent of patients with stricture.

2. **Altered bowel habit** due to bacterial overgrowth, associated with malabsorption, malnutrition and weight loss (see also Chapter 8)
3. **Abdominal mass** in 30–35 per cent of patients with ileocaecal or colonic tuberculosis,
4. **Perforation** occurs in 1–10 per cent of patients with intestinal disease and may manifest as an acute abdomen or more silently in immunocompromised patients.
5. **Colitis**: diffuse colonic involvement due to tuberculosis may mimic ulcerative colitis,
6. **Acute appendicitis** due to appendicular involvement.
7. Rarely **dysphagia, gastrointestinal bleeding or obstruction** due to oesophageal, duodenal or colonic tuberculosis. **Intestinal fistula** is also very rare.

Peritoneal tuberculosis

There are two common presentations of peritoneal tuberculosis.

1. Ascitic type – in endemic areas peritoneal tuberculosis is the commonest cause of exudative ascites.
2. The fibroadhesive type invariably presents with an abdominal mass, frequently in the periumbilical or epigastric area. Abdominal pain is frequent with or without subacute intestinal obstruction.

Glandular tuberculosis

Isolated involvement of mesenteric lymph nodes is common in children. The dominant clinical manifestation is persistent abdominal pain due to involvement of the adjacent peritoneum. Infrequently the glands may compress the intestinal lumen causing subacute intestinal obstruction. Mesenteric lymph node involvement was rare in adults until the HIV epidemic began but is being encountered more frequently (Chapter 10 p 172).

Other forms of abdominal tuberculosis

Infrequently other organs such as the liver, spleen or pancreas can be involved.

Granulomatous hepatitis presents with gross hepatomegaly, fever and weight loss. Liver histology invariably reveals granulomatous lesions. Jaundice is rare and occurs only when a tubercle ruptures into a bile duct resulting in cholangitis or when a tuberculoma compresses one of the larger bile ducts. Pancreatic tuberculosis mimics pancreatic neoplasm and is diagnosed only by histology. Splenic tuberculosis presents with splenomegaly and fever. The diagnosis in such patients is usually made by splenectomy for unexplained splenomegaly (see pp 173–4).

Diagnosis

Investigations

The diagnosis of abdominal tuberculosis in the presence of pulmonary tuberculosis is not difficult (Figure 6.4). However, a definitive diagnosis of primary intestinal tuberculosis is difficult, and is based on finding one or more of the following:

1. Positive guinea pig inoculation or culture.
2. Demonstration of acid fast bacillus on smear or histological specimen.
3. Histological evidence of tubercle with caseation necrosis.
4. Combination of a typical gross appearance with the lymph nodes showing granulomata or caseation.
5. The bowel wall showing non-specific changes and caseation present in the mesenteric lymph nodes.

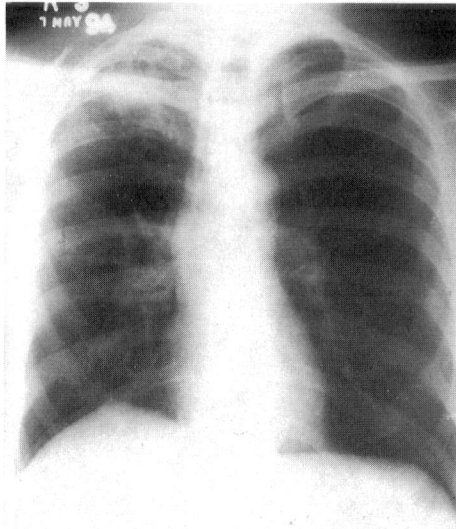

Figure 6.4   Intestinal TB in a patient with pulmonary TB.

6. A non-caseating granuloma with tuberculosis elsewhere responding to antitubercular treatment.

It is obvious that demonstration of a characteristic granuloma and/or identifying AFB in the tissue involved is the gold standard for diagnosis. For this purpose tissue must be obtained from the involved organ. Investigations should aim first to establish the site of involvement and then achieve a tissue.

Radiology

Plain X-ray of abdomen

Patients presenting with features of subacute intestinal obstruction reveal dilated small bowel loops with or without air fluids levels in a plain X-ray of the abdomen taken in an erect position. Demonstration of dilated bowel loops is adequate evidence of small bowel involvement. It may also reveal calcified lymph nodes in the retroperitoneum. Barium follow-through or small bowel enema in such patients after the obstruction is relieved, do not improve the chances of determining the site of obstruction. However, a contrast study may be necessary to exclude other pathological conditions such as neoplasm. A barium study revealing a contracted caecum and ascending colon with a deformed ileocecal angle is highly suggestive of tuberculosis in endemic areas (Figure 6.5). If the small bowel is suspected to be the site of disease then a barium meal follow-through or small bowel enema is preferred. A small bowel enema is likely to yield better results than a conventional follow through, because, it prevents overlapping of small bowel loops and distends the intestinal lumen, thus making incomplete strictures more prominent. A barium enema is preferred if colonic or ileocaecal tuberculosis is suspected.

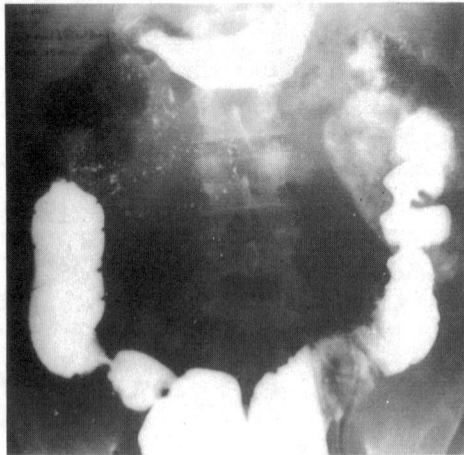

Figure 6.5   Barium meal follow through showing ileal stricture.

Ultrasonography

Detection of lymph nodes in the mesentery or retroperitoneum as well as mass lesions in ulcerohypertrophic tuberculosis is often possible, particularly in those with a painful abdomen or abdominal mass. An ultrasound-guided fine needle aspiration biopsy enables a tissue diagnosis to be made at the same time.

Computed tomography CT scan of the abdomen

CT scan of the abdomen may be necessary to detect retroperitonel lesions and to rule out neoplastic conditions in the abdomen. CT-guided fine needle aspiration biopsy is helpful if there are enlarged retroperitoneal or mesenteric lymph nodes.

Ascitic fluid examination

In places where ascites may be due to peritoneal tuberculosis, analysis of ascitic fluid is mandatory. It confirms the exudative nature of the ascitic fluid and may demonstrate acid-fast bacilli. Raised levels of adenine deaminase (ADA) in ascitic fluid helps confirm the diagnosis of tubercular ascites.

Tissue diagnosis

Fine needle aspiration biopsy (FNAB)
FNAB using imaging modalities like ultrasonography or CT (if available) is the first step to achieving a tissue diagnosis, particularly in patients with retroperitoneal lymphadenopathy or an abdominal mass. In about 50–85 per cent of patients presenting with an abdominal mass or lymphadenopathy the presence of an epitheloid or caseating granuloma will be found. The complication rate is less than 1 per cent.

Endoscopic biopsy
In colonic and ileocaecal tuberculosis, characteristic colonoscopic appearances of transverse/linear ulcers, skip areas, strictures, mucosal nodules and deformed iliocecal valve have been described. A biopsy from the site of involvement, should be simultaneously processed for histology, AFB staining, and culture. A definitive diagnosis can be achieved in about 60 per cent of the patients.

Similarly upper gastrointestinal endoscopy for suspected oesophageal, gastric and duodenal tuberculosis is helpful in achieving tissue diagnosis. In proximal small bowel lesions enteroscopy may be helpful.

Peritoneoscopy or laparoscopy
Peritoneoscopy is the diagnostic procedure of choice in patients suspected to have peritoneal tuberculosis. It provides visualisation of the peritoneal surface and documentation of characteristic nodules, adhesions and thickened perito-

neum. A punch biopsy from the peritoneum provides a diagnostic yield of more than 85 per cent. It also provides opportunity for inspecting the liver surface and taking biopsies simultaneously. Percutaneous blind peritoneal biopsy using a Cope's or Abraham's needle has been gradually replaced by peritoneoscopy.

Liver biopsy

Liver biopsy is only helpful in patients with miliary tuberculosis. Over 90 per cent of these patients will be found to have a hepatic granuloma.

Serodiagnosis

Serological diagnosis for active tubercular infection has been recently introduced and is used for:

- rapid diagnosis,
- epidemiological surveys to devise control strategies,
- monitoring of patients for reactivation of disease,
- information on immune response of an individual to tubercular infection.

Serodiagnostic methods to detect both the antibody and antigen of *M. tuberculosis* have been reported. However antigen and antibody detection, particularly the IgG fraction in the sera using enzyme-linked immunosorbent assay (ELISA) or radioimmunoassay, has a low specificity in endemic areas so is not popular. Certain modified techniques to detect specific antigen or antibody fraction of *M. tuberculosis* seem promising but await reproducibility in further trials:

1. Sandwich ELISA adaptation of **solid phase antibody competition test (SACT-SE)**. In this method a monoclonal antibody known as mouse anti-IgG TB 72 monoclonal antibody is used on a solid phase to bind specific *M. tuberculosis* antigen (Antigen-5). Its sensitivity and specificity in active tuberculosis has been shown to be 78 per cent and 98 per cent, respectively.
2. **Soluble antigen fluorescence antibody test (SAFA)** – A saline extract of crude *M. tuberculosis* antigen is used to detect the antibody in patients sera by using immunofluorescence technique. However it carries a false positive rate of 4 per cent and cross reacts with antigens of fungi.
3. **Detection of tuberculostearic acid** – Tuberculostearic acid is a fatty acid present only in mycobacteria which can be detected by gas chromatography or mass spectrometry. Even though its sensitivity and specificity has been claimed to be more than 90 per cent, its use has been limited by the expensive equipment required and the complexity of the procedure.
4. **Adenosine deaminase (ADA) activity** – ADA is released by lymphocytes and macrophages during cellular immune response. Estimation of ADA in sera, CSF and ascitic fluid has been found to be highly specific and sensitive (>95 per cent specificity and sensitivity) in the diagnosis of active tuberculosis.

Polymerase chain reaction (PCR)

Recently amplification of a 240 base pair region in the MPB-64 protein coding gene, followed by starch gel electrophoresis has been shown to detect as few as 10 AFB/ml fluid. Normally a conventional smear positive for AFB will have over 10 000 AFB/ml. However cost and accessibility limit the use of polymerase chain reaction in developing countries particularly in peripheral medical centres most in need of a rapid diagnostic test.

Differential diagnosis

Intestinal tuberculosis

The differential diagnosis of intestinal tuberculosis depends upon its presenting features such as subacute intestinal obstruction, small bowel diarrhoea, gastrointestinal bleeding, or an abdominal mass. Each of these presenting symptoms can be encountered in a number of other intestinal disorders and are discussed in detail elsewhere in this book. The most important intestinal disease that shares many clinical, radiological and pathological features of intestinal tuberculosis is Crohn's disease. Fortunately the latter is infrequently encountered in the countries where intestinal tuberculosis is common. The similarities and dissimilarities between intestinal tuberculosis and Crohn's disease are listed in Tables 6.1 and 6.2.

Table 6.1   Similarities between intestinal tuberculosis and Crohn's disease.

Clinical
1. Peak age of presentation: 20–40 years
2. Typical presentation: Pain in right lower quadrant of abdomen with fever, anorexia, weight loss.
3. Recurrent attacks of pain with a relatively asymptomatic interval between attacks.

Pathology
1. Site of involvement: Most patients have small bowel involvement; predominant site of disease is ileocaecal region. There may be multiple sites of lesion with normal intervening areas (skip lesions).
2. Gross appearance: The mesentery is thickened with enlarged matted lymph nodes, dilated lymphatics are seen on the serosal surface, small bowel is thickened and there are linear mucosal ulcers.
3. Microscopic examination: Transmural involvement of the bowel with multiple granulomas.

Investigations
1. Endoscopic: Mucosal folds are swollen and oedematous, linear ulcers are present and multiple pseudopolyps (inflammatory) may be seen.
2. Radiological: Mucosal irregularity, filling defects and stricture formation may be observed in both the diseases.

Table 6.2 Differentiation between intestinal tuberculosis and Crohn's disease.

Criteria of differentiation	Intestinal tuberculosis	Crohn's disease
Epidemiological and racial factor	Asians & Africans	Europeans & Jews
Clinical features		
Diarrhoea	30%	80–90%
Intestinal obstruction	40–60%	< 10%
Anal lesions	< 5%	30%
Extraintestinal manifestation	< 5%	25%
Fistulae	< 10%	30%
Pathology		
Gross appearance		
Serosal nodules	Common	Never
Ulcers	Superficial transversely located	Longitudinal, oblique or serpiginious
Microscopy		
Caseation necrosis	Common	Never
Acid fast bacilli	Detected but infrequent	Never
Granulomas	Confluent	Discrete
Muscularis mucosae fibrosis	Common	Rare
Submucosal oedema	Rare	Common
Laboratory parameters		
Immunological		
Tuberuculin test (+ve)	90%	< 5%
SAFA/ELISA (+ve)	80%	< 5%
Endoscopic appearance	Mucosal nodules scattered over involved areas	Cobblestone pattern
Bacteriological		
AFB isolation	40–50%	Never
Radiological		
Chest X-ray (+ve)	25–40%	Never
Therapeutic challenge	Response to antitubercular	Response to steroids
Course and prognosis	Complete cure with therapy	Multiple relapses despite therapy

Peritoneal tuberculosis

Since exudative ascites is the commonest form of peritoneal tuberculosis, its differential diagnosis includes other causes of exudative ascites prevalent in the region. It needs to be differentiated from malignant ascites and hepatic venous outflow tract obstruction. The differentiating points between these three conditions are listed in Table 6.3.

Table 6.3   The differential diagnosis of exudative ascites: features of peritoneal tuberculosis, malignant ascites and hepatic vein obstruction.

Criteria of differentiation	Peritoneal tuberculosis	Malignant ascites	Hepatic vein obstruction
Clinical			
Constitutional symptoms (anorexia, weight loss)	30–50%	> 90%	< 30%
Dependent oedema & back veins	Rare	Rare	Frequent
Other sites of involvement	30% (pulmonary TB)	primary site frequently in GI tract	Nil
Laboratory parameters			
Ascitic fluid			
Cell	Lymphocyte predominant	Malignant cells present	Few mesothelial cells and lymphocytes
Laparoscopy	Characteristic finding of nodules, adhesions thickening	Nodules of varying size present in clumps	Collaterals lymphatic cysts, with congested liver oesophageal varices
Endoscopy	–	–	
Histology			
Peritoneal histology	Granuloma	Adenocarcinoma	Non-specific
Liver biopsy	Rarely granuloma	May show metastatic lesions	Characteristic sinusoidal dilatation

Glandular tuberculosis

Isolated mesenteric or retroperitoneal lymphadenopathy in any age group in developing nations is normally caused by tuberculosis, lymphoma or HIV infection. The diagnosis is confirmed by lymph node biopsy or fine needle aspiration cytology can sometimes be facilitated by ultrasound and CT. Otherwise a mini-laparotomy or laparoscopy may need to be performed. Often, when guided biopsy seems risky due to proximity of vessels and bowels to the target lesion, it is safer to undertake a mini-laparotomy. In one of the tertiary care centres in India, the diagnostic yield of mini-laparotomy in patients with retroperitoneal lymphodenopathy was 95 per cent.

Management

Anti-tubercular drugs

Medical therapy using specific antitubercular drugs should be used in all patients with abdominal tuberculosis. Both short-course chemotherapy and conventional chemotherapy are effective. Six month regimens initially using three to four drugs are preferred to reduce drug resistance and improve compliance. A commonly used regimen is isoniazid (INH), rifampicin and pyrazinamide for 2 months, then isoniazid and rifampicin for another 4 months. In HIV infected persons, isoniazid and rifampicin are continued for a further 7 months.

Treatment with isoniazid, rifampicin, pyrazinamide and ethambutol three times a week for 6 months is another highly effective regimen. Administration of isoniazid and rifampicin for 9 months is effective when drug resistance rates are low. The above treatment regimens have cure rates of over 95 per cent. The actual doses are shown in Table 6.4.

Table 6.4   Doses of anti-tubercular drugs.

Drugs	Adult	Children
Isoniazid	5–10 mg/kg	10–20 mg/kg
Rifampicin	10 mg/kg	10–20 mg/kg
Ethambutol	15–25 mg/kg	10–15 mg/kg
Pyrazinamide	20–40 mg/kg	30 mg/kg
Streptomycin	15 mg/kg	20 mg/kg

Not only do over 95 per cent of patients respond, but also 70–75 per cent of intestinal strictures resolve on anti-tubercular therapy. Side effects occur in up to 10 per cent. Hepatotoxicity is the major adverse effect of isoniazid, rifampicin and pyrazinamide; optic neuritis can result from ethambutol at dosages of 25 mg/kg per day. Late relapse after discontinuation of therapy is rare, being reported in less than 1 per cent. The response to chemotherapy is assessed by monitoring constitutional symptoms and by radiology. Clinical recovery usually occurs in 3–9 months. Patient compliance is an extremely important aspect affecting the outcome of therapy so that drug therapy must be closely supervised.

Drug resistant abdominal tuberculosis

Reports on drug resistant abdominal tuberculosis are lacking. About 10–30 per cent of all tubercular infections in developing countries have multiple drug resistance. Drug resistance is assessed by persistence of disease activity and lack of clinical and laboratory response after at least 3–6 months of adequate therapy. When drug resistant infection is proven the regimen should be changed. Individualised drug regimes, based on sensitivity testing, generally include at least three drugs to which the organism is likely to be susceptible. A single drug should never be added to the previous regimen. Re-treatment should be done in the hospital under supervision.

Surgical intervention

Surgery is indicated for acute, or persistent subacute, intestinal obstruction, perforation, uncontrolled gastrointestinal bleeding, or persistent fistulae. Long (greater than 12 cm) and multiple strictures are the most likely to require surgery, particularly if the presentation is delayed or there is a poor response to medical therapy. Laparotomy may be indicated for diagnostic uncertainty about an abdominal mass.

When abdominal tuberculosis is discovered inadvertently at laparotomy, dissection should be kept to a minimum to avoid injury to the bowel. Surgery should be restricted to biopsy and dealing with any life-threatening problem such as acute intestinal obstruction or perforation.

Prevention and control

The indications for preventive therapy are:

1. household members or close contacts of a infectious tubercular patient;
2. immunocompromised patients with history of tuberculosis or inactive chest lesion on chest X-ray;
3. HIV infection.

Isoniazid daily (5–10 mg/kg) for 6 to 12 months is recommended for those requiring preventive therapy for tuberculosis.

Further reading

Anand BS. Distinguishing Crohn's disease from intestinal tuberculosis. Natl Med J Ind 1989;2:131–75.

Anand SS. Hypertrophic ileocaecal tuberculosis in India with a record of fifty hemicolectomies. Ann R Coll Surg Engl 1956;19:205–22.

Anon. Drug treatment of tuberculosis – 1992. Drug 1992; 42:651–73.

Bhansali SK. Abdominal tuberculosis: Experience with 300 cases. Am J Gastronenterol 1977;67:324–37.

Bhargava DK. Intestinal tuberculosis. In: Tandon B N, Nundy S editors. Recent advances in tropical gastroenterology. New Delhi: Leipzig Press, 1982.

Bhargava DK, Shriniwas, Chawala TC. Intestinal tuberculosis: Bacteriologic study of tissue obtained by colonoscopy and during surgery. J Trop Med Hyg 1985;88:249–52.

Crawford PM, Sawyer HP. Intestinal tuberculosis in 1400 autopsies. Am Rev Tuberc 1934;30:568–83.

Das P, Shukla HS. Clinical diagnosis of abdominal tuberculosis. Br J Surg 1976; 63:941–6.

Granet E. Intestinal tuberculosis: A clinical roentological and pathological study of 2086 patients affected with pulmonary tuberculosis. Am J Dig Dis 1935;2:209–14.

Paustian FP, Bockus HL. So called primary ulcerhypertropic ileocaecal tuberculosis. Am J Med 1959;27:509.

Paustian FF, Monto GL. Tuberculosis of the intestines. In Bockus HL, editor. Gastroenterology. Philadelphia: Saunders, 1976:750–77.

Prakash A. Ulceroconstrictive tuberculosis of the bowel. Int Surg 1978;63:23–9.

Tandon HD, Prakash A. Pathology of intestinal tuberculosis and its distinction from Crohn's disease. Gut 1972;13:260–9.

7

Other Specific Gastrointestinal Infections

Intestinal and hepatosplenic schistosomiasis

Schistosomiasis is a parasitic infestation (trematode). The intestinal and hepatosplenic form is often caused by *Schistosoma mansoni* and *japonicum*. Very rarely it is caused by *Schistosoma intercalatum* and *haematobium*.

Schistosomiasis is predominately a disease of rural and agricultural communities. In some countries programmes for developing water resources in endemic areas have worsened the situation.

It has been estimated that over 200 million people in the world suffer from schistosomiasis and several more millions have been exposed to infection. Schistosomiasis is endemic in 72 countries. *Schistosoma mansoni* is endemic in some countries of Africa especially Egypt and Sudan, the Middle East and some parts of Latin America. *Schistosoma japonicum* is endemic in the Far East, particularly in Japan, China and Korea.

Pathogenesis

Infection occurs in areas where water is contaminated by ova from stools and urine. The ova then develop in the intermediate snail host from which cercariae emerge to penetrate human skin and subsequently develop into adult worms in the venous plexuses.

Schistosoma mansoni adult worms normally live in the tributaries of the inferior mesenteric vein where they lay eggs, usually resulting in involvement of the large bowel. Embolisation of ova, into the portal vein leads to hepatic involvement. This may result in the formation of hepatic granuloma and periportal fibrosis leading to portal hypertension. At this stage ova may also lodge into tributaries of the superior mesenteric vein and may result in involvement of the stomach and small intestine.

Schistosoma japonicum adult worms usually live in the tributaries of the superior mesenteric vein and to a lesser extent in the inferior mesenteric vein tributaries. The adult worm is relatively well tolerated by the host compared with *Schistosoma mansoni* and this results in less irritation, inflammation, fibrosis and obstruction of the portal venous system.

The association between *Schistosoma haematobium* and carcinoma of the urinary bladder is well known. However there is no definite association between *Schistosoma mansoni* and colorectal carcinoma or liver cancer.

Clinical manifestations

Schistosoma mansoni and *japonicum* infection can be divided into acute and chronic forms. The clinical manifestation is mainly due to the presence of ova and depends on the intensity of infection, frequency and severity of exposure and the immunological status of the person. The host granulomatous response to the egg is a form of delayed hypersensitivity and plays an essential role in the pathogenesis of schistosomiasis.

Acute infection

This can be subdivided into three types:

1. **Cercarial dermatitis** (stage of invasion). This occurs within 24 h after cercarial penetration of the skin (swimmer's itch)
2. **Katayama syndrome** (toxaemic phase). This is the hypersensitivity stage and occurs 4–6 weeks after exposure. It coincides with maturation of the schistosomes resulting in ova deposition. It is an acute febrile illness with diarrhoea and eosinophilia.
3. **Acute intestinal disease** (bilharzia dysentery). This results from egg deposition in the bowel wall. It starts about 2 months after infection with dysenteric like symptoms, fever, anorexia and abdominal tenderness. Exacerbations occur every few weeks. It may last 6–12 months and if not treated may progress to a chronic form.

Chronic infection

Two types of chronic infection occur.

Chronic intestinal infection

This usually involves the large bowel and to lesser extent the stomach, small bowel or the appendix. Other organs such as the gallbladder and pancreas may also be involved. In the large intestine viable ova produce an inflammatory reaction, granuloma formation, ulceration, bleeding, papillomata and fibrosis which give rise to abdominal pain, diarrhoea, bleeding, anaemia and protein losing enteropathy.

The stomach and small intestine may rarely be involved. If the small intestine is involved stunting of the villi may cause a malabsorption-like syndrome.

Hepatosplenic form

Hepatosplenic involvement occurs late in the disease process and usually develops 5–10 years after the initial infestation in about 10 per cent of patients. Embolisation of ova to the liver results in a hypersensitivity reaction with granuloma formation and later fibrosis. The resultant periportal fibrosis (Symmers' fibrosis) may lead to portal hypertension and oesophageal or gastric varices in about one-third of patients. Variceal bleeding is the leading cause of death in these patients.

Hepatocellular function is usually well preserved until late in the disease. Portal hypertension becomes evident long before any deterioration of liver function. Hypersplenism may develop.

Diagnosis

The diagnosis of schistosomiasis is easy to establish in endemic areas and is usually based on finding the ova in the stool by simple smear examination, concentration methods or quantitative techniques such as the Kato/Kazt methods. However in the chronic form the passage of ova is not constant and in this situation the diagnosis can be made by:

1. **Rectal or colonoscopic biopsy.** This is very useful especially in the chronic forms of intestinal schistosomiasis. However, in endemic areas, schistosomiasis may co-exist with other pathologies.
2. **Radiology.** Ultrasound of the liver demonstrates periportal fibrosis. A barium swallow may show oesophageal varices and portal venography and hepatic angiography may show evidence of portal hypertension. A barium enema may reveal the presence of schistosomal colonic polyps.
3. **Liver biopsy.** The biopsy will show characteristic ova and granuloma but the procedure may be complicated by bleeding due to hypoprothrombinaemia or thrombocytopenia due to hypersplenism. The clotting time should be checked before biopsy.
4. **Serology.** Haemagglutination tests are not always positive nor specific. The new developments in immunodiagnosis, radioimmunoassay and enzyme-linked immunosorbent assay (ELISA) are promising.

Management

Different antimonial compounds including hycanthone and niridazole were originally used. Newer antischistosomal drugs are are now available which are safe and effective in treating both acute schistosomiasis and halting the progress of the disease in chronic forms.

Praziquantel (40 mg/kg as a single dose) eradicates ova from the stool in over 90 per cent. Levopraziquantel (which is the active isomer) is equally effective at a single dose of 20 mg/kg. Oxamniquine is also highly effective, particularly against *Schistosoma mansoni*, and egg output is reduced by 80–90 per cent. Oltripraz has also been found to be effective in *Schistosoma mansoni* infection.

Visceral leishmaniasis

Visceral leishmaniasis (kala azar) is a disease caused by a protozoon called *Leishmania donovani* which is widely distributed around the Mediterranean basin, tropical Africa, parts of South America and Central and Eastern Asia.

Visceral leishmaniasis is also known as kala azar which is a Hindi word for 'black sickness' because of the skin pigmentation which is a feature of the disease.

Epidemiology

The epidemiology varies in different parts of the world. All sandflies breed in dark, moist habitats, such as cracks in masonry, piles of rubble, caves and dark, protected sites such as holes in termite mounds. The sandflies have a short flight range, being seldom found more than 200 m from their breeding place. They do not fly very high and seldom bite people sleeping on the first floor of a building. They normally bite at dawn, dusk and during the night.

The usual reservoirs of infection are: canines in the Mediterranean basin, the Middle East, Central Asia and South America (the relative importance of domestic dogs and wild canines, such as jackals and foxes, varies with each area), rodents in sub-Saharan Africa and man in India.

Mediterranean kala azar tends to affect young children more than adults. Epidemics occur in India, but in Africa the infection is usually sporadic.

Pathogenesis

The organs affected are the bone marrow, liver, spleen and the reticuloendothelial system which become infiltrated by infected (parasitised) macrophages. There is a general hyperplasia of lymphoid tissue. Splenic enlargement may lead to hypersplenism which may present with anaemia and thrombocytopenia. The Kupffer's cells enlarge due to infiltration by the amastigotes. The bone marrow is also infiltrated by infected macrophages, and both the IgG and total protein levels are elevated. Immune complex levels rise and it is deposited in the kidneys. In the skin a macular rash may follow chemotherapy. It is called post-kala-azar dermal leishmaniasis (PKDL). These lesions are teeming with parasites and this makes the patient a reservoir of infection.

There is impaired cellular immunity which facilitates uncontrolled parasitisation of the phagocytes. The IgM and IgG levels are elevated. This impaired cellular immunity reverts to normal after successful chemotherapy.

Clinical recognition

The incubation period is weeks to a few months. Patients usually present with anaemia, splenomegaly (which is often massive), hepatomegaly and wasting. Skin pigmentation may occur. Thus the combination of anaemia with splenomegaly or hepatosplenomegaly should always raise the possibility of visceral leishmaniasis.

The essential laboratory findings include pancytopenia, normocytic normochronic anaemia, the presence of LD (leishmania Donovan) bodies in splenic aspirate (which is the best site to identify them), liver aspirate and bone marrow aspirate. The aspirate is stained in leishmania stain while some of it is cultured in Novy, MacNeal and Nicolle (NNN) media and Schneider medium.

Management

Sodium stibogluconate (Pentostam)

Pentavalent antimonials have been the mainstay of the treatment of visceral, cutaneous and mucocutaneous leishmaniasis for approximately half a century. Pentostam (sodium stibogluconate) is the pentavalent antimony compound used. In the 1950s a dose of 10 mg/kg body weight per day for 30 days was found to be the most effective with minimal toxicity. However, relapses occurred and some cases proved refractory. Studies on the pharmacokinetics of sodium stibogluconate revealed that the drug is rapidly excreted by the kidney. Blood levels fall to less than 1 per cent of the peak 6 h after intravenous administration.

As dosage regimes for treating leishmaniasis evolved, the daily dose of antimony has been progressively increased to improve response, decreasing the duration of treatment, but without significantly increasing toxicity. Three dosage schedules of 10 mg/kg body weight were compared. Once daily for 31 days, twice daily for 15 days or thrice daily for 10 days. The parasites were cleared most rapidly from the spleen and haemoglobin levels rose most quickly in those treated with the highest daily dose although the differences were not significant.

A higher dose of 15 mg/kg body weight twice daily for 30 days resulted in a good response without serious side effects. Two other dosage regimes –

10 mg/kg and 20 mg/kg once daily until two consecutive weekly splenic aspirates are negative – have been compared. Only 60 per cent of patients less than 20 years of age responded to 10 mg/kg as compared to 100 per cent of those receiving 20 mg/kg per day. Such differences in response were not observed in adults who responded well to both treatments. This suggests that children require more antimony to achieve cure than adults. The rate of relapse was similar in both treatment regimes in adults and children.

In the 1980s, the use of 20 mg/kg per day (instead of 10 mg/kg per day) of antimony became standard therapy but only up to a maximum daily dose of 850 mg. This has recently been adjusted to exceed the 850 mg daily limit without increased toxicity. Given the status of treatment of leishmaniasis and the fact that the drug of choice sodium stibogluconate (Pentostam) is a heavy metal compound which is potentially toxic, it is clear that new anti-leishmanial drugs are required. Treatment of leishmaniasis is also expensive.

Aminosidine

Aminosidine has been used widely as an aminoglucoide antibiotic of wide spectrum for a long time. It is poorly absorbed in the gut and is more effective parenterally. Chunge found aminosidine (14–16 mg/kg daily) alone or in combination with sodium stibogluconate (20 mg/kg daily) to be superior to sodium stibogluconate alone.

Toxicity of treatment

1. Bleeding may occur from the gums and nose.
2. Secondary pneumonia, dysentry and tuberculosis may occur due to impaired cellular immunity and granulocytopaenia.

Control

Peridomestic sandfly can be destroyed by residual insecticides around the houses and the elimination of breeding sites. The methods that can be used depend on the epidemiological situation. Most success has been achieved where the domestic dog is the main reservoir, efforts being directed at catching and destroying infected dogs. Where man is the main reservoir, such as India, successful control was achieved when widespread insecticide spraying of houses for malaria control was in use. Sandflies are not resistant to DDT, so their 'hopping' flight pattern renders them particularly vulnerable.

In the sporadic kala azar of Africa, where rodents are the main reservoir, there are no practical control measures available. Individual protection against sandfly bite is difficult because repellents have only a brief effect and sandflies can pass through the mesh of normal mosquito nets. Good protection against night biting is given by sleeping on the first floor of the house. Efforts to produce a leishmania vaccine are in progress. Recovery from a natural attack leads to life-long immunity to attack by the same parasites.

Hydatid disease

Hydatid disease is due to the larval stage of a small tape worm of dogs and other canines developing in man. The infection is a zoonosis, normally maintained in dogs and sheep or cattle in close association with man (*Echinococcus granulosus*) or in a wild cycle such as in wild canines and rodents (*Echinococus multiclocularis*). Most human infections are with *E. granulosus* and are associated with the rearing of sheep and cattle in climatic conditions varying from tropical to subarctic.

Infection is usually acquired in childhood but the cysts grow slowly and usually present after some years. In endemic areas such as Turkey, northern Kenya and Libya childhood hydatid disease is common. The host is usually a dog which carries the adult parasite in its intestines. Ova are excreted into water, grass or vegetables and ingested by sheep, cattle or man. After ingestion the ovum enters the portal system and then may lodge anywhere in the body, most commonly the liver (70 per cent), but sometimes the kidneys or pancreas. The lung and brain are the most common extra-abdominal sites. Approximately two-thirds of cysts are single and the rest multiple. Rarely a cyst may rupture into the peritoneal cavity or the bile duct. This may result in anaphylactoid-like reactions and widespread echinococcosis.

Life cycle

E. granulosus

Infected dogs harbour the minute, adult tapeworms 3–6 mm long in the small intestine. The worms possess only three proglottides, the end of one being mature. The eggs are liberated either before or after the proglottid escapes in the faeces and contaminate pasture. When ingested by the normal intermediate host, the oncospheres liberated in the gut enter the circulation and are trapped in the capillaries of various viscera, where they develop into cysts. A cyst is composed of a sphere of germinal epithelium containing protruding invaginations (brood capsules) and fluid. From the inner surface of the brood capsules, protoscolices develop. The whole structure is a hydatid cyst, and it becomes surrounded by a fibrous capsule derived from host tissue. The cyst may develop large 'daughter cysts' in its cavity, each containing more brood capsules. The cyst continues growing for years. Brood capsules which break free from the cyst wall, and the individual scolices in the cyst cavity, are called the hydatid sand.

Dogs become infected by eating the contents of hydatid cysts in infected carcases. Sheep and other herbivores become infected by swallowing the taenia-like eggs passed in dog faeces.

E. multilocularis

This is similar but different hosts are involved. The cyst produces daughter cysts by external and not internal budding, so it tends to extend like a malignant tumour. It is not contained in well-defined, fibrous capsule. Man becomes infected by swallowing the eggs passed by foxes and other canines, possibly mainly from contaminated, wild, ground fruits. Various rodents are the intermediate hosts.

Clinical presentation

Cysts commonly develop in the liver (70 per cent) and lungs (20 per cent). The spleen, kidneys or pancreas may also be affected. The clinical features depend on three processes:

1. **Mechanical effects** such as painful enlargement of the liver (commonest presentation), cough and breathlessness (cyst may compress bronchi and cause collapse of a lobe), symptoms suggesting a brain tumour (intracerebral cysts), bone pain or spontaneous fractures (medullary cysts of bone).
2. **Hypersensitivity** reactions such as urticaria and anaphylaxis due to the escape of allergenic hydatid material into the circulation or peritoneum.
3. **Complications** due to:
   - rupture causing anaphylatic shock and sudden death,
   - spread to other organs or across serous cavities due to seeding with viable germinal epithelium,
   - secondary infection of the cyst.

In endemic areas, hydatid cysts are a common cause of intra-abdominal mass or pulmonary opacity.

Diagnosis

The diagnosis can be made by ultrasound examination (Figure 3.7, p 52) (or CT scanning if available), which reveals the typical grape-like, intracystic brood capsules with daughter cysts. Needle biopsy is contraindicated, but fine-needle aspiration (22 gauge or smaller) is safe.

Practice point
- *Wide-bore aspiration of the cyst contents should not be carried out for diagnostic purposes, because subsequent leakage may cause anaphylaxis or the development of widespread metastatic cysts.*

Other diagnostic tests

1. The Casoni test: this involves injecting 0.1 ml of standardised Seitz-filtered hydatid fluid intradermally. A positive result is the development of a wheal, at least twice the diameter of the initial bleb and usually surrounded by a pronounced flare, within 20 min of the injection. The test remains positive long after all cysts have been removed.
2. The detection of anti-hydatid antibodies using either counter immuno-electrophoresis (CIE) or ELISA. The CIE method may give false positive results in other conditions such as lung cancer.
3. The detection of circulating antigen. This may be positive even when the antibody tests are negative.

Management

Albendazole

The drug of choice is albendazole, an absorbable relative of mebendazole. A dose of 10 mg/kg per day in 2 divided doses for 7–60 days has been followed by spontaneous regression of the cyst in many cases. Surgery may still be needed to remove the dead cyst contents.

Surgery

The objective of surgical treatment includes removal of all parasitic elements including the germinative membrane, avoidance of spillage of cyst contents, closure of any communication with adjacent anatomical structures such as the bile duct, and management of the residual cavity.

At surgery care should be taken to protect the rest of the abdominal cavity from cyst spillage by placing towels around the operating field. After aspirating the cyst contents hypertonic saline (20 per cent) is injected into the cavity for 10 min. Then the saline is aspirated and the endocyst delivered. The cavity is inspected for open biliary channels which should be closed. Further management depends upon the anatomy of the pericyst. Excision of the pericyst can be performed if damage to major structures can be avoided and haemostasis easily achieved, particularly for peripheral and pedunculated cysts. An external drain should be always left. An alternative is to pack the pericyst cavity with omentum and close without drainage. Hepatic lobectomy may be required for multiple cysts confined to one lobe.

Secondary infection of the cavity can be treated by antibiotics, continued drainage and irrigation. If there is a persistent bile leak in a patient with external drainage the possibility of distal bile duct obstruction should be excluded by cholangiogram. Close follow-up of the patient by ultrasound is necessary because recurrence rates are in the order of 20 per cent.

Endoscopic retrograde cholangiopancreatography (ERCP) has been successfully used for internal drainage of biliary cysts.

Control

Very high levels of human infection persist in areas where sheep and cattle rearing and the presence of domestic dogs coexist in the absence of health education, such as the Turkana region of Northern Kenya. There the close association of dogs and children ensures that children are exposed to the eggs and infections develop at an early age. The disease is also prevalent in some countries in the Middle East. One of the main control measures recommended is the periodic deworming of dogs.

Further reading

Schistosomiasis

Amino T. Clinicopathological studies on gastrointestinal schistosomiasis. Jpn J Parasitol 1981;30:135–49.

Bella H, Abdel Rahim A, Mustafa D, Ahmed MA, Wasfi S, Bennett JL. Oltipraz – antischistosomal efficacy in Sudanese infected with *Schistosoma mansoni*. Am J Trop Med Hyg 1982;31:775–8.

Cevallos AM, Farthing MJG. Parasitic infections of the gastrointestinal tract. Curr Opin Gastroenterol 1993;9:96–102.

Da Silva LC *et al*. Hepatosplenic schistosomiasis. Pathophysiology and treatment. Gastroenterol Clin North Am 1992;21:163.

Doehring E. Schistosomiasis in childhood. Eur J Paediatr 1988;47:2–9.

Kipatrick ME, Farid Z, Bassily S, El Masry NA, Trabdisi B, Watten RH. Treatment of schistosomiasis mansoni with oxamniquine – five years experience. Am J Trop Med Hyg 1981;30:1219–22.

Webb G. Schistosomiasis, some advances. BMJ 1981;283: 1104–6.

Visceral leishmaniasis

Anabwani GM, Ngira JA, Dimity G, Bryceson DAM. Comparison of two dosage schedule of sodium stibogluconate in the treatment of visceral leishmaniasis in Kenya. Lancet 1983;i:201–13.

Chunge CN, Gachihi G, Mugambi M, Chulay JD, Spencer HC. Treatment of visceral leishmaniasis using sodium stibogluconate in a dose of 15mg/kg body weight twice daily for 30 days: preliminary report. East Afr Med J 1984;61:570–4.

Chunge CN, Owate J, Pamba HO, Donno L. Treatment of visceral leishmaniasis in Kenya by aminosidine alone or combined with sodium stibogluconate. Trans R Soc Trop Med Hyg 1990;84:221–5.

Chulay JD, Bryceson ADM. Quantitation of amastigotes of *Leishmania donovani* in smears of splenic aspirates from patients with visceral leishmaniasis. Am J Trop Med Hyg, 1983;32:475–9.

Chulay JD, Bhartt SM, Muigai R, Ho M, Gachihi G, Were JBO, Chunge C, Bryceson ADM. Comparison of three dosage regimens of sodium stibogluconate in the treatment of visceral leishmaniasis in Kenya. J Infect Dis 1983;148:148–55.

Herwald BL, Berman JD. Recommendations for treating leishmaniasis with sodium stibogluconate (Pentostam) and review of pertinent clinical studies. Am J Trop Med Hyg, 1992;46:296–306.

Oster CN. Advances in clinical diagnosis and chemotherapy of visceral leishmaniasis in Kenya. Insect Sci and its Applicat 1986;7:235–40.

Siddig M, Ghalib H, Shillington DC, Peterson EA, Khidir S. Visceral leishmaniasis in Sudan. Clinical features. 1990;42:107–12.

WHO (1984). The leishmaniases. Report of a WHO Expert Committee. Geneva, Switzerland. World Health Organization Technical Report Series 1984;No. 701.

Hydatid disease

Can Basaklar A. Hydatid cysts in children: report of 88 cases. J R Coll Surg Edinb 1991; 36:166–9.

Cotton M, Amuso M, Cotton PB. Endoscopic retrograde cholangiography in hepatic hydatid disease. Br J Surg 1978;65:107–8.

Gahukamble DB, Khamage AS, El Gadi M, Shatwan F. An effective and safe surgical method for the treatment of hydatid cysts in children. Trop Geogr Med 1991;43:7–11.

Lewis JW, Koss N, Kerstein MD. A review of echinococcal disease. Ann Surg 1975; 182:390 6.

Morris DL. The use of albendazole in human hydatid disease. Ann Trop Med Parasitol 1984;78(3):204–5.

Morris DL, Skene-Smith H, Haynes A, Burrows GO. Abdominal hydatid disease: computed tomographic and ultrasound changes during albendazole therapy. Clin Radiol 1984;35:297–300.

Nelson GS. Hydatid disease: research and control in Turkana, Kenya. I. Epidemiological observations. Trans R Soc Trop Med Hyg 1986;80:177–82.

8

Malnutrition and Weight Loss

The importance of nutrition and weight loss in tropical gastroenterology cannot be understated in view of the extremely high mortality associated with malnutrition and diarrhoea in developing countries. The chief function of the bowel is to absorb nutrients and consequently chronic gastrointestinal disease is invariably associated with weight loss. However, equally important is the fact that chronic inflammatory bowel diseases produce anorexia, due to the secretion of inflammatory mediators such as cytokines (Table 8.1), and diminished food intake may be the chief explanation for weight loss. It is important therefore to decide which is the cause, as treatment will be quite different. For example, weight gain may be achieved in anorexic patients by supplemental feeding or nasoenteric feeding, whereas nutrition may only be improved by intravenous means when intestinal obstruction is the cause. It must also be remembered that malnutrition in itself is the cause of intestinal failure as both digestive enzymes and absorptive cells depend upon an adequate supply of dietary amino acids to maintain function. Consequently a vicious cycle of malnutrition and malabsorption may intercede (Figure 8.1). In this situation intravenous feeding may be life-saving.

Table 8.1 Symptoms during cytokine infusion.

Nausea
Anorexia
Fatigue, lethargy
Weight loss
Fevers
Muscle cramps
Flu-like symptoms
Diarrhoea
Anaemia
Leukopenia
Headache
Confusion
Tachycardia
Hypotension

114

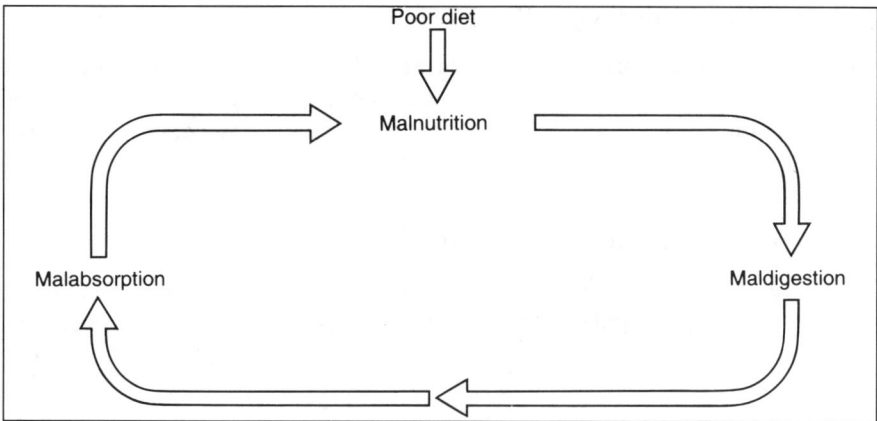

Figure 8.1   The vicious cycle of malnutrition and malabsorption.

Definition of weight loss

It is important to differentiate acute from chronic weight loss. Thus a weight loss of 10 kg in 3 months is of significance whereas the loss of 10 kg in 2 years is less so. Knowledge of the pre-morbid, or 'usual' weight, is also important, as a loss in weight of 20 kg in someone weighing 100 kg is well tolerated, whereas a loss of this amount of weight in someone weighing 50 kg might be life-threatening. An accurate assessment of weight loss is also only possible in patients who have home facilities for measuring weight change. Indirect assessment, such as loosening of clothes, might be the only clue as to the degree of weight loss in less privileged societies.

Recognition and investigation of malnutrition and weight loss

Assessment of nutritional status

Body weight

Body weight is measured as routine in most hospitals and outpatient clinics and therefore records are usually available. However, it must be remembered that the sensitivity of the measurements as indicators of nutritional status will decrease in dehydrated and oedematous patients. Furthermore, weight will depend upon the size of the patient and therefore some correction factor needs to be made. The most currently accepted measure is the body mass index (BMI):

$$\text{BMI} = \frac{\text{Weight (in kg)}^2}{\text{Height (in m)}^2}$$

the normal range being 21–26. In general, patients with a BMI less than 17 need urgent nutritional help.

Triceps skinfold thickness (TSF)

This is the simplest, practical index of body fat stores. In many comparative studies, it has performed remarkably well in comparison to more sophisticated methods of measurement such as underwater weighing, impedance plethysmography and dual X-ray absorptiometry.

Midarm muscle circumference (MMC)

When allowance for skinfold thickness (and therefore fatness) is made, an assessment of upper midarm muscle circumference (MAC) can be calculated from:

$$MMC = MAC(mm) - TSF(mm) \times \pi$$

Biochemical markers

The most commonly used blood test is the **plasma albumin concentration**. This is used, often wrongly, as an index of body protein status. In hospital practice, its use as a measurement of nutrition is invalidated by changes in concentration resulting from hydrational status and 'third space losses' – or extravascular sequestration – as commonly observed in critically-ill patients with septicaemia. For this reason, it forms a more useful index of the degree of 'sickness' and is directly correlated with expected mortality. The same argument goes for the other plasma proteins such as transferrin and **retinol-binding protein**, which have been considered more sensitive markers of protein nutrition, in view of their shorter half-lives.

Vitamin concentrations

Biochemical analyses of the vitamins A, E, C, D, pyridoxine, riboflavin and nicotinic acid are available, but are more often used as research tools in view of the low demand for measurements and difficulties in analysis. Furthermore, interpretation of the meaning of concentration levels is often difficult. For example, a low plasma value does not necessarily imply tissue or functional deficiency. Consequently, functional measurements are more useful – such as the use of **prothrombin time** as an assessment of vitamin K sufficiency, and **transketolase activity**, for thiamine. Alternatively, tissue levels may be more closely related to **white cell concentrations** – as commonly used for vitamins C, B_{12} and folate.

Dietary history

Possibly one of the most difficult things to measure accurately in clinical practice is dietary intake. Accurate assessment is only possible when patients are observed in a metabolic ward when a weighed diet is provided, or when a specific diet is fed via feeding-tube. In all other situations, we have to rely on the patient's memory and assessment of quantity of food taken. This is where inaccuracy enters and the best one can expect to achieve is a measure of the types of foods eaten and their frequency. Consequently, the only safe way of determining the inadequacy of dietary intake is to prove that the weight loss was not due to malabsorption or hypermetabolism.

Metabolic expenditure

Hypermetabolism is a relatively minor cause of weight loss – unless dietary intake is also defective as, for example, in critically-ill patients. It may be measured at the bedside by indirect calorimetry i.e. the measurement of oxygen consumption and CO_2 production. In addition, the rate of protein catabolism can be measured by analysing the quantity of nitrogen excreted in the urine over a 24-h period. The nitrogen can then be converted into 'protein equivalents' by multiplying by 6.25. Catabolism will be present if urinary losses exclude dietary intakes.

Nutrient absorption

Despite its unpopularity with patients, nursing staff and laboratory technicians, the **72-h faecal collection** remains the gold standard for overall assessment of intestinal function. Shorter collections are often invalidated because of the delay in intestinal transit. However, it is critical to perform the test correctly as knowledge of the rate of excretion of nutrients, such as fat or nitrogen, is meaningless if an accurate simultaneous assessment of dietary intake was not known. For example, it is not uncommon for doctors to state that 'steatorrhea was not detected' and therefore malabsorption did not exist – despite the fact that the patient was not eating! Consequently, all patients should be placed on a standard diet containing between 80 g and 100 g of fat and protein throughout the 3-day period (i.e. a normal diet). Sometimes patients are unable to take this quantity of food. In this situation, the help of a dietitian must be sought to measure the actual quantity of food eaten and express stool outputs as **percentages** of dietary intake. For example, if only 50 g of fat were eaten and 10 g of fat appeared in the stool, the efficiency of absorption would have been 80 per cent i.e. the same as a faecal excretion of 20 g in a patient who consumed a normal diet.

The 72-h stool collection is also important for the measurement of stool weight, which should be less than 300 g per day, and also for electrolyte content in order to differentiate 'secretory' from 'osmotic' diarrhoea. Normally the efficiency of fluid and electrolyte absorption is so great that only small quantities of electrolytes appear in the stools. For example, of the approximately 600 mmol of sodium chloride and 10 litres of fluid that enter the duodenum each day, only 10 mmol of NaCl and 200 ml of water will be excreted in stools. A practical aid for the estimation of stool osmolarity will be to add the sodium and potassium concentrations together and multiply them by 2, to make allowance for the cations. The total figure should be considerably less than the plasma osmolarity of approximately 250 mOsm/l. In practice, any value over 100 will suggest an element of secretory diarrhoea.

Stool nitrogen may also be measured and compared with dietary intake in the same manner. The efficiency of absorption of both fat and protein is very high, usually greater than 95 per cent. Finally, **total energy absorption** can be assessed by bomb calorimetry measurement of stool samples. However, the equipment required for the analysis is not commonly available and therefore restricted to research studies.

Shorter, more convenient, measures of absorption are also available but provide less information on overall absorptive function. For example, fat absorption can be specifically measured by giving the patient a drink of triglycerides labelled with ^{14}C-triolein. If absorption is normal, the labelled triglyceride is absorbed and metabolized to $^{14}CO_2$. The labelled CO_2 is then excreted in the breath, where it can be detected. The greater the degree of malabsorption, the lower the breath $^{14}CO_2$ (Figure 8.2).

Carbohydrate absorption can be measured by **xylose absorption**. Xylose is normally absorbed by the small intestine but cannot be metabolised by humans and is therefore excreted quantitatively in the urine, where it can be measured. Reduced, or absent, urine excretion will be seen in patients with malabsorption.

Investigation of the cause of malabsorption

Diseases that cause malabsorption can be generally divided into those that affect **absorptive cell function** and those that interfere with the **digestive**

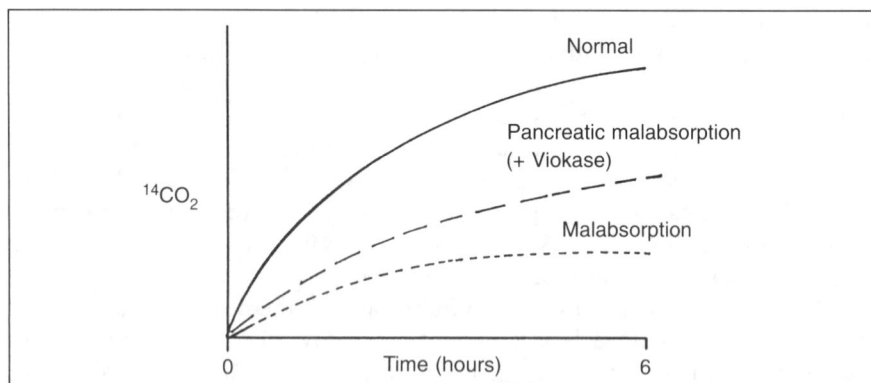

Figure 8.2   The ^{14}C triolein fat absorption test. The figure illustrates that $^{14}CO_2$ production in the breath is reduced after a drink containing ^{14}C-labelled fat in patients with malabsorption. Those with pancreatic malabsorption can be differentiated by showing an improvement with commercial pancreatic supplements (Viokase).

process. A good example of the former is coeliac or tropical sprue, and of the latter, pancreatic insufficiency. The 72-h stool fat excretion can be used as a rough initial guide as to which of the two conditions prevails (Figure 8.3). In general, intestinal diseases produce relatively mild steatorrhea, not exceeding 20 g/day. In contrast, steatorrhea associated with pancreatic insufficiency is far greater and may exceed 40 g/day. The next line of investigation for the former group is upper GI endoscopy with aspiration of duodenal juice for microscopy and culture and duodenal mucosal biopsy to examine the villi and absorptive mucosa. In the latter group, a straight abdominal X-ray needs to be taken to rule out pancreatic calcification, followed by computed tomography (CT) or ultrasound scanning of the pancreas, if negative. Exocrine function is most accurately assessed by measuring the quantities of pancreatic enzymes secreted into the duodenum in response to intravenous cholecystokinin. If the test is unavailable, a therapeutic trial of pancreatic enzymes would be indicated.

Common GI causes of weight loss

Infective or inflammatory disease

Tuberculosis

In Westernized communities the most common cause of chronic GI disability and weight loss is Crohn's disease. In the tropics, the counterpart is intestinal tuberculosis (TB) which might present with identical features. Most commonly, the terminal ileum and cecum are involved and radiological appearance

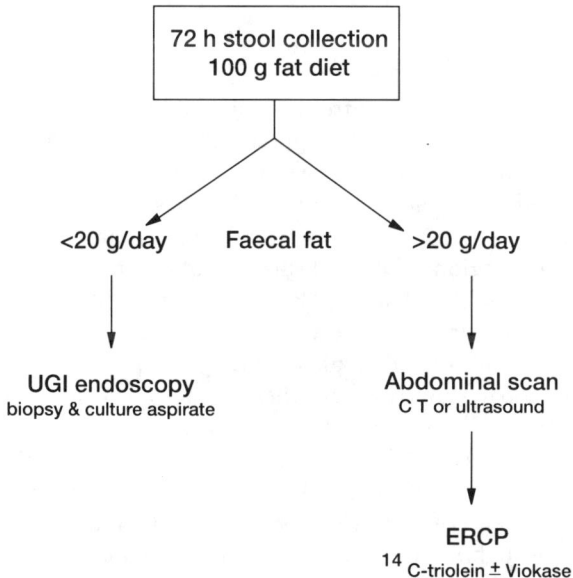

Figure 8.3 Algorithm for work-up of malabsorption based on 72-h stool collection.

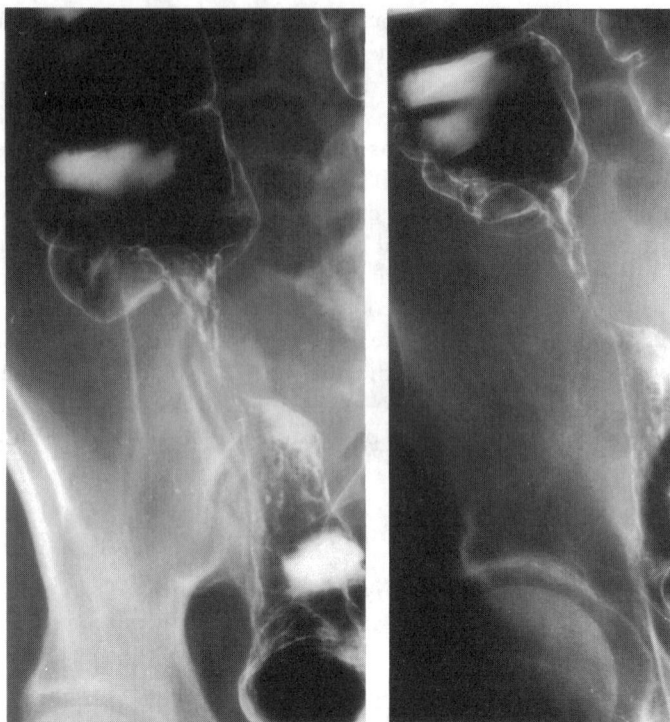

Figure 8.4   The terminal ileum of a patient with tuberculosis visualised by small bowel enema technique. The terminal ileum is contracted and ulcerated with pre-stenotic dilatation, distortion and indrawing of the caecum. Note that the ileal stream enters directly into the ascending colon rather than into the side. This is characteristic of tuberculosis rather than Crohn's disease.

may be difficult to differentiate from Crohn's disease, although caecal distortion is more common with TB (Figures 8.4 and 8.5). Diagnosis will then depend upon the history of exposure to tuberculosis, and histological proof of infection obtained by endoscopic biopsy techniques. Consequently, colonoscopy is essential in order to take biopsies from ulcerated areas and from the cecal and terminal ileal regions. The pick-up rate of positive tissue with caseating granulomata and acid-fast bacilli (AFBs) has been high in some centres, but is frustratingly low in our own experience. We are often therefore forced to use a therapeutic trial of anti-tuberculosis therapy in patients coming from high risk populations, particularly where there is radiological evidence of iliocecal disease in patients with progressive weight loss. In populations where Crohn's disease is also common, it is often safer to provide anti-tuberculosis cover should corticosteroid therapy be prescribed. (See Case history 3, page 137.)

Since the advent of the AIDS epidemic, TB infections have increased dramatically throughout the world. The combination is particularly catastrophic in Central Africa where reports from some hospitals record that 70 per cent of patients admitted with pulmonary TB are HIV positive.

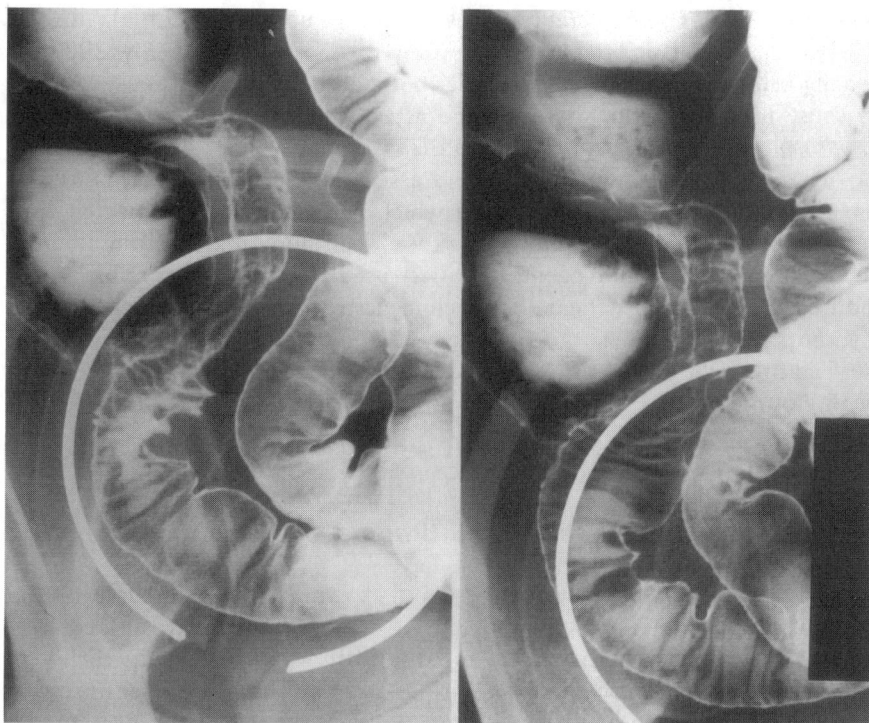

Figure 8.5 Another example of terminal ileal disease but this time due to Crohn's disease rather than tuberculosis. Note on this occasion, in contrast to Figure 8.4, the diseased terminal ileum enters the side of the caecum and ascending colon with no significant distortion of the caecum.

Immunodeficiency disease

Human immunodeficiency virus (HIV) infection is an important cause of clinical malnutrition, with weight loss occurring in 60–90 per cent of patients by the time AIDS develops. Even in asymptomatic patients with early disease weight loss is evident in 30 per cent. In Central Africa, 'slim disease' (weight loss and diarrhoea) is the most important AIDS-defining event.

Malnutrition in HIV patients is caused or aggravated by a wide range of factors which can be broadly categorised into increased energy needs, reduced energy intake and enteral nutrient losses. Fever, either due to HIV infection itself, or to opportunistic disease may be responsible for a catabolic state with high resting energy expenditure. Anorexia is almost universal in advanced disease, probably due to the effects of inflammatory cytokines (Table 8.1), but intake is also affected by odynophagia (oral candidiasis, apthous ulcers, herpes simplex (HSV), necrotising gingivitis) and dysphagia (oesophageal candidiasis, Kaposi's sarcoma, and oesophageal ulcers caused by HSV and cytomegalovirus). The incidence of diarrhoea in AIDS is reported as 30–60 per cent. The causative organism varies according to the degree of immunosuppression; virulent organisms such as *Salmonella* can cause diarrhoea at any stage of HIV disease whereas opportunistic infections occur only with CD4 counts below 200, and usually below 50. Organisms infecting the small bowel are particularly likely to cause malabsorption, these include *Mycobacterium avium-intracellulare*, *Cryptosporidium*, *Microsporidium* and *Isospora* (see Chapter 5).

Protein and energy malnutrition is associated with a decreased survival time in AIDS (Figure 8.6). Studies in which patients are supplemented with defined formula diets have shown increased lean body mass, serum albumin and total body fat. Several agents have been used in an attempt to reduce AIDS induced anorexia and cachexia of which megestrol acetate is the most promising, but the effect on survival is less well demonstrated. With improved survival in AIDS, malnutrition will have a growing impact on morbidity and quality of life and effective treatment strategies need to be sought.

Coeliac and tropical sprue, small bowel bacterial overgrowth

Sprue is characterised by weight loss and diarrhoea due to malabsorption resulting from villous atrophy and loss of mucosal absorptive surface area. Coeliac disease is rare in the tropics and results from hypersensitivity to gluten, a protein contained in the germ of various cereals. The protein sensitises the mucosa to produce an intense inflammation with the production of α gliadin antibodies which can be detected in the blood-stream and used in diagnosis. Diagnosis is more commonly made by endoscopic biopsy of the duodenum where a flat surface with absent villi is characteristically found, in addition to intense inflammation. Other forms of villous atrophy include subclinical or tropical partial villous atrophy and tropical sprue, the aetiology of which is unclear but may be related to bacterial overgrowth and chronic malnutrition. Treatment for coeliac disease will be based on the provision of a gluten-free diet, which is now commercially available. Tropical sprue on the other hand might respond to broad-spectrum antibiotic therapy and reinstatement of a good balanced diet.

The small intestinal bacterial overgrowth may, on its own, interfere with nutrient absorption. The condition may be secondary to a variety of immunodeficiency diseases (congenital and acquired) and a loss of gastric acid secretion as in atrophic gastritis and after proton-pump inhibitor therapy. It may be detected either directly by aspiration of duodenal contents during upper GI endoscopy with culture of aspirated fluid, or indirectly with the use of the 1 g ^{14}C-xylose breath test. This test is based on the fact that xylose is normally absorbed in the upper small intestine and because it cannot be metabolised by humans, it is excreted in the urine. Consequently no ^{14}C carbon dioxide will appear in the breath. In contrast, patients with small intestinal bacterial overgrowth show a rapid increase in breath $^{14}CO_2$ as a result of metabolism of the xylose by bacteria in the small intestine before it is absorbed (Figure 8.7).

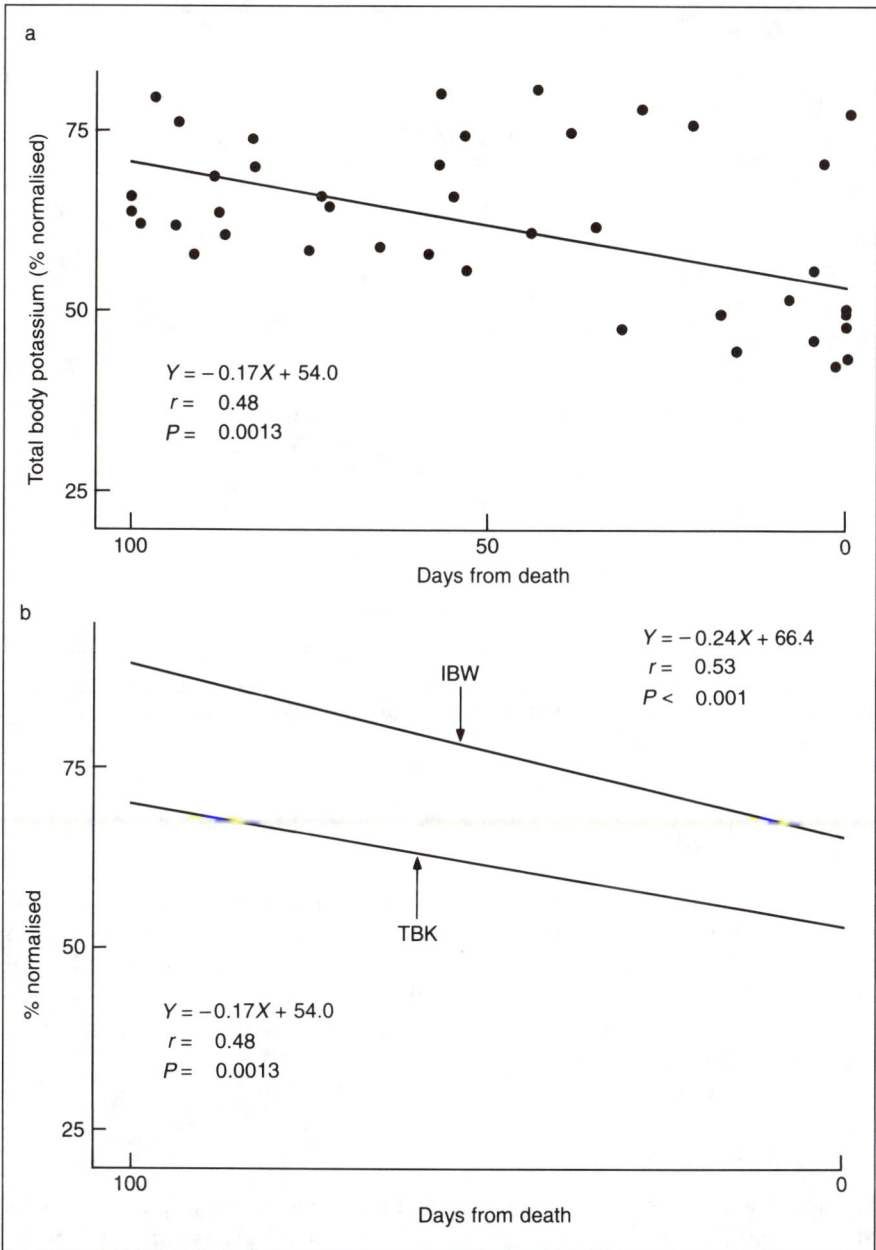

Figure 8.6(a)   The relationship between total body potassium content and survival in patients with HIV disease. **(b)** Total body potassium content and body weight had similar relationships to time before death. Reproduced with permission from: Kotler DP (ed.). In: Gastrointestinal and nutritional manifestations of the acquired immuno-deficiency syndrome. New York: Raven Press, 1991.

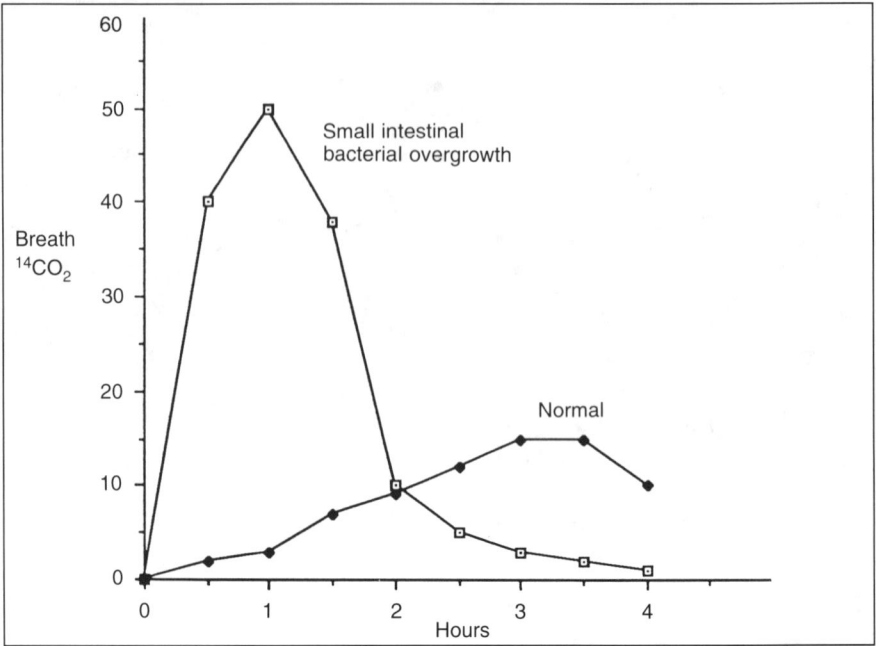

Figure 8.7   The ^{14}C xylose breath test demonstrating an abnormally high breath $^{14}CO_2$ excretion in a patient with small intestinal bacterial overgrowth in comparison to a normal healthy control.

Digestive diseases

Malabsorption and weight loss can result from the loss of the ability to digest food, as in pancreatic insufficiency – or in the loss of the ability to absorb digested food – as in the short bowel syndrome. However, the reserve capacity of the bowel is great and a loss of greater than 90 per cent of pancreatic enzyme production and a loss of greater than 75 per cent of bowel is required before steatorrhoea develops.

Pancreatic insufficiency

Pancreatic insufficiency is a late result of chronic pancreatitis. In most regions of the world chronic alcohol abuse is the most common cause of pancreatitis, but gallstones and biliary obstruction can also result in chronic pancreatic damage. Steatorrhea, the result of pancreatic insufficiency, is usually only seen after many years of heavy alcohol abuse i.e. 15–20 years. It is often preceded by repeated attacks of acute pancreatitis and may be preceded, or followed, by the development of pancreatic endocrine dysfunction with diabetes mellitus. The onset of either diabetes or steatorrhea is usually accompanied by a sudden deterioration in body weight due to the combined effects of chronic disease, maldigestion and metabolic instability. Insulin is the most powerful anabolic hormone in the body and defective secretion will result in loss of fat, glycogen and protein stores. (See Case history 1, page 131.)

Non-alcoholic tropical pancreatitis consists of a heterogeneous group of diseases identified in Africa, Malaysia and India. The disease appears to primarily affect young men, with a history of attacks of abdominal pain starting in the second decade of life. Calcification is an early feature and in a study in Nigeria, the frequency of pancreatic calcification among diabetics under the age of 20 was shown to be as high as 78 per cent. The aetiology is unclear but usually associated with chronic malnutrition and low-protein diets.

Diagnosis of chronic end-stage pancreatitis is commonly made by straight abdominal X-ray, where pancreatic calcification may be evident. A swollen and enlarged gland may be detected by ultrasound or CT imaging techniques. Finally, endoscopic retrograde cholangiopancreatography (ERCP) may be used to show abnormalities in ductular structure. The specific investigation for pancreatic exocrine dysfunction will, however, be a **pancreatic function test** consisting of the measurement of the amount of enzymes secreted into the duodenum in response to a hormonal secretogogue, such as CCK. Proof of malabsorption will, as discussed above, be obtained from the results of a 72-h stool fat collection. Alternatively, pancreatic steatorrhea can be differentiated from other forms of malabsorption by employing the two-phase ^{14}C triolene breath test. Proof that fat malabsorption is secondary to pancreatic enzyme insufficiency is obtained when the breath test improves with the co-administration of commercial enzyme supplements (Figure 8.2).

Treatment of pancreatic insufficiency with commercial enzyme supplements is never perfect, as it is impossible to reproduce the physiological integration of enzyme secretion in response to food. However steatorrhea is generally decreased, with symptomatic improvement, lower stool output and some improvement in weight gain. The value of co-treatment with H_2 antagonists to reduce acid degradation of pancreatic enzyme supplements is controversial as it adds to the expense, and is unnecessary in many patients who have low gastric acid secretion.

Short bowel syndrome

As mentioned above, nutrient absorption will only suffer when more than 50 per cent of the small intestine is lost. However, this assumes that the remaining intestine is normal and healthy, and patients with diseases that affect the entire gastrointestinal tract might well suffer from resections of considerably less length. The common example of this is Crohn's disease which may leave behind diseased bowel and areas of stenosis with poor motility. Secondary bacterial overgrowth might also occur, particularly with the loss of the ileocaecal valve, further compromising absorption. In general terms however, nutrient absorption is not affected by loss of the colon or loss of sections of ileum or jejunum. Retention of the colon is extremely important as fluid and electrolyte deficiency is the first problem that occurs in patients with short bowel and the colon can adapt to prevent much of the loss. Loss of the colon and ileum can, on the other hand, have disastrous effects and patients with end-jejunostomy syndrome become chronically salt and fluid depleted. The kidneys attempt to diminish the deficits by reducing volume to less than 1 litre/day with almost complete reabsorption of sodium chloride. However potassium and magnesium losses continue and intermittent or permanent intravenous supplementation may be required. Only when there is less than 100 cm remaining does nutrient malabsorption become inevitable. Nutritional status will then deteriorate rapidly and the patient will soon die unless full intravenous nutrition is commenced.

Treatment for fluid, electrolyte and nutrient depletion in short bowel should follow the general lines given below for weight loss due to any cause. Hyperphagia is a normal adaptive response and food should not be restricted. Although some worsening of diarrhoea can be expected with increased food intake, the net absorption will increase. It must be remembered, however, that nutrient requirements may change with time as the gut has a considerable ability to adapt to losses in length. There is an increase in villus length, and therefore mucosal absorptive surface, as well as changes in enzyme secretion, gut motility and blood flow which together result in improved absorption. The whole process of adaptation can continue for up to 6 months following resection. Consequently every effort should be made to maintain nutritional status with the judicious parenteral supplementation of nutrients in the expectation that such supplements will become less necessary in the future. (See Case history 4, page 139.)

Neoplastic disorders

Intestinal lymphoma

A wide variety of different lymphomas can affect the intestinal tract. These will include nodal lymphomas (e.g. Hodgkin's) that invade the GI tract and lymphomas that originate from the gut mucosa (e.g. mucosa associated lymphoid tissue (MALT)-lymphomas). Furthermore they may involve only one segment of the bowel or most of the mucosal surface. Regional lymph glands may, or may not, be involved. Weight loss is one of the early features of MALT-lymphomas and the diagnosis of nodal lymphomas can be difficult to differentiate from tuberculosis, as X-ray changes are often similar. The final diagnosis will depend upon histological proof, proof obtained either at endoscopy or open laparotomy.

Included under intestinal lymphomas are the **immunoproliferative small-intestinal diseases** – or IPSIDs. These are somewhat unusual in that they have primarily been described in patients coming from impoverished Third World communities and because of their association with bacterial overgrowth and response to (and sometime cure by) simple antibiotic therapy. The disease often presents with severe weight loss (as described in the case history below) and diarrhoea which is uncontrollable. The diagnosis is made by endoscopic biopsy of the upper small intestine where immunoproliferation is identified with the secretion of abnormal immunoglobulin A (IgA) α-heavy chains with light chain restriction, both into the mucosa and the blood stream, where they can be detected and used to confirm diagnosis. Diagnosis and differentiation from the other lymphomas now depends upon immunohistochemical staining techniques. Recent investigations have suggested that IPSID and α-heavy chain disease are members of the MALT-lymphomas. However, as mentioned above, treatment with broad spectrum antibiotics and nutrition during the early stages of the disease may reverse the condition. However, if the disease is not treated, it may progress to a high grade B-cell lymphoma which will only respond to radiotherapy or combined chemotherapy. The response to antibiotic therapy has led to the hypothesis that the disease results from an abnormal reaction to small bowel bacterial overgrowth, the bacterial antigens provoking a 'neoplastic' immunological response. (See Case history 2, page 132.)

More recently it has been suggested that chronic *Helicobacter pylori* infection also predisposes to the development of gastric MALT lymphomas. This concept is supported by the fact that *H. pylori* infection is far more common in impoverished communities, such as those in which the IPSID group of diseases prevail.

Abdominal carcinoma

Oesophagus
Oesophageal stenosis due to either benign or malignant disease is one of the most common causes for rapid weight loss in GI patients. Information on the aetiology will be obtained by endoscopic biopsy techniques. Unfortunately the prognosis of oesophageal carcinoma is extremely poor, most patients dying within the year. As metastatic spread is common at initial presentation, curative surgery is often not possible. Consequently palliation, such as dilatation or stenting of the stenosis, will be indicated. If this is not possible a surgical gastrostomy will be needed to maintain nutrition and hydration.

Carcinoma of the stomach
Possibly the most useful method of differentiating gastric ulceration from gastric cancer is the association of rapid weight loss in the latter. Gastric ulceration is often associated with pain after eating and therefore some diminution in food intake can be expected, but the degree of weight loss is far less than observed in cancer patients who, in addition, become anorexic. The diagnosis of gastric cancer is again dependent upon endoscopy and biopsy. As with oesophageal carcinoma, the prognosis of gastric carcinoma is poor unless the lesion is detected early, in which case a total gastrectomy might be lifesaving. With obstructing lesions, it is often possible to pass a feeding tube through into the duodenum to maintain nutrition. Otherwise surgical enterostomy will be needed, together with gastric decompression.

Colon cancer

Colon cancer is thankfully rare in developing countries, possibly due to the protective effect of a high carbohydrate, and low animal protein and fat diet. The same is true for other colonic diseases, such diverticulitis, ulcerative colitis and adenomatous polyps. Colon cancer has far less effect upon appetite, and weight loss is, therefore, a late feature in this disease. Once weight loss has occurred the prognosis is likely to be poor, as dissemination of the disease has almost certainly occurred.

Pancreatic and liver cancer

The combination of epigastric pain, jaundice, anorexia and weight loss in elderly patients raises the strong possibility of pancreatic or biliary carcinoma. Weight loss may be associated with steatorrhea due to interference with the pancreatic enzyme secretion, or more commonly due to anorexia and gastric outlet obstruction due to compression of the duodenum by tumour. Diagnosis will be made by CT or ultrasound examination with fine needle biopsy confirmation. Unfortunately the prognosis is extremely poor as the disease is usually advanced by the time of its diagnosis. The same follows for hepatic cancer due to either secondaries or primary hepatocellular carcinoma.

Treatment and management of weight loss

Treatment will depend upon the type and severity of the underlying condition. Thus improvement in weight might be achieved by simple dietary advice or, in a situation of intestinal failure, by the use of specialised feeding techniques such as intravenous nutrition. The principles of management are the same, irrespective of the cause of weight loss. Although parenteral feeding is relatively easy to implement, it is costly and has major side-effects and is less efficiently utilised than enteral feeding. Consequently every attempt must be made to devise a satisfactory form of enteral feeding and, only if this fails, should parenteral feeding be entertained. The following is a **step-wise approach to nutritional support.**

Step 1   Normal food

The initial approach to patients with weight loss is to assess whether their normal dietary intake cannot simply be increased. This is often achieved by adding in snacks in between meals and at bedtime and, in addition, encouraging patients to eat larger portions during their main meals.

Step 2   Oral supplements

When the above approach fails, use can be made of energy-dense commercial liquid supplements. These can be taken as drinks between normal meals and at bedtime.

Step 3   Tube feeding

If supplemental feeding fails, then a more dramatic change is required. Many patients with anorexia have normal intestinal function and nutrition can be improved if the diet is infused into the stomach or duodenum. Infusions should start at **a slow rate using a full-strength formula** providing one calorie per ml. Initial infusion rate should be 20–40 ml/h, increasing to approximately 80 ml/h over 48 h. For the vast majority of hospital patients, the goal should be to provide a total of 25–35 Kcal/kg per day of energy and 0.8 – 1.5 g/kg per day of protein.

Enteral feeding often makes diarrhoea initially worse, but, with time, tolerance increases. An improvement can be expected by day 4. Refeeding diarrhoea is especially common in malnourished patients who have not eaten for some time, because disuse of the bowel results in mucosal villus atrophy and bacterial overgrowth. Both of these abnormalities are reversed by the passage of food through the bowel. Consequently diarrhoea should **not** be an indication to avoid or discontinue tube feeding. Tube-feeding associated diarrhoea is common and of complex aetiology, involving **host-factors** such as the presence of intestinal disease or mucosal atrophy, small-bowel bacterial overgrowth and changes in gut flora related to the use of broad-spectrum antibiotics, *Clostridium difficile* infection, and also due to **feed-associated factors** such as osmolarity, rate of infusion and the presence of lactose in lactase-deficient patients. The initial diarrhoea can be controlled by the use of anti-motility drugs (such as loperamide) but usually this is not necessary. Other factors, such as medications, must also be scrutinised for the presence of osmotic substances, such as sorbitol, which is often used as a vehicle ('syrup') in liquid medications. If tolerance to tube-feeding is good i.e. 100–120 ml/h is tolerated, consideration should be given to converting tube-feeding to a cyclical, nocturnal infusion of approximately 1 litre of a liquid formula, allowing greater mobility and normal eating during the day.

Step 4   Elemental diets

For tube-feeding it is best to start with the **normal commercial liquid formula diets which are polymeric and inexpensive.** If the patient does not tolerate these diets, consideration needs to be given to converting them to an 'elemental formula' i.e. one that is pre-digested, with proteins hydrolysed to amino acids and starch to glucose. These diets are particularly effective in patients with digestive abnormalities, and may be used in patients with pancreatic insufficiency without the need for pancreatic enzyme supplements. Because elemental diets are also more rapidly absorbed, they might also have advantages in patients with absorptive defects. Their chief drawback is that they are, unfortunately, more expensive.

Step 5   Total parenteral feeding (TPN)

If all the above approaches fail, then a state of **gut failure** is present, and intravenous feeding will be the only alternative remaining. The problem with intravenous feeding is that the nutrients are now infused directly into the systemic circulation without the filtering and sterilising effect of the gut mucosal barrier. Furthermore, the metabolic regulation by the pancreas and liver are lost (Figure 8.8). Consequently, the **complications of TPN** are related (1) to catheter sepsis, (2) metabolic instability, particularly hyperglycaemia and (3) to venous thrombosis due to the infusion of concentrated nutrients into the venous circulation. Because of the loss of enteropancreatic and hepatic regulation, the **efficiency of utilisation of intravenous nutrients** is always **lower** than that for enteral feeding.

The complications of TPN can, however, be minimised if:

1. A central vein catheter (e.g. subclavian/superior vena cava) is used so that the nutrients are rapidly diluted by the bloodstream.
2. Infusions are supervised by an **experienced team** to ensure a protocolised approach to catheter insertion, catheter-care and TPN administration. The central line must be dedicated to intravenous feeding and not contaminated

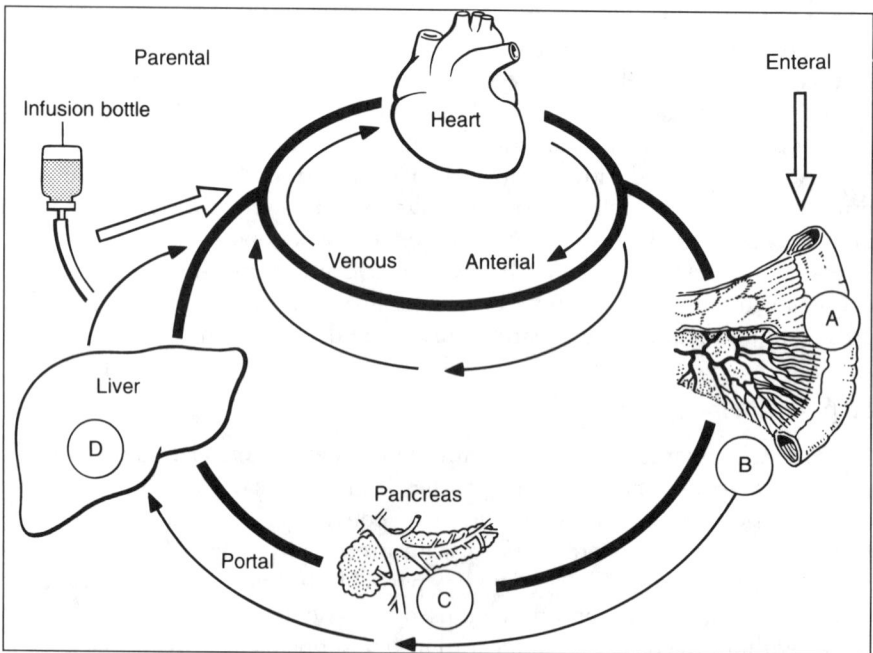

Figure 8.8 Side-effects of total parenteral nutrition are related to the fact that the route of nutrient infusion has been changed from the portal to the systemic circulation. Thus hepatic(D) and pancreatic regulation(C) is lost and concentrated nutrients are infused into the venous circulation, potentiating metabolic instability. Furthermore, the sterilising (A) (i.e. acid secretion, enzymic digestion and solubilisation) and filtration (B) (mucosal barrier) effects of the GI tract and the gut immune system (IgA, Peyer's patches) are lost, increasing the risk of septicaemia.

by other infusions. Infections most commonly arise from contamination of the catheter insertion site and infusion line.

3. Infusion rates are regulated to provide no more than 25 Kcal/kg per day of energy and 0.8–1 g/kg per day of amino acids. Ideally 25 per cent of calories should be in the form of lipid emulsion.
4. Fluid and electrolyte infusions are regulated to maintain a urine output of at least 1 litre per day, with a sodium and potassium excretion of between 40 and 80 mmol/day.
5. Monitor blood glucose and keep levels below 15 mmol/l by reducing glucose infusion, provide insulin coverage in diabetic patients, initially via sliding-scale and then by direct addition to the TPN solution.

Case history 1. Chronic pancreatitis

A 38-year-old male farm worker was admitted with a 6-month history of weight loss amounting to 10 kg. He had always been slim, his usual weight being 60 kg, the weight loss representing a drop in body mass index from 20 to 17. He denied any loss of appetite although he had intermittent attacks of abdominal pain associated with nausea and vomiting, approximately once per month. His chief complaint was that of weight loss, weakness and inability to perform his work. In addition, he had noted a recent worsening of his bowel function with almost persistent diarrhoea. He also complained of thirst. Stools were bulky, pale and occasionally he noted free oil floating in the toilet. Another complaint was numbness in his hands and feet and occasional cramps in the fingers and hands when trying to perform delicate tasks. Of importance in his history was the admission to heavy alcohol abuse for many years. As he was working on a wine farm, he had free access to cheap alcoholic beverages. Due to his present illness his alcohol intake was down, but he would normally drink at least one bottle of wine a day and, in addition, brandy at weekends. His attacks of abdominal pain, nausea and vomiting often proceeded heavy alcohol abuse, most attacks occurring on Monday mornings. He smoked 50 cigarettes per day. He had a good work record until 3 months ago when the pains and weakness prevented him from performing manual labour. He was then referred to hospital for investigation and treatment.

His past health was reasonably good, apart from the attacks of nausea and vomiting described above, and three more severe bouts of illness which necessitated admission to hospital. His symptoms in hospital had settled after bed-rest and intravenous fluids for a 3-day period. Examination of records demonstrated mild liver function test abnormalities, including an alkaline phosphatase and AST both increased to approximately twice normal. In addition his plasma amylase was noted on two occasions to be markedly elevated. He had been discharged with strong advice to stop drinking.

Dietary intake was irregular, probably disturbed by his drinking habits. As mentioned above he had always been slim, but his present weight was the lowest it had ever been in adulthood.

On admission, physical examination revealed slight dehydration in a wasted man. Body mass index was reduced to 17 (i.e. 75 per cent of normal). Mid-arm muscle circumference was reduced to 80 per cent of standard and triceps skin-fold thickness was only 40 per cent of standard, indicating loss of muscle and fat mass. Abdominal examination revealed epigastric tenderness and a slightly enlarged liver, and a diffuse loss of sensation was detected in both feet. Blood tests revealed a normal haemoglobin, but red cells were macrocytic (110). Blood chemistry revealed a low potassium of 3.0 mmol/l (3.5–5.5 mmol/l) and magnesium 0.6 mmol/l (0.7–1.0 mmol/l) and an alkaline phosphatase of 240 units/l (30–115 units/l), an AST of 100 units (0–40 units/l), an amylase of 380 units (170–300 units/l), and a reduced albumin concentration of 28 g/l (35–50 g/l). Blood glucose was elevated at 12 mmol/l (3.9–5.6 mmol/l). Blood levels of the fat-soluble vitamins A and E were particularly low (reduced to 20 per cent of normal), with milder deficiencies of vitamins C and thiamine (i.e. transketolase activity). Straight abdominal X-ray revealed pancreatic calcification and ultrasound scan a 5 mm pseudocyst in the head of the pancreas.

A diagnosis of chronic calcific pancreatitis with pseudocyst formation was made, with intestinal malabsorption particularly affecting fat and fat soluble vitamins. In addition, the presence of increased blood glucose in this patient suggested pancreatic endocrine dysfunction. He was treated with intravenous fluids in order to correct hydration and potassium and magnesium concentrations. After 3 days his nausea and vomiting settled and oral liquids were introduced and well tolerated. After 5 days he could tolerate a normal diet, permitting the measurement of fat absorption based on a 72-h stool collection. Results demonstrated gross steatorrhea with 45 g appearing in the stool per day indicating an absorption of only 45 per cent. Measurement of two-phase-^{14}C-triolein breath test demonstrated that triolein absorption improved markedly when pancreatic enzyme supplements were given, confirming that the cause of steatorrhea was pancreatic enzyme deficiency. He was therefore commenced on pancreatic enzyme supplements (Viokase 4 tablets t.d.s. with meals) with marked symptomatic improvement including a reduced stool volume from 800 g/day to 300 g/day and a reduction in stool fat to 20 g/day. His weight increased slowly by 2 kg per week, and he gradually regained strength. However with the improvement in absorption, his blood sugar rose dramatically, confirming pancreatic endocrine dysfunction. He was finally discharged on pancreatic enzyme supplements and long acting insulin (30 units/day) and strong advice to avoid all alcohol consumption. At outpatient follow-up 3 months later, he had put back all his lost weight and was fully rehabilitated.

Case history 2. α-Heavy-Chain Disease: MALT-lymphoma

A 20-year-old black male was transferred from a rural area with a 5-month history of severe diarrhoea and weight loss of 30 kg. Stools were watery (10–15/day) and yellow, but contained no blood or mucus. On admission he was emaciated, weak and unable to walk (Figure 8.9). He was mentally obtunded, pale but lacked finger clubbing and no lymph glands were felt. No masses were felt from the abdomen and rectal examination revealed a mildly inflamed mucosa with watery stool, but no blood.

Investigations revealed a macrocytic (mean corpuscular volume (MCV) 101 fl) anaemia (8.4 g/dl), high white cell count (11.4 × 10^9/l), polymorph (85 per cent), and platelet count (602 × 10^9/l). Prothrombin time was prolonged (International normalised ratio 2.1), as was erythrocyte sedimentation rate (ESR) (72 mm/1st h). The multiple

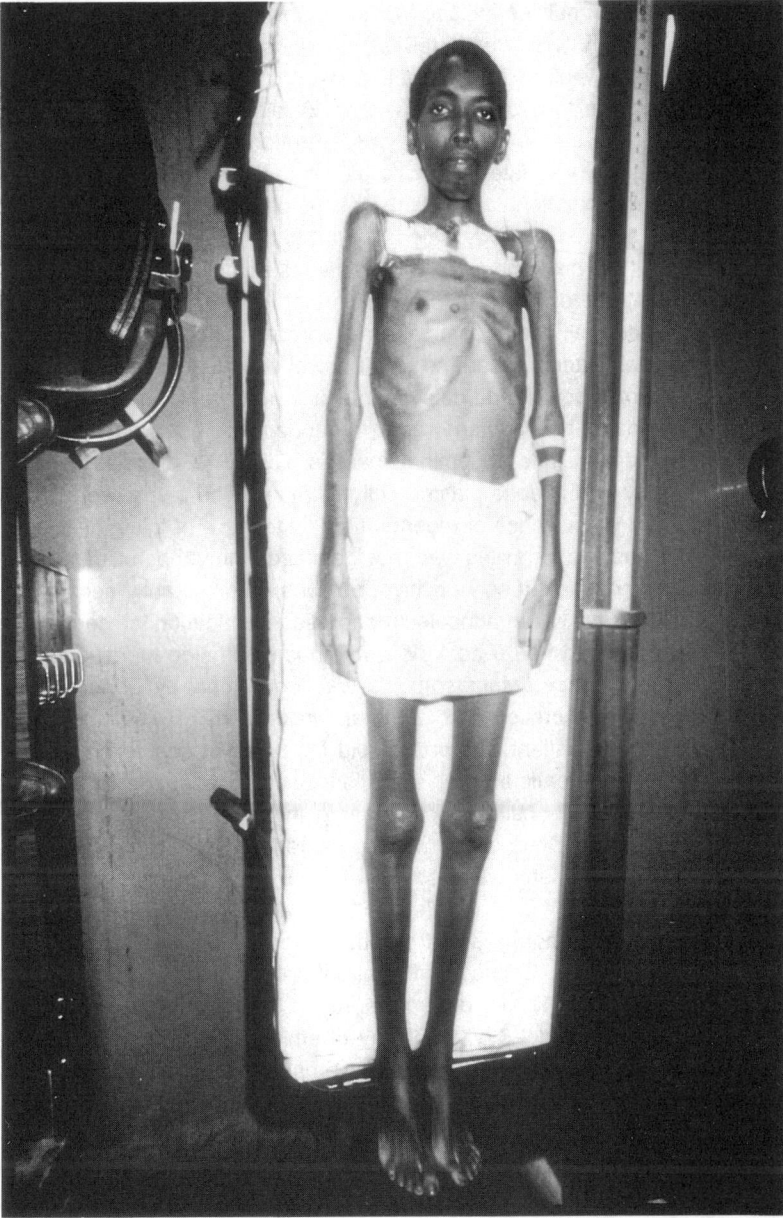

Figure 8.9 A young adult patient admitted with α-heavy-chain disease – immunoproliferative small-intestinal disease (IPSID) having lost 60 per cent of his body weight. Attempts at oral refeeding failed because of digestion and malabsorption failure secondary to severe protein deficiency, necessitating intravenous feeding.

plasma biochemical abnormalities included a low potassium (2.8 mmol/l), albumin (18 g/l), transferrin (1.0 g/l), total protein (50 g/l), magnesium (0.6 mmol/l), and iron (4 mg/l) concentration, as well as iron saturation (14 per cent). Serum and red cell folate concentrations were low, but serum vitamin B levels were normal. Thyroid function, as assessed by serum T_3 and T_4 concentrations, was low, but thyroid-stimulatory hormone assay was later shown to be within the normal limits.

The severity of his nutritional depletion was emphasised by anthropometric measurements which showed his body weight (24 kg) to be 38 per cent, his mid-arm circumference (13.2 cm) to be 45 per cent and his triceps skinfold thickness (2.6 mm) to be 21 per cent of standard.

Chest X-ray was normal, and abdominal X-ray showed multiple air fluid levels in non-dilated large bowel. Barium meal and small bowel examinations revealed mild dilation of the entire small bowel, and delayed intestinal transit. No focal lesion was demonstrated. Gastroduodenoscopy showed mild duodenitis. Abdominal ultrasound and CT scans revealed no intra-abdominal masses. Duodenal biopsies revealed subtotal villous atrophy and intense plasma cell infiltration. The crypts were widely separated and showed no evidence of regeneration, suggestive of folate deficiency. Lymphoepithelial lesions and parasites were not identified. Immunoperoxidase staining for IgA heavy chains was strongly positive, but was predominantly negative for κ- and λ-light chains. Finally, immunoelectrophoretic examination of serum and duodenal juice demonstrated free α-heavy chains, thus confirming the diagnosis of IPSID/α-heavy chain disease. Malabsorption was confirmed by abnormal 5-g D-xylose absorption (urine excretion < 0.5 g/5 h) and increased 3-day stool fat excretion of 20 g/day, while the patient was on a liquid formula diet containing approximately 68 g of fat/day. Pancreatic enzyme secretion was also measured in response to CCK demonstrating a 48 per cent reduction in trypsin, an 80 per cent reduction in amylase, and an 86 per cent reduction in lipase secretion. Resting metabolic rate determined by indirect calorimetry was also low at 1048 kcal/24 h.

Initial treatment included IV fluid and electrolyte replacement. As his appetite was good, he was first offered a normal ward diet but unfortunately this worsened his diarrhoea and malabsorption. Consequently parenteral feeding was commenced initially at a slow rate (25 kcal/kg per day) of energy in the form of glucose (70 per cent) and fat (30 per cent) and 1.5 g/kg per day of amino acid. In addition he was started on oral tetracycline 250 mg b.d. His improvement was dramatic, and by day seven, his diarrhoea had stopped allowing the reintroduction of a soft diet. Stool output increased slightly but to only three times per day enabling progression to a full normal diet by day 14, permitting discontinuation of TPN. His appetite thereafter was voracious and within 6 weeks his weight had doubled from 22 kg to 45 kg! Likewise his plasma albumin had increased from 18 g/l to 35 g/l and triceps skin-fold thickness measurements from 2.8 mm to 6.2 mm, with an increase in mid-arm circumference from 14 cm to 19 cm. The patient then underwent an elective laparotomy, which revealed a thickened white jejunum, enlarged mesenteric lymph nodes, and a normal spleen. Histological examination of the full-thickness jejunal biopsy and lymph node specimens excluded large-cell lymphoma. The patient made an uneventful recovery, and was well at the time of discharge on a normal diet and tetracycline 250 g/day. He was readmitted for review 2 months later, and on this occasion looked, if anything, obese, weighing 60 kg (Figure 8.10). All blood tests were normal, except for a persistently elevated alkaline phosphatase of 615 units/l (normal, 30–85 units/l). Upper gastrointestinal endoscopy was macroscopically normal, and histological examination of the biopsies showed complete resolution of disease.

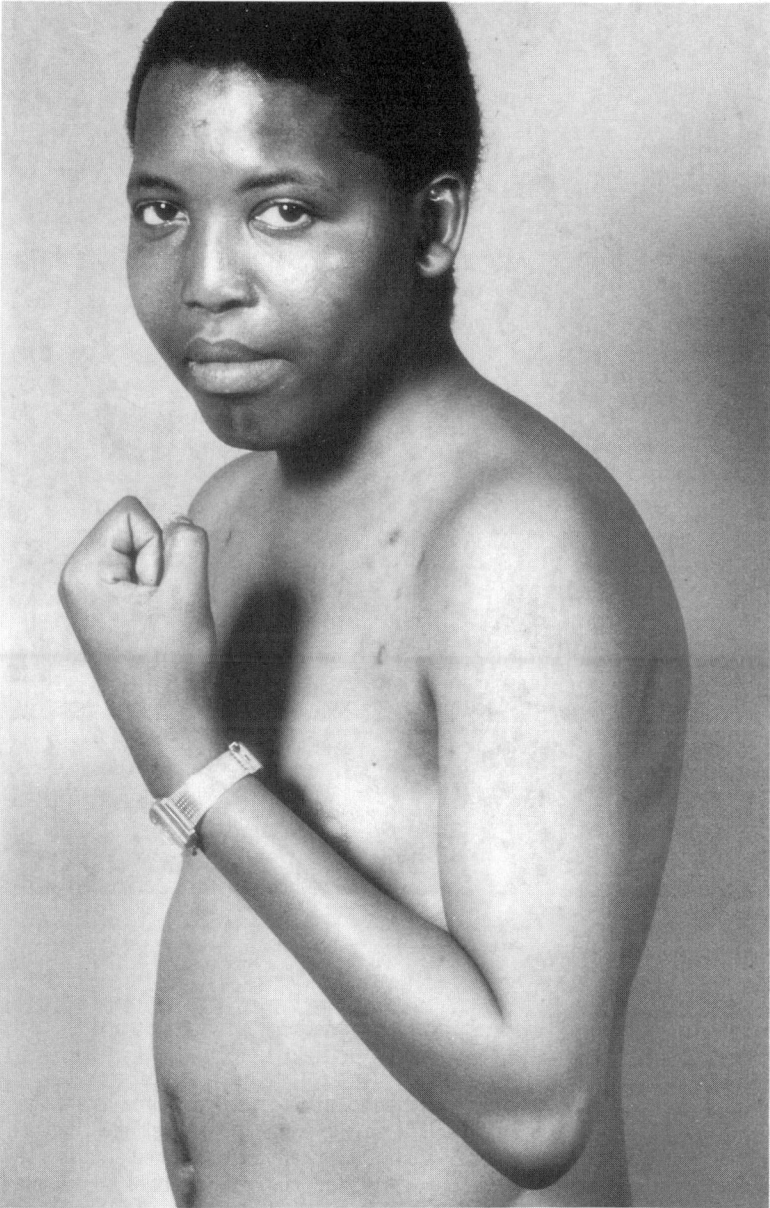

Figure 8.10   The same patient as shown in Figure 8.9 following 4 months of treatment consisting of intravenous feeding followed by enteral nutrition in conjunction with oral tetracycline 250 mg b.d.

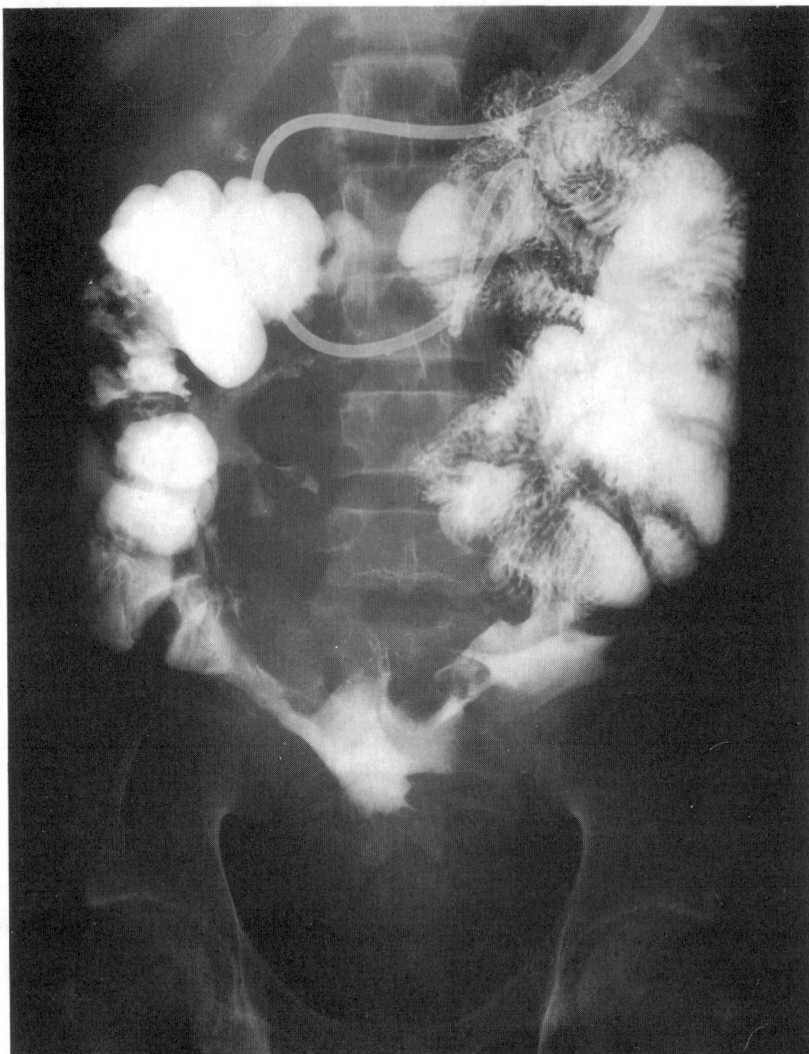

Figure 8.11   *Above* A small bowel enema performed in a patient with severe weight loss and diarrhoea (case 3) demonstrating short-circuiting of half of the small intestine via a large abscess in the lower abdomen to the caecum. Chest X-ray demonstrated an apical lesion and sputum was positive for acid fast bacilli. Following commencement of intravenous feeding and intravenous anti-tuberculosis therapy his diarrhoea decreased dramatically enabling recommencement of oral feeding. *Right* After 4 weeks repeat barium study demonstrated visualisation of the whole of the small intestine for the first time indicating spontaneous healing of the entero-caecal fistula and restoration of intestinal continuity.

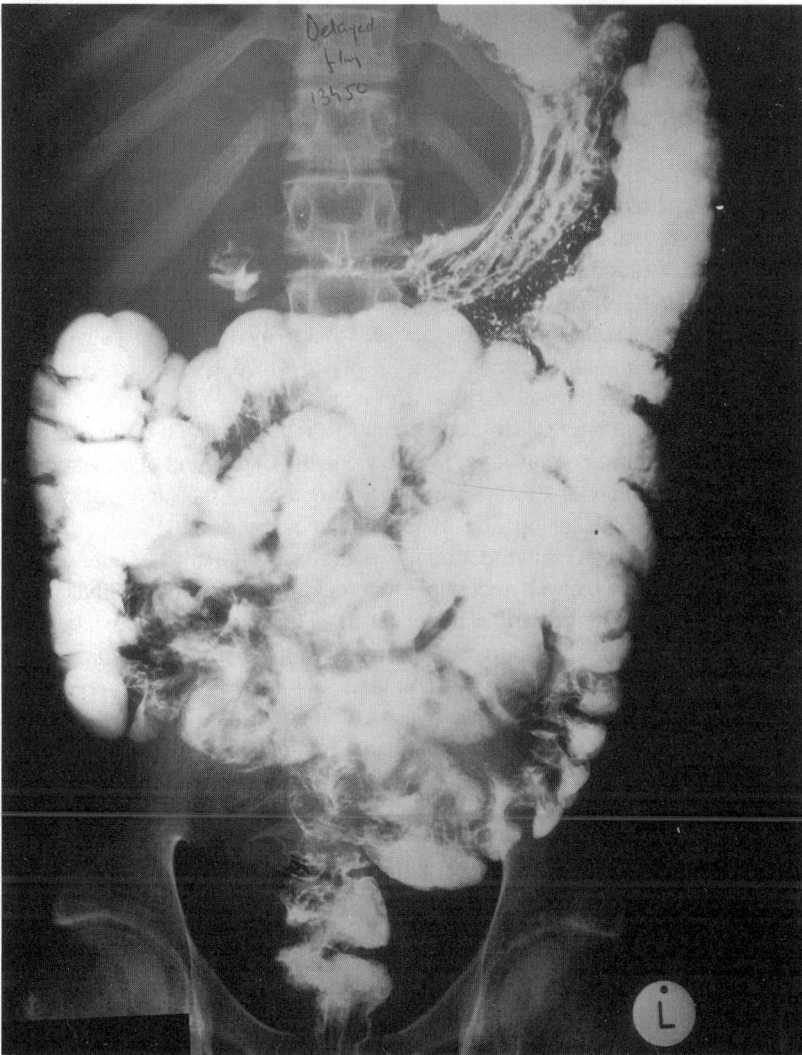

Case history 3. Abdominal tuberculosis

A 19-year-old boy was transferred from a rural district with a 4-month history of episodic watery diarrhoea and severe weight loss down to 35 kg (body mass index 13). Stools were pale in colour and on no occasion was blood noticed. He also complained of intermittent abdominal pain which was diffuse and cramping in nature. His dietary intake was impaired, with vomiting after the consumption of large meals.

On examination he was emaciated and dehydrated. He looked ill, was jaundiced and pyrexial with peripheral oedema. There was no evidence of clubbing or lymphadenopathy. Right leg was more oedematous than the left with a possible deep vein thrombosis (DVT). No specific abnormalities were found in cardiovascular or respiratory systems. Abdominal examination revealed generalised guarding with a doughy abdomen, but no ascites or visceromegaly. Rectal examination revealed pale stool that was occult blood negative.

Investigations revealed a microcytic anaemia of 7.4 g, a white count of 3.2 and an ESR of 76 mm/1st h. Blood chemistry revealed a low sodium of 126 mmol/l, a urea of 5 mmol/l and creatinine of 60 mmol/l. Total protein was also low at 66 g/l, as was albumin at only 20 g/l. Alkaline phosphatase was slightly elevated at 165 units/l. Blood glucose and magnesium were normal. Chest X-ray revealed apical disease on the right and sputum confirmed positive AFBs and active tuberculosis. Venogram confirmed a DVT in the right leg. Xylose absorption was reduced with a urine excretion of 2.6 g over 5 h. Blood was negative for α-heavy chains. Ultrasound of the abdomen suggested fatty infiltration of the liver with no pancreatic or biliary abnormality. Evidence of peritoneal thickening and abnormal tissue between distended bowel loops was seen on the scan, with moderately severe mesenteric lymphadenopathy. The findings were compatible with abdominal tuberculosis or lymphoma. Small bowel enema demonstrated short-circuiting of the distal small bowel with spillage of contrast into a large irregular cavity which then communicated with the caecum (Figure 8.11a). Duodenal biopsy showed blunting of the duodenal villi and inflammatory infiltration with numerous giardia present along the epithelial brush border.

In view of his confirmed diagnosis of pulmonary tuberculosis, it was assumed that he had disseminated abdominal tuberculosis and was commenced on anti-tuberculosis therapy. Because of his degree of gut failure, he was converted to intravenous feeding and IV anti-tuberculosis therapy. His progress thereafter was extremely good with significant weight gain of 6 kg in 2 weeks. In addition he felt symptomatically better and regained strength. After one week, a soft diet was reintroduced and tolerated remarkably well. By the third week he had advanced to a normal diet with a dramatic decrease in diarrhoea. A repeat small bowel barium study demonstrated closure of the internal fistula with visualisation of the whole of the small intestine for the first time (Figure 8.11b). The subclavian catheter was then withdrawn, the TPN discontinued, and the anti-tuberculosis drugs converted to oral. Despite his continued improvement on anti-tuberculosis therapy, there was still some concern that his problem was complicated by intra-abdominal lymphoma. Consequently a laparotomy was performed 2 months later which revealed a 'frozen abdomen'. Biopsy specimens revealed only chronic inflammatory tissue. At the time of discharge he weighed 50 kg. Review in outpatients 6 months later showed continued improvement with a body weight of 55 kg (BMI 20) and no specific abdominal complaints.

Case history 4. Short bowel syndrome

A 50-year-old woman was involved in a road traffic accident resulting in abdominal trauma. At laparotomy the ileum and the distal jejunum had to be removed necessitating formation of a jejunostomy and defunctioned colon. Measurement of her remaining small intestine at the time of surgery was 180 cm. Her postoperative course was extremely stormy with high jejunostomy outputs requiring intravenous fluid, electrolytes and nutrition. Her progress was complicated by repeated attacks of abdominal sepsis requiring further laparotomy and drainage and of two episodes of catheter-associated sepsis.

One month later, she was finally sufficiently stable to permit transfer to a general ward. Throughout her time in the intensive care her chief form of nutrition had been TPN as attempts at oral feeding had resulted in massive increases in stomal output up to 5 l/day. Despite intravenous feeding her weight had dropped by 15 kg. After 5 days in the general ward she again developed septicaemia necessitating withdrawal of her central line. In view of her poor venous access, attempts at supplemented oral feeding were instituted. Once again this failed as she became gradually more dehydrated and developed multiple electrolyte deficiencies. Enteral tube-feeding was then attempted with a semi-elemental diet. Initial infusion rate was 20 ml/h after which the rate was gradually increased up to 80 ml/h. There appeared to be a threshold limit for tolerance at 60 ml/h and so infusions were kept at this rate for 7 days. During this period her stomal output gradually decreased to under 2 l/day. Further improvement was seen the next week with a reduction to 1500 ml per 24 h despite the increased nasoenteric infusion-rate of 80 ml/h. The formula was then converted to a polymeric composition, with no resultant change in stomal output. At this stage the decision was made to give her tube-feeding of 1 litre at night with encouragement to eat normal food during the day. Progress was slow but steady and by the time of discharge 4 weeks later she was managed on normal food alone given in the form of multiple small meals. After discharge unfortunately she ran into further hydration problems and was readmitted dehydrated and electrolyte deficient once again. The decision was then made to take her back to surgery in order to reconnect her colon. Postoperative course was uneventful and by day 7 she was back on to a full normal diet with the passage of only two stools per day. Her 24-h urine output improved to over 1½ litres/day and her electrolytes and urea and renal function normalised by the time of discharge 2 weeks later. At 1 month follow-up in outpatients she had put on 10 kg in weight and was able to return to work. Her only parenteral supplement now remains vitamin B_{12} intramuscular injections once per month.

Further reading

Jelliffe DB. Assessment of the nutritional status of a community. World Health Organization Monograph Series, No 53 Geneva: WHO, 1966.

Kotler DP, editor. Gastrointestinal and nutritional manifestations of the acquired immuno-deficiency syndrome. New York: Raven Press, 1991.

O'Keefe SJD, Kelly DG. Nutrition and gastroenterology. Current Gastroenterology 1992;12:351–81.

O'Keefe SJD, Rosser BG. Nutrition in inflammatory bowel disease. In: Targan SR, Shanahan, editors. Inflammatory bowel disease: from the bench to the bedside. Maryland, USA: Williams & Wilkins, 1994.

Rombeau JL, Caldwell MD, editors. Clinical nutrition, parenteral nutrition and clinical nutrition, enteral and tube feeding. 2nd ed. Philadelphia: WB Saunders, 1993.

9

Malabsorption

Malabsorption is a relatively common clinical problem in the tropics. Malabsorption can result from defective digestion of foodstuffs within the lumen of the bowel, structural changes in the bowel wall or anatomical abnormalities in the lymphatic drainage of the bowel. There are a large number of causes of malabsorption which are listed in Table 9.1.

Table 9.1 The causes of malabsorption.

---

1. **Infective**
   Acute enteritis
   Intestinal tuberculosis
   Parasitic disease of the intestine
   Travellers' diarrhoea
   Whipple's disease
   Contaminated small bowel
      Anatomical:
         blind loops, diverticula, strictures, fistulae
      Motility disturbance:
         systemic sclerosis, diabetes mellitus, pseudo-obstruction, radiotherapy

2. **Defective luminal digestion**
   Pancreatic
      Chronic pancreatitis
      Cystic fibrosis
      Malnutrition
      Defective stimulation: gastric/intestinal surgery
      Zollinger–Ellison syndrome
      Pancreatectomy
   Bite-salt mediated
      Biliary obstruction
      Terminal ileum disease/resection
      Parenchymal liver disease
      Bacterial overgrowth/contaminated small bowel

3. **Mucosal**
   Food sensitivities:
      Gluten-sensitive enteropathy
      Tropical sprue
      Cows' milk sensitivity in infants
      Dermatitis herpetiformis
   Alactasia
   Abetalipoproteinaemia
   Whipple's disease
   Intestinal lymphangiectasia
   Mast cell disease

4. **Structural**
   Gastric surgery
   Crohn's disease
   Intestinal resection
   Small intestine lymphoma
   Idiopathic chronic ulcerative enteritis
   Amyloidosis
   Blind loops, fistulae, strictures, diverticula

5. **Lymphatic obstruction**
   Congenital lymphangiectasia
   Acquired lymphangiectasia: tuberculosis, lymphoma, cardiac disease.

6. **Specific biochemical defects**
   Disaccharidase deficiency
   Vitamin B_{12} malabsorption
   Folate malabsorption
   Cystinuria
   Hartnup disease
   Pancreatic enzyme deficiencies

7. **Drugs**
   Neomycin
   Cholestyramine
   Metformin
   Methydopa
   Alcohol
   Liquid paraffin
   Antacids
   Irritant purgative abuse
   Para-amino salicylic acid

8. **Disease outside the gastrointestinal tract**
   Endocrine disorders
      Hyperthyroidism
      Hypothyroidism
      Addison's disease
      Hyperparathyroidism
      Hypoparathyroidism
   Collagen diseases

Clinical presentation

Malabsorption may present with a wide range of symptoms including bulky stools, abdominal distension, flatulence, weight loss, anorexia, generalised weakness, bleeding, paraesthesia and bone pain. A careful history should include bowel habit in childhood, medical history, previous surgery, family history and dietary habits including alcohol. A knowledge of diseases that commonly cause malabsorption in the patient's environment will ensure the history is taken thoroughly.

The key symptoms and signs of the malabsorption syndrome are:

1. **Diarrhoea.** The stools are typically loose, bulky, offensive, greasy, light coloured and difficult to flush away. Stool frequency is often increased.
2. **Abdominal symptoms.** These include abdominal discomfort, distension and boborygmi.
3. **Nutritional deficiency** (Chapter 8). Malabsorption may result in an apparently isolated nutritional deficiency or electrolyte deficiencies. Such deficiencies may be reflected by a variety of symptoms and signs including glossitis, pallor, muscle pain, petechiae and bruising of the skin, hyperpigmentation, neurological abnormalities and skeletal abnormalities.
4. **Features of general ill health.** These include anorexia, weight loss, lethargy, dyspnoea and easy fatiguability. Finger clubbing may occur. Hypoalbuminaemia, oedema, dehydration and electrolyte deficiencies may occur in severe or prolonged disease.
5. **Features related to the underlying cause.** These are features that give a clue to the underlying disease such as an abdominal mass, previous operation scars etc.

Investigation of the patient suspected of malabsorption

Faecal fat (p 117)

The quantity of fat in the stool depends on the intake of fat in the diet. Thus for interpretation of the faecal fat, dietary fat intake must be known. The faeces need to be collected over several days, preferably at least three, and the result expressed as an average daily excretion. Although there is a small quantity of endogenous fat in the stool, of the order of 1–2 g per day, much higher levels are obtained in patients with steatorrhea. Indirect methods of fat absorption have also been devised and these include the use of radioactive fats, macroscopic or microscopic examination of faeces and fat tolerance tests.

Carbohydrate absorption

The glucose tolerance test, which measures the blood levels after a standard oral dose of glucose, tends to give a lower than normal rise in most cases of malabsorption but a higher than normal in patients with pancreatic disease.

The test that is usually used to assess carbohydrate absorption is the xylose absorption test. An oral dose of xylose is given and the excretion in urine measured for the ensuing 5 h. Excretion of greater than 22 per cent of a 5-g dose and greater than 17 per cent of a 25-g dose may be regarded as normal. Besides intestinal malabsorption, abnormal results can occur due to delayed gastric emptying, low urine flow or poor renal function.

A lactose tolerance test can be performed in a similar manner to the glucose tolerance test. In patients with lactase deficiency oral lactose is followed by little rise in the blood glucose. However direct measurement of lactase in mucosal biopsy specimens is a better test for alactasia than lactose tolerance test.

Protein absorption

Faecal nitrogen is a measure of protein malabsorption particularly in pancreatic disease. It is however rarely used. Excessive loss of protein (protein losing enteropathy) can be assessed by measuring faecal radioactivity after intravenous injection of radioactive protein.

Vitamin B_{12} absorption

In the absence of other reasons for it to be malabsorbed, the absorption of vitamin B_{12} may be used as a test of ileal function. The Schilling test consists of an oral dose of radioactive vitamin B_{12} followed by a large intramuscular 'flushing' dose of non-radioactive B_{12}. The 24-h urinary B_{12} radioactivity is then measured.

If a low level is obtained, the test should be repeated by giving intrinsic factor with the oral dose of B_{12}. If the result remains low, this is indicative that the malabsorption is due to ileal disease. On the other hand if the repeat test with intrinsic factor results in a normal result, this would suggest the diagnosis of pernicious anaemia or some other gastric pathology.

Small bowel biopsy

The most widely used is the Crosby–Krugler capsule in which a spring-located blade is activated by suction through a fine tube. The main disadvantage is the fact that only a single specimen can be obtained. An advance on the Crosby–Krugler capsule is a hydraulic capsule which enables multiple biopsy specimens to be taken.

Endoscopic biopsy

With the ready availability of upper gastrointestinal endoscopy, small biopsy samples from the duodenum are frequently taken. Although endoscopic biopsies may reliably suggest or refute conditions such as coeliac disease, it should be pointed out that there are a number of pitfalls in the interpretation of duodenal biopsies.

Enzyme measurements

Estimation of enzyme activity in biopsy tissue may reveal multiple deficiencies associated with histological abnormalities. Isolated deficiency of lactose is diagnostic of primary alactasia.

Small bowel radiology

This may reveal anatomical lesions that are responsible for the malabsorption. It may also indicate gross defects of motility.

A definitive diagnosis of a cause of malabsorption such as diverticula, blind loops or strictures may be revealed by radiology. Alternatively the findings may be non-specific such as dilatation, thickened folds (suggesting oedema) and poor motility. Flocculation of the contrast medium is minimised by the technique of small bowel enema.

Nutritional status

Deficiencies of major nutrients are reflected mainly by the loss of body weight and a low serum albumin. Deficiencies of haematinic factors (iron, folic acid, and vitamin B_{12}) and fat soluble vitamins (A, D and K) are common.

In cases of severe diarrhoea, water and electrolyte deficiencies need to be recognised and treated. Hypokalaemia is common. Magnesium deficiency may be suspected from low plasma and urine magnesium levels. Hypocalcaemia can also occur.

Some causes of malabsorption which are important in the tropics

The recognition and management of malabsorption, malnutrition and weight loss is discussed in detail in Chapter 8. Some causes of chronic diarrhoea and malabsorption are discussed below.

Disccharidase deficiency and malabsorption

The enzymes reponsible for splitting disaccharidases into monosaccharides are found in the brush border of the intestinal epithelium. The highest concentration is found in the proximal small intestine. Deficiencies of these disaccharides may occur as an isolated deficiency of the enzyme (primary deficiency) or as a result of small intestinal disease (secondary deficiency).

Hypolactasia

This condition is rare in Europe and UK but affects over 90 per cent in certain African and Oriental races. There is a genetic factor but it is not clear to what degree villous abnormalities caused by infections and parasites contribute to the lactase deficiency.

Pathogenesis

The inability to split disaccharides results in defective absorption of these sugars which now pass into the colon. Diarrhoea is partly caused by the increased osmotic load and partly by products of bacterial fermentation resulting in lactic acid production and gaseous distension.

Clinical features

These vary from mild to severe symptoms. This relates to dietary lactose intake and the extent to which the colon is able to absorb fluid and electrolytes. Important features include loose or watery diarrhoea, intermittent abdominal distension, colic, audible boborygmi and passage of excess flatus.

Diagnosis

The definitive test is the measurement of lactase in a jejunal biopsy. Other tests include the lactose tolerance test and the measurement of breath hydrogen following an oral dose of lactose.

Treatment

In primary hypolactasia, lactose-free diets usually bring marked improvement in symptoms.

Post-infective malabsorption syndrome (tropical sprue)

This is a chronic malabsorption syndrome of greater than 2 months duration which is common in tropical countries in which abnormal bacterial flora is present in the small intestinal lumen. The disease is common in India and South-East Asia and the Carribean. There is a relative sparing of Africa although there have been reports from Southern and West Africa.

Aetiology and pathogenesis

The vast majority of cases start with an acute diarrhoea, which presumably is of infective origin. The initiating infections presumably differ from place to place and these could include bacteria, viruses and parasites.

This results in mucosal damage of the jejunum and ileum. By 4–6 months the serum folate levels will have fallen to low levels resulting in further mucosal damage. Hypochlorhydria, which is common in this condition, as well as the slowing of small intestinal transit time due to the high levels of enteroglucagon, provide the setting for secondary bacterial colonisation.

Clinical features

The disease can present as an isolated case or in epidemics. It usually starts with an acute attack of diarrhoea which may be occassionally bloody. It is associated with abdominal distension and flatulence. Lactose intolerance may occur. Physical examination may reveal weight loss and abdominal distension. Pallor and glossitis occur after several months in untreated cases and this is due to folate deficiency. Later vitamin B_{12} deficiency may also develop in long standing chronic cases.

Investigations

D-xylose, fat and vitamin B_{12} malabsorption are present. Secondary hypolactasia (lactose intolerance) may be present. Megaloblastic anaemia caused by folate depletion and later vitamin B_{12} deficiency is also a feature.

Treatment

It is probable that the milder cases recover spontaneously. In those with moderate and severe disease, folic acid 15 mg/daily is given daily for at least 1 month. This is given together with tetracycline 250 mg four times daily and there is prompt clinical improvement in most cases treated with this combination. If vitamin B_{12} deficiency co-exists, 1000 mg vitamin B_{12} is given for several days followed by 1000 mg monthly for several months. The experience with antibiotics in India has been disappointing but this may be because viruses rather that bacteria could be the important aetiological agents in that region.

Giardiasis is the commonest cause of malabsorption and is diagnosed by examining the stools or smearing of mucus from jejunal biopsies on to a microscopic slide. Villous atrophy can occur. The treatment is metronidazole 400 mg t.d.s. for 3–7 days or tinidazole which can be given as a single dose. If bacterial overgrowth is considered to be a factor in causing malabsorption tetracycline can be given.

Tropical calcific pancreatitis

Tropical calcific pancreatitis may cause malabsorption, weight loss and diabetes and is discussed on pages 125 and 364.

Other causes of malabsorption

Coeliac disease, bacterial overgrowth (p 122), short bowel syndrome (p 125) and small bowel lymphoma (p 126) are discussed briefly in Chapter 8. Previous gastric surgery is discussed in Chapter 15 (p 287).

Drug-induced malabsorption

Numerous drugs have been implicated some of which are listed in Table 9.2. The different mechanisms of action include structural damage to the mucosa, inhibition of mucosal and luminal enzymes, precipitation of bile acids and fatty acids, physico-chemical factors and alteration of bowel flora.

Malabsorption produced by drugs is reversible and dose-related. The treatment is to stop the drug.

Table 9.2 Examples of drugs causing malabsorption.

Drug	Mechanism	Results
Cholestyramine	Binds bile acids	Steatorrhoea Gall stones Malabsorption of fat soluble vitamins
Colchicine and cytotoxics	Arrest enterocyte mitosis	Steatorrhoea
Neomycin	Partial villous atrophy and enzyme inhibition	Steatorrhoea Iron, B_{12}, glucose malabsorption
Ferrous sulphate	Binds with tetracycline	Malabsorption of both drugs
Methyldopa	Partial villous atrophy	Steatorrhoea
Ethanol	Damage to enterocyte subcellular organelles	Folate deficiency Steatorrhoea

Primary hypogammaglobulinaemia

The syndrome of severe combined immune deficiency may have malabsorption as a feature in about a quarter of cases. Malabsorption is rarely severe and tends to affect adults rather than children.

Protein-losing enteropathy

Inflammatory, infective, allergic or neoplastic conditions may give rise to a protein-losing enteropathy. Often the protein loss is mild and incidental but can be severe in Ménétrièr's disease and lymphatic disorders. Severe cases present with peripheral oedema, and hypoalbuminaemia in the absence of liver or renal disease. Diarrhoea, often with steatorrhoea is a feature of lymphatic disorders. The diagnosis requires the technology to measure the rate of ^{51}Cr-labelled protein loss into the small intestine or the ability to measure faecal α-1-antitrypsin. The management involves nutritional support and treatment of the underlying disorder.

Whipple's disease

This disease is rare and characterised by large, foamy periodic acid-Schiff (PAS) positive macrophages containing glycoprotein within the lamina propria of the small intestine. Most patients present with malabsorption, steatorrhoea and episodes of migratory polyarthritis affecting the large joints without causing residual deformity. Fever, lymphadenopathy, finger clubbing, cardiac and neurological manifestations may occur. Antibiotic therapy is rapidly effective and involves intramuscular penicillin and streptomycin for 2 weeks and tetracycline for 1 year. About 30 per cent of patients will relapse.

Lymphangiectasia

Dilated lacteals develop in the villi due to hypoplasia of the lymphatics. It is normally idiopathic but can arise secondary to abdominal malignancy. The patient presents with peripheral oedema secondary to hypoproteinaemia due to protein-losing enteropathy. The diagnosis is established by small bowel biopsy and the treatment involves a low-fat diet and possibly substitution of dietary fat by medium chain triglycerides. If a short segment of bowel is affected it can be resected.

Abetalipoproteinaemia

This rare autosomal recessive disorder results in defective transport of triglyceride from the liver and the gut. It usually presents in childhood with mild diarrhoea and steatorrhoea. Later neurological deficits develop with peripheral neuropathy and cerebellar ataxia. Plasma betalipoproteins are absent and plasma cholesterol, triglycerides and phospholipids are low. The red cells show spiked acanthocytes. The diagnosis is confirmed by small bowel biopsy which shows cytoplasmic fatty vacuolation of the enterocytes at the apex of the villi. There is no curative treatment. A low-fat diet should be given and deficiencies of fat soluble vitamins corrected.

Further reading

Alpers DH, Seetharam B. Pathophysiology of diseases involving intestinal brush border proteins. New Engl J Med 1977; 296:1047–50.

Cook GC. Aetiology and pathogenesis of post-infective tropical malabsorption (tropical sprue). Lancet 1984; i:721–3.

Gray GM. Intestinal disaccharidase deficiencies and glucose–galactose malabsorption. In: Stanbury JB, Wyngaarden JB, Fredrickson DS, Goldstein JL, Brown MS, editors. The metabolic basis of inherited disease. 5th ed. New York: McGraw-Hill, 1983: 1729–42.

Lowosky MS. In: Bouchier IAD, Allan RN, Hodgson HJE, Keighley MRB, editors. Textbook of Gastroenterelogy. London: Ballière Tindall, 1984:441–7.

Losowsky MS, Walker BE, Kelleher J. Malabsorption in clinical practice. Edinburgh: Churchill Livingstone, 1974.

10

Abdominal Masses:
a practical approach

Abdominal masses may arise from:

1. The **abdominal walls,** which anteriorly and laterally include the skin, subcutaneous fat, fascia and muscle, and posteriorly include the vertebral
   bodies and the paravertebral muscles. Inferiorly, the posterior and lateral
   walls are formed by the sacrum, iliac bones and iliacus muscles, and the
   anterior wall by the pubic bones.
2. The **peritoneal cavity,** within which lie the intraperitoneal organs which
   either hang freely from a mesentery (e.g. liver, spleen, small bowel, ovary,
   uterus) or become attached to the posterior abdominal wall by congenital
   fusion of their mesentery with the posterior peritoneal lining (e.g. duodenum, ascending and descending colon) (Figure 10.1).
3. The **retroperitoneal organs,** (renal system, adrenals, pancreas, great vessels,
   lymphatics and autonomic nervous system) which lie between the peritoneal
   cavity and the posterior abdominal wall (Figure 10.2).
4. The **bladder,** which as it fills with urine, strips the peritoneum away from
   the lower, anterior abdominal wall.

Clinical assessment

History

An abdominal swelling may form part of the patient's presenting symptomatology, but is more commonly discovered during clinical examination. In
all cases the history must include gastrointestinal, urinary and gynaecological
symptoms, together with social, residential and family history. The latter may
reveal:

1. heavy alcohol intake and therefore the possibility of hepatomegaly due to
   hepatic cirrhosis, splenomegaly due to portal hypertension or pancreatic
   pseudocyst complicating pancreatitis;

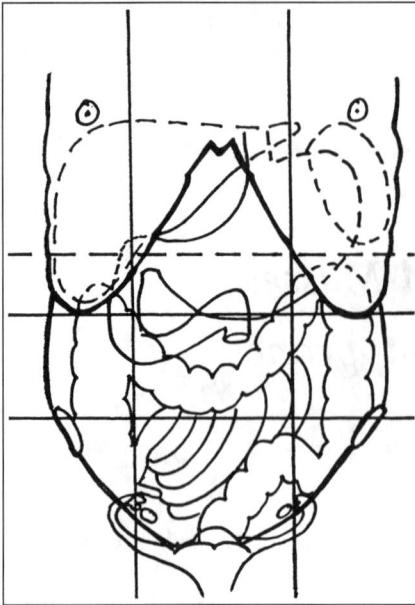

Figure 10.1 Organs in the peritoneal cavity in which disease may cause an abdominal mass.

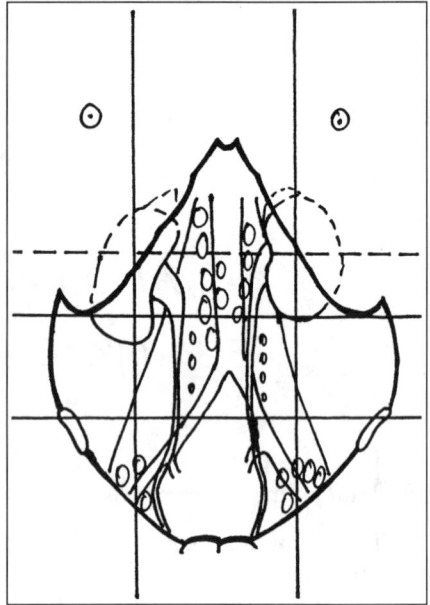

Figure 10.2 Structures in the retroperitoneum which may give rise to an abdominal mass.

2. heavy smoking and the possibility of hepatomegaly caused by metastatic bronchial carcinoma;
3. previous residence in areas with risk of specific geographical disease (schistosomiasis, amoebiasis, hydatid disease (Chapters 3 and 7);
4. a familial disorder such as polycystic disease (p 172).

Symptoms usually point to the primary organ of involvement but may also result from pressure, malignant infiltration or inflammation of organs adjacent to the mass, and mislead the clinician. For example, hepatomegaly or splenomegaly may interfere with appetite by pressure on the stomach; a lower abdominal mass may lead to frequency of micturition by pressure on the bladder or constipation by pressure on the rectum; an inflammatory mass may cause frequency of micturition or diarrhoea by irritation of the bladder or distal bowel respectively.

Examination

Thorough examination is particularly important where facilities for investigations are limited as it frequently reveals the likely cause of an abdominal mass and always encourages the economic and rational use of investigations. Clues to the diagnosis of an abdominal mass may be found in any part of the body and therefore the patient must, routinely, be examined naked on a bed with a sheet being used to preserve dignity.

General examination

Begin with examination of the hands, feel the elbows for epitrochlear nodes and the axilla for axillary nodes, look at the face and examine the sclerae, conjunctivae and oral cavity, feel the neck anteriorly for abnormal masses. Ask the patient to sit forward, palpate the neck for nodes from behind, feel the patient's back with your hands, test for chest expansion, auscultate and percuss the chest posteriorly. Palpate the spine and look for differential enlargement of the flanks. Ask the patient to lie down again. Observe, percuss and auscultate the chest from the front. Examine the breasts. Examine the feet and ankles and run your hands up both legs to the thighs. Expose the groins, ask the patient to cough and look for cough impulses. Examine the groins and external genitalia.

Practice points

- *Feeling the skin of the arms, torso and legs allows detection of subcutaneous nodules, such as metastases, more easily than by relying on sight alone.*
- *Examination of all lymph node groups as a preliminary to examining the abdomen is important, because superficial lymphadenopathy may be associated with palpable para-aortic nodes or splenomegaly or suggest background HIV infection. Discovery of a node or nodes confined to the left supraclavicular fossa (Virchow's node, Troisier's sign) suggests an intra-abdominal malignancy that has metastasised along the thoracic duct.*
- *Enlarged iliac lymph nodes are felt just above the inguinal ligament, and disappear when the patient tenses his abdominal muscles. Enlarged iliac nodes can be biopsied extraperitoneally.*
- *Examination of the external genitalia is especially important in the male where an abnormally enlarged testis may suggest that the abdominal mass is a para-aortic node involved by metastatic testicular tumour; bilateral atrophic testes that the mass is a cirrhotic liver with or without hepatoma; an absent testis that the abdominal mass is a malignancy arising in an undescended intra-abdominal gonad.*

Abdominal examination

The patient should be lying comfortably on a flat surface, preferably with his head slightly raised on a pillow and his arms by his side. Ideally, the whole abdomen and groins should be exposed. Human dignity does not always allow this, but the importance of proper exposure should not be forgotten since pathology in the groin and genitalia is easily missed.

Firstly, inspect the abdomen and look for abnormal contours, visible peristalsis, bulging of one or other of the flanks or distended veins. Ask the patient to cough and observe for cough impulses indicating the presence of a hernia.

Secondly, palpate the abdomen with the right hand from the right side of the patient.

1. Carry out light 'reconnaissance' palpation.
2. Carry out deep palpation.
3. Turn your attention to defining the characteristics of any palpated mass(es), namely exact location, shape, size (measured accurately with a ruler or tape measure), consistency, the presence of fluctuation or pulsation, mobility and percussion note.
4. Carry out specific manoeuvres to make the liver, spleen and kidneys more prominent.

Test all upper abdominal masses for movement with respiration. Attempt to ballot all lateral masses. Try to move the mass in the lateral and vertical planes and observe if the mass changes position with posture. A fluctuant, distended abdomen is likely to contain ascites. Large cysts and a large bladder are also fluctuant. Additional tests that may be of value are testing the direction of flow in veins that are visible, listening for a succussion splash, auscultating the mass (a venous hum may be present with a hepatoma, a friction rub may be present over an inflamed liver or spleen), and testing for pain or restriction of hip movement if a psoas mass is suspected. Rectal and vaginal examination complete the clinical assessment and are important even if a mass is outside the pelvis. An abdominal mass may represent metastatic lymphadenopathy or metastatic hepatic nodules from a primary pelvic malignancy. Conversely, the finding of multiple pelvic masses or fixed, immobile pelvic organs ('frozen pelvis') suggests transcoelomic metastases to the pelvis. In males, attention is paid to the contour and consistency of the prostate and in females, to the feel of the cervix.

Where patients report abnormalities of stool or urine, these should be examined personally if possible, as should the vomitus in those with vomiting.

Practice points
- *Failure to detect abdominal masses often results because the patient cannot be made to relax his abdomen. A relaxed, considerate manner on the part of the clinician helps the patient to relax but where this fails, ask the patient to flex the hips and knees and to breathe in and out deeply and slowly.*
- *The spleen, liver, gallbladder and kidneys all move with deep inspiration. Masses arising from the stomach or transverse colon may also move with respiration unless tethered by malignant or inflammatory adhesions.*
- *Ballottement describes the manoeuvre in which the mass can be bounced back and forth from one hand held behind the loin to the other hand palpating the mass from the front. Ballotable masses are usually retroperitoneal (and most commonly renal in origin) although a very large spleen may also be ballotable.*
- *Where it is suspected that a mass is within, or superficial, to the abdominal wall, examine for the mass with the abdominal muscles tensed. Abdominal*

wall muscles are made tense by having the patient raise both legs in the air or raise his torso off the bed without the use of his arms.

- A *pulsatile mass* may be an aneurysm, though the normal aorta is palpable in many thin individuals and masses overlying the aorta can transmit pulsation from the normal aorta.

Case history 1

A 40-year-old woman presented with abdominal pain and was referred by the casualty officer for a surgical opinion on account of a tender right lumbar mass. Careful clinical examination revealed an additional sign, namely slight local tenderness of the thoracolumbar spine. Plain abdominal radiology showed loss of T12–L1 joint space with destruction of the adjacent vertebrae compatible with tuberculosis of the spine. At surgery, a cold psoas abscess was drained. The patient recovered completely on antituberculous therapy.

Case history 2

A 42-year-old woman presented with anorexia and weight loss and was referred for investigation of a right upper abdominal mass. On examination there was nodular hepatomegaly compatible with metastatic disease. Examination of the patient's right breast revealed a mobile mass which was proved to be malignant on biopsy.

Investigations

Not all abdominal masses require immediate or extensive investigation. Most non-inflammatory abdominal masses will require surgery, some exceptions being hepatomegaly, splenomegaly, asymptomatic fibroids and advanced tumours.

Inflammatory masses benefit from a non-operative approach in the absence of generalised peritonitis, intestinal obstruction or a deterioration in the patient's general condition. Thus if it is not possible to perform many investigations the decision as to whether or not to proceed to laparatomy can usually be made by a surgeon on clinical grounds alone.

Examination under anaesthesia may provide useful information on the relationship of a lower abdominal mass to the bladder, gynaecological organs and rectum, especially if combined with sigmoidoscopy and/or cystoscopy.

General investigations

Urinalysis should be performed in every case. A white cell count is indicated for possible inflammatory masses. The choice of other blood tests including liver function tests, coagulation profile, urea and electrolytes will be determined according to the likely site of origin and complications of the mass.

Plain radiographs

A plain abdominal radiograph of a solid tumour may show a soft-tissue mass or calcification in a tumour (Figure 10.3), chronically inflammed pancreas or aneurysm. An abscess may have a mottled, irregular appearance similar to faeces or even a fluid level, in the case of subphrenic abscess. A chest radiograph should be taken for all cases of abdominal mass.

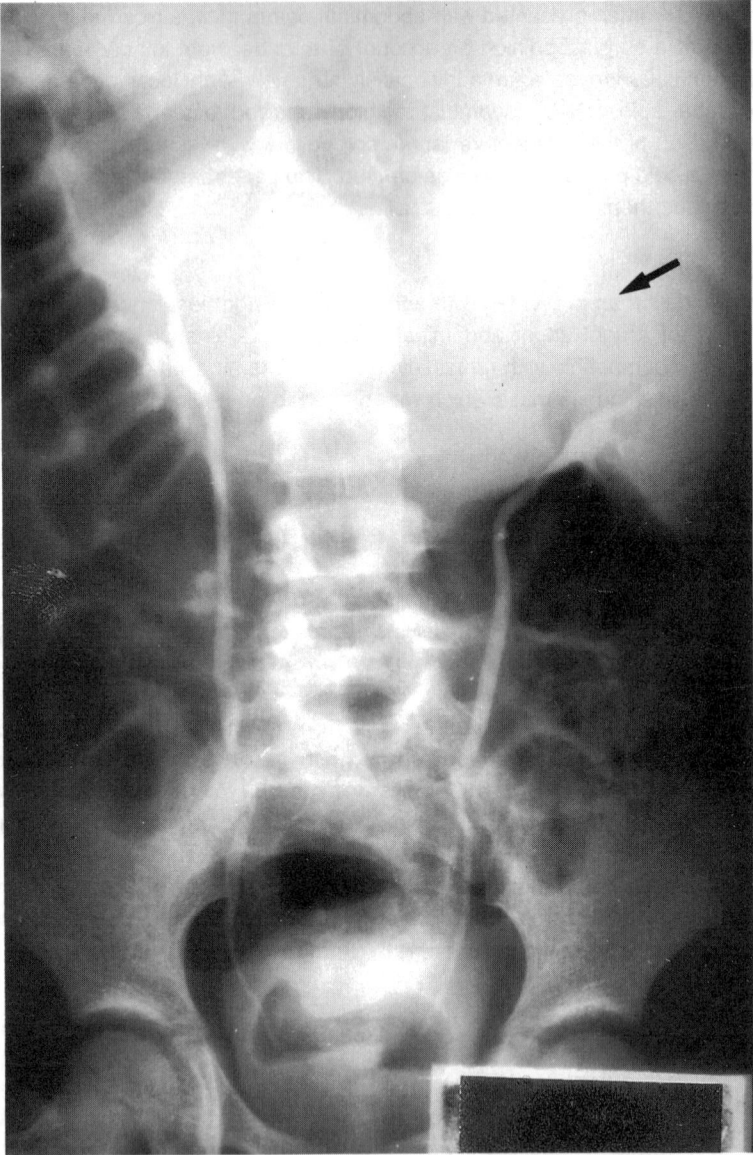

Figure 10.3 Soft tissue calcification in a neuroblastoma in a 5-year-old boy. The kidney is displaced downwards.

Ultrasound

The most valuable and readily available investigation is an ultrasound scan which may show the organ from which the mass arises and determine its consistency, particularly whether it is solid or cystic. It is particularly useful for liver, biliary tract and renal masses and will demonstrate whether or not a retroperitoneal mass is obstructing or involving the ureters. It is unlikely to be diagnostic for masses arising from the gastrointestinal tract or when distended bowel loops are interposed between mass and skin.

Endoscopy

Gastroduodenal and colorectal lesions are best visualised at endoscopy which also facilitates biopsy. Cystoscopy is indicated for bladder masses.

Contrast radiology

Intravenous urography is indicated for suspected urinary tract lesions. It will demonstrate the ureters and any displacement, obstruction or involvement of the ureters by a mass. It is important to exclude an ectopic or horseshoe kidney and to demonstrate renal function on the opposite side of the abdomen, particularly where a kidney might be at risk of inadvertent removal at laparotomy. Gastrointestinal lesions will benefit from a barium meal and follow-through or barium enema. Since colonoscopy is often not available in the tropics a barium enema may be, in many hospitals, the investigation of choice for right iliac fossa masses.

Fine-needle aspiration (FNA) and biopsy

This is indicated for solid tumours, particularly in childhood where chemotherapy may be indicated before surgery for advanced neuroblastomas (Figure 10.3) or Burkitt's lymphoma. In the case of suspected hepatocellular carcinoma FNA or Tru-Cut biopsy may enable a tissue diagnosis to be made without extensive investigation. Needle aspiration will confirm the presence of a cyst. Any enlarged superficial lymph nodes or subcutaneous mass suspicious of metastasis should be biopsied.

Tumour markers

α-Fetoprotein is raised in hepatocellular carcinoma and helps provide confirmation of the diagnosis in the absence of histology. Since hepatitis B surface antigen is strongly associated with hepatocellular carcinoma, patients with suspected liver masses should have a hepatitis screen.

Carcino-embryonic antigen (CEA) is raised in colonic cancer but detection of raised levels has failed to alter the outcome in large groups of patients so that its use should be restricted to areas with a high incidence of colorectal cancer.

Diagnostic laparotomy

In the presence of limited resources, the clinician in the tropics and subtropics is often unable to make a firm pathological diagnosis on the basis of the investigations available to him. In these circumstances, the value of an exploratory, 'diagnostic' laparotomy cannot be underestimated if anaesthetic services are available. Many masses are found to be amenable to surgical excision, and others which require medical treatment, especially tuberculosis, can be identified. Where advanced intra-abdominal malignancy is discovered, the patient and his family, can be truthfully informed of the prognosis. Such surgery can even on occasion be carried out under local anaesthetic (local infiltrative with sedation or spinal) through a conveniently sited midline incision that admits one hand.

Diagnostic laparotomy should normally be carried out by a surgeon capable of proceeding to resection. Pathology can often be confidently diagnosed by macroscopic examination but should later be confirmed by histology with the exception of masses arising in the pancreas (as pancreatic biopsy is frequently complicated by pancreatic fistula) and highly vascular tumours (because of the danger of uncontrollable bleeding). Where diagnostic laparotomy or biopsy is being performed for a suspected hepatic tumour, the clotting time (normal 8–14 min) should be checked before operation and if prolonged, surgery preceded by vitamin K, 10 mg twice daily, for 5 days. Diagnostic laparotomy should not be carried out for splenomegaly (pp 173–5) unless splenectomy is indicated for hyperspenism or malignancy. A lower abdominal mass originating in the bladder is best diagnosed by cystoscopy.

Laparoscopy

In the future increasing use will be made of laparoscopy to visualise and biopsy tumours and determine resectability. This may be combined with endocavity ultrasound. Many hospitals now have a laparoscope to perform tubal ligations and laparoscopy is likely to become widely available in the tropics.

Other investigations

In major centres computed tomography (CT) and nuclear magnetic resonance (NMR) scanning, and angiography may be available to determine the site, extension and vascularity of a mass. These investigations help the privileged surgeon to advise the patient and his family about the necessity and likely outcome of laparotomy. In some advanced inoperable tumours embolisation may be performed at angiography. However, in the tropics one often has to proceed to a trial of dissection, whether or not resection is possible. In centres attempting liver resection for the small proportion of hepatocellular carcinomas which are resectable, intraoperative ultrasound helps to determine resectability.

Presenting problems

This section emphasises a diagnostic approach based largely on clinical findings. The choice of investigations depends on the site of the mass, the structure involved and the likely pathology.

Abdominal wall mass

Superficial abdominal wall mass

A mass superficial to the abdominal wall muscles moves freely when the abdominal muscles are tensed and may be a lipoma, fibroma, subcutaneous metastatic deposit or any of the benign or malignant skin lesions. If multiple, they may represent multiple neurofibromata, multiple lipomas, metastatic deposits, or nodules of Kaposi's disease. The diagnosis is made by surgical biopsy.

Tender deep abdominal wall mass

A mass arising from, or attached to, the abdominal wall muscles or their covering fascia becomes fixed when the abdominal muscles are tensed. If it is painful or tender, such a mass may be a:

1. strangulated abdominal wall hernia (see Table 10.1);
2. pyomyositis of the abdominal wall musculature which is normally accompanied by fever;
3. rectus muscle haematoma – results from rupture of an inferior epigastric artery (less commonly a superior epigastric artery) which can follow trauma, sudden muscular exertion or paroxysm of coughing.

If there is any chance that a tender abdominal wall mass could be a strangulated hernia, it should be explored under anaesthesia, as blind incision of a strangulated hernia in the mistaken belief that it is an abscess will cause an intestinal fistula.

Table 10.1   Abdominal wall hernias.

Hernia	Position
Epigastric hernia	Midline, upper abdomen
Umbilical hernia (congenital)	Umbilicus
Paraumbilical hernia (acquired)	Umbilical but acquired in life
Spigelian hernia	Lateral edge of the rectus sheath
Intermuscular hernia	Lateral abdominal wall
Incisional hernia	Scar of previous laparotomy incision

Non-tender deep abdominal wall mass

The differential diagnosis of a non-tender mass arising from the abdominal wall musculature includes a reducible abdominal wall hernia, a 'burnt-out', quiescent abscess, a desmoid tumour, a sarcoma of the abdominal wall and infiltration of the abdominal wall by intra-abdominal malignancy. Reducible hernias of the abdominal wall are usually easily diagnosed (Table 10.1).

Umbilical and paraumbilical hernias

Umbilical hernias should be distinguished from paraumbilical hernias. Clinically, both are umbilical in position but have a different natural history. Umbilical hernias are present at birth and though they usually close spontaneously before 5 years of age, may persist into old age. Umbilical hernias do not increase in size (except in the presence of ascites) and rarely cause problems. Surgery in older children and adults is indicated for cosmetic reasons. Paraumbilical hernias occur in adults and originate as a protrusion of fat along a small blood vessel penetrating through the linea alba, adjacent to the closed umbilical scar. By the time a true peritoneal hernia is present, the paraumbilical hernia clinically resembles an umbilical hernia, but paraumbilical hernias may continue to increase in size and can be complicated by obstruction so herniorrhaphy is advised.

Epigastric hernia

The patient with an early epigastric hernia does not usually complain of a lump, only of intermittent pain. At this stage, there is a small protrusion of peritoneal fat through the linea alba, which is painful when compressed by rectus muscle contraction. The early epigastric hernia is an important differential diagnosis in the patient with dyspeptic-like pain. At this stage, the small fatty hernia is palpable only with the patient's abdominal musculature tensed. With time, peritoneum follows the protrusion of fat and a true peritoneal hernia develops.

Other hernias (Table 10.1)

Lateral abdominal hernias should be distinguished from local bulges of the abdominal wall resulting from paralysis of abdominal wall myotomes by surgical division of their nerve supply (e.g. during nephrectomy) or, less commonly, by neuropathy. Midline abdominal hernias should be distinguished from divarification of the recti, in which the linea alba becomes thinned, widened and weakened and allows the intra-abdominal contents to bulge through the midline.

Desmoid tumour

A desmoid tumour is a peculiar, uncommon, locally infiltrative, solid tumour arising from abdominal wall muscle and fascia. It most commonly occurs in women in their second to fourth decade during or following pregnancy. Histologically, it resembles a low grade fibrosarcoma but does not metastasise, though does recur locally if not excised with adequate margins. For this reason, following diagnosis by incision biopsy, the tumour is best excised by a surgeon able to carry out reconstructive surgery to the abdominal wall. True sarcomas of the abdominal wall muscles or fascia are rare.

Umbilical mass

The differential diagnosis of a lump at the umbilicus includes a hernia (see above), a metastatic malignant deposit, adenoma, endometrioma, pyogenic granuloma, an omphalolith, omphalitis, a distended periumbilical vein and eversion of the umbilicus due to ascites. The umbilicus is a classical site for an abdominal wall metastasis. Such a malignant umbilical deposit is known as a Sister Mary Joseph nodule, after the nurse in whom the condition was first recognised. Any solid umbilical mass needs to be biopsied and confirmation of malignancy indicates advanced disease. An adenoma may arise in ectopic epithelium left behind after embryonic closure of the vitellointestinal duct. An umbilical endometrioma is a rare presentation of endometriosis. An omphalolith is a concretion of desquamated skin and hair within the umbilicus. Omphalitis (periumbilical cellulitis) may complicate an omphalolith or local trauma. Distended umbilical veins occur in portal hypertension and usually radiate out from the umbilicus but may present as a solitary, compressible umbilical mass. Such an umbilical vein can bleed heavily when traumatised and, obviously, should not be subjected to incision biopsy.

Case history 3

A 52-year-old woman presented with vague abdominal pain, weight loss and constipation. On abdominal examination, there was a hard umbilical nodule, and on rectovaginal examination, multiple, hard, extra-vaginal and extra-rectal masses. Laparotomy revealed widespread inoperable peritoneal malignancy. Histology of the umbilicus and peritoneum showed an undifferentiated carcinoma. Gastric and ovarian carcinoma are the two common causes of widespread peritoneal metastases.

Generalised abdominal swelling

Generalised abdominal swelling may be due to fat, fluid, faeces, flatus or fetus (the five 'F's'). Massive fibroids occasionally produce a similar appearance.

Obstruction and paralytic ileus (see also pp 310–16)

In obstruction there is usually a typical history including pain, vomiting and constipation. A painful, massively swollen tympanitic abdomen suggests the gas-filled loop of acute sigmoid volvulus, or less commonly pneumoperitoneum. The latter occurs when gastrointestinal perforation results in release of gas, rather than liquid and faecal material into the peritoneal cavity. The actual diagnosis can usually be confirmed on plain radiology.

Megacolon (see also p 316)

Chronic or recurrent distension of the abdomen by faeces and flatus suggests the possibility of subacute intestinal obstruction due to distal bowel obstruction, late onset Hirschsprung's disease, Chagas' disease or idiopathic chronic constipation, and needs to be evaluated by sigmoidoscopy, rectal biopsy and barium enema.

Ascites

Ascites is the presence of fluid in the abdominal cavity (Table 10.2). Ascites is sometimes difficult to differentiate clinically from a massive ovarian cyst distending the whole abdomen. Less frequently, a massive retroperitoneal cyst mimics ascites. A paracentesis (21 gauge needle) will confirm the presence of fluid. Differentiation between ascites and a cyst can be made on ultrasound where there is doubt. Peritonitis, resulting from infection of ascitic fluid, can also present as a painful, tender, distended abdomen.

Fat

A large amount of adipose fat may in itself lead to a large abdomen, but care must be taken that subcutaneous fat is not hiding a more sinister cause of abdominal swelling.

Case history 4

A 45-year-old woman was mistakenly diagnosed as having ascites and underwent repeated abdominal aspiration. Aspiration was eventually complicated by abdominal pain and fever, for which she underwent laparotomy. Surgery revealed a massive ovarian cystadenoma, filling and distending the whole abdomen, with secondary infection. The cystadenoma was removed.

Table 10.2   Causes of ascites.

Peritoneal cavity (malignancy or tuberculosis)
Liver (cirrhosis)
Pancreas (acute pancreatitis)
Kidney (nephrotic syndrome)
Intestinal tract (malnutrition, protein losing enteropathy)
Heart (right sided heart failure, especially pericarditis).

Character of ascitic fluid
   Exudate (high protein content): malignancy, tuberculosis, pancreatitis, infection of
      transudate
   Transudate (low protein content): pathology associated with increased hydrostatic pressure
      and hypoproteinaemia
   Blood stained: malignancy, acute pancreatitis
   Fatty (chylous ascites) (rare): blockage of the thoracic duct by lymphoma or tuberculous
      lymphadenitis

Intra-abdominal mass

Decide whether an intra-abdominal mass is normal or not. Although the liver is not normally palpable in healthy adults, its lower edge becomes palpable on deep inspiration, especially in the epigastrium, in many individuals. If a full urinary bladder is palpable, re-examine the patient after micturition (or catheterisation if this is not possible). A menstrual history and pregnancy test avoids a pregnant uterus being diagnosed as an abnormal mass. In a thin patient with a relaxed abdominal wall, the vertebral column, aorta, and sometimes the kidneys (especially the right) are palpable. In a muscular person, the upper intermuscular septum of the rectus abdominis muscle may be mistaken for the liver edge.

Faeces
Faeces may be palpable in the normal colon in a patient with constipation. Faeces may indent on palpation, but this is not usually appreciable on abdominal examination. The presence of faeces can be confirmed by plain abdominal X-ray, on which faeces have a characteristic mottled appearance. A mass due to faeces disappears after administration of a laxative, suppositories or enema or with spontaneous bowel motion. It is important to re-examine the patient in order not to miss a subacute obstruction.

Masses which require urgent evaluation and treatment
Abdominal masses that are obviously tender, associated with obstruction, jaundice, weight loss or fever warrant emergency admission. Abdominal masses in patients who are otherwise healthy can be investigated less urgently.

Abdominal abscesses and inflammatory masses
Abdominal organs develop tenderness if they become inflamed, infarcted or are suddenly distended. An inflamed, oedematous organ may become palpable and tender in itself. More commonly, it becomes palpable by inducing an inflammatory mass which includes adjacent structures, most commonly the omentum, small bowel and sigmoid colon. Inflammatory masses also occur around intra-abdominal abscesses (see below) and small, self-healing gastrointestinal perforations. Examples of acute inflammatory masses include the appendix mass, the tubo-ovarian mass, amoeboma. Chronic inflammatory masses most frequently occur in the right iliac fossa and include ileocaecal tuberculosis and actinomycosis.

Intra-abdominal abscesses are common in tropical and subtropical countries (Table 10.3). Clinical differentiation from an inflammatory mass can be difficult, especially as the latter often form around a small abscess or, even with antibiotic treatment, an inflammatory mass can evolve into an abscess. An abscess should be suspected in the presence of exquisite tenderness, marked toxaemia, swinging pyrexia or fluctuation and can be confirmed by needle aspiration or ultrasound examination. Rupture of an intra-abdominal

Table 10.3 Abdominal abscesses.

Site	Predisposing factor
Hepatic	Pyogenic portal pylephlebitis, cholangitis, systemic bacteraemia, infection of hepatic cyst or haematoma Amoebic
Splenic	Infection of splenic cyst, haematoma or infarct Systemic bacteraemia
Pancreatic	Necrotising pancreatitis Infection of pancreatic pseudocyst
Subhepatic	Empyema of gallbladder (due to cholelithiasis) Perforated duodenal or gastric ulcer (usually peptic, but latter may be malignant) Renal Colonic perforation (amoebic, malignant)
Subphrenic	Peritonitis or any intra-abdominal infection see p 324
Paracaecal	Appendicitis Gynaecological
Paracolic	Colonic perforation (amoebic, malignant) Diverticulitis
Interileal (interloop)	Typhoid perforation
Renal	Systemic bacteraemia Pyonephrosis (infected hydronephrosis)
Psoas	Pyomyositis Septic spondylitis
Gynaecological	Tubo-ovarian abscess (pyosalpinx) Pyometra (puerperal or post-abortal)
Pouch of Douglas (rectovesical pouch)	Pelvic abscess

abscess with development of generalised peritonitis has a high mortality in the tropics.

Infarction of a mass

Infarction presents with acute pain and may occur when a pedicled cyst or neoplasm undergoes torsion. Most pedicled tumours are ovarian in origin; other examples may arise from the uterus (pedicled subserous fibroids) or liver (pedicled neoplasms). Infarction of an intra-abdominal mass can also result from vascular thrombosis, as may occur spontaneously in part of the enlarged spleen. Infarction leads to reflex guarding of the abdominal wall and therefore a distinct mass is not commonly palpable in these circumstances, but sometimes the patient may present less acutely with recurrent, intermittent pain on account of repeated twisting and untwisting of a palpable, pedicled mass.

Ultrasound will be the most helpful investigation in those patients who are not subjected to emergency laparotomy.

Rapid distension

Sudden distension of an organ results in pain. The distended organ is usually easily recognised clinically as it retains its normal, though enlarged, shape and form, e.g. the urinary bladder distended by acute urinary obstruction, the liver enlarged by sudden congestion by inflammation or right-sided heart failure, the spleen by inflammation or splenic vein thrombosis. Rapid distension of a cyst or tumour by haemorrhage is also painful, as is the rapidly expanding and leaking aortic aneurysm. A rapidly growing tumour may be tender, though pain, unaccompanied by excessive tenderness, in a tumour, suggests malignant infiltration of nerves.

Intestinal masses

An abdominal mass with subacute intestinal obstruction is likely to be ileocaecal tuberculosis or a colonic neoplasm. A palpable mass arising from large bowel may be malignant (carcinoma, lymphoma), inflammatory (tuberculous, amoebiasis, schistosomiasis, diverticulitis, Crohn's disease), intussusception or impacted faeces proximal to an obstruction. A palpable mass arising from small bowel is less common and most likely to be a mass of *Ascaris* worms, lymphoma or an intussusception. Intestinal obstruction can also arise from adhesions to an inflammatory or malignant mass.

Jaundice

A mass associated with jaundice is likely to be an enlarged liver or gallbladder, though severe sepsis, and therefore intra-abdominal inflammatory masses and abscesses at any site, can be accompanied by jaundice. Irregular, knobbly hepatomegaly usually indicates advanced malignant disease. An enlarged gallbladder in the presence of jaundice indicates obstruction of the common bile duct (usually by pancreatic malignancy) for which palliative surgery, such as cholecystojejunostomy, is possible. Urinalysis, liver function tests, and especially abdominal ultrasound are the most important investigations.

Intra-abdominal masses in specific sites

Right upper abdominal masses

Liver

The most common cause of a right upper quadrant mass is an enlarged liver (Table 10.4). The clinical characteristics of a hepatomegaly are that it emerges from under the costal margin, moves with respiration, is dull to percussion and has a sharp lower edge unless distorted by nodular disease. A focal swelling in the liver may be an amoebic or pyogenic liver abscess, a hepatoma, metastasis or the most palpable nodule in a cirrhotic liver. A tender right upper quadrant

Table 10.4 Causes of an enlarged liver.

Diffuse enlargement
  Malignant neoplastic infiltration (primary or secondary)
  Benign infiltration (e.g. fatty infiltration, amyloidosis, storage disease)
  Micronodular cirrhosis
  Inflammatory oedema (e.g. viral hepatitis, amoebic hepatitis)
  Venous congestion (right-sided heart failure, hepatic vein thrombosis)

Multinodular enlargement
  Malignant neoplastic nodules (primary or secondary)
  Macronodular cirrhosis
  Multiple abscesses
  Multiple cysts

Single nodule
  Malignant neoplasm (primary or secondary)
  Abscess
  Cyst
  Benign neoplasm (e.g. haemangioma, hamartoma, adenoma)
  Riedel's lobe

---

or epigastric mass in the liver that has recently enlarged is most likely to be an amoebic or pyogenic liver abscess or a bleed into a hepatoma. Therapeutic response to antibiotics including metronidazole and a diagnostic aspiration will allow these to be distinguished. A liver abscess mass is often stuck to the abdominal wall so that it is not obliterated by abdominal wall contraction.

Gallbladder

The enlarged gallbladder presents as a globular mass emerging from under the sharp edge of the liver or from under the mid right costal margin, that moves with respiration. The gallbladder may be enlarged by pus (empyema of the gallbladder), mucus (mucocoele of the gallbladder) or bile (in association with obstruction of the common bile duct). A single hepatic nodule can be mistaken, clinically, for an enlarged gallbladder, but can be excluded by ultrasound. Carcinoma of the gallbladder is uncommon and if associated with a mass, the mass is usually due to hepatic metastasis. Sometimes a normal right lobe projects down from under the lateral right costal margin. This is known as a Riedel's lobe and is an anatomical variant, requiring no treatment once diagnosed as such.

Nodes in the porta hepatis

Deeper in the right upper quadrant enlarged lymph nodes around the porta hepatis may be palpable and can be associated with jaundice through pressure on the hepatic duct.

Retroperitoneum

A mass originating in the kidney, pancreas and other retroperitoneal organs and hepatic flexure of the colon can also present as a right upper abdominal mass. If cystic, the mass is most likely to be a pancreatic pseudocyst; less common is a renal cyst and very uncommon is a choledochal cyst (see p 435).

Epigastric mass

The commonest cause of an epigastric mass is enlargement of the left lobe of the liver due to hepatoma or amoebic liver abscess (see above). The differential diagnosis of a solid mass includes malignancy of the stomach, pancreas, transverse colon and omentum, or more rarely enlarged para-aortic lymph nodes and aortic aneurysm. Such masses may, or may not, disappear under the costal margins.

Cystic and fluid-filled masses

A tender fluctuant mass in the epigastrium is likely to be an amoebic liver abscess in endemic areas. A large cystic mass filling the whole of the epigastrium is either a pancreatic pseudocyst (see Table 10.5) or massive gastric distension due to gastric outlet obstruction. Gastric outlet obstruction is often missed clinically. Gastric outlet obstruction is suspected from a history of repeated vomiting, no bile in the vomit and eliciting a succussion splash; occasionally gastric peristalsis is seen. Gastric outlet obstruction can be confirmed by relief of epigastric distension with nasogastric aspiration. A wide bore nasogastric tube may not enable large lumps of food residue, blood clot or bezoars to be removed. If obstruction is due to a gastric malignancy, a smaller, hard residual mass may then become palpable. Other causes of gastric distension include duodenal scarring by chronic peptic ulceration pyloroantral scarring following corrosive ingestion or bezoars. Good clinical examination often enables the correct decision regarding surgery to be made even if barium meal or endoscopy are not available. Figure 10.4 shows a barium meal with an irregular mass indenting the lesser curve of the gastric antrum. The differential diagnosis includes malignancy and an inflammatory mass.

Inflammatory masses

An epigastric abscess or inflammatory mass may complicate pancreatitis or gastric perforation. The latter is usually benign but may complicate gastric carcinoma and surgery for gastric perforation must always include gastric biopsy. In the tropics it is not uncommon for a perforated gastric ulcer to be contained by adacent tissues such as the liver or pancreas so that the patient presents late with abdominal pain, anaemia and sometimes an inflammatory mass. The appearance of a perforated benign ulcer on endoscopy is punched out, deep and large, usually greater than 3 cm.

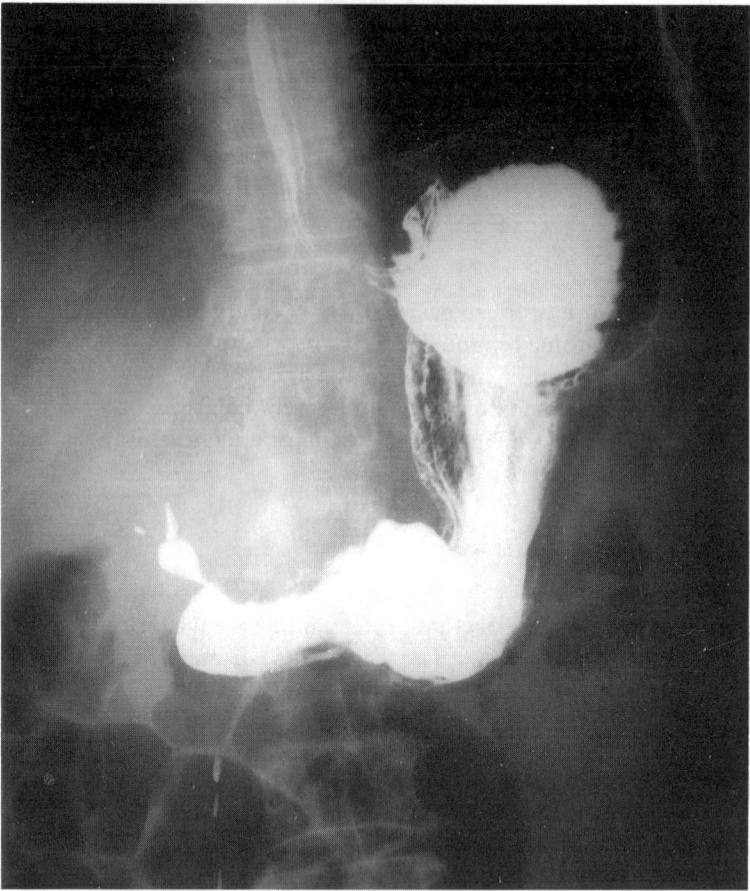

Figure10.4   Barium meal showing an irregular mass indenting the gastric antrum on the lesser curve. In this case the diagnosis was an abscess but gastric malignancy should also be considered in the diagnosis.

Left upper abdominal masses

A mass emerging from under the left costal margin is most commonly the spleen. It normally undergoes diffuse enlargement with preservation of its characteristic shape with a well defined, curved edge and splenic notch. Unusual, confusing shapes may, however, arise from uncommon, focal lesions of the spleen (Table 10.5). The spleen enlarges transversely across the abdomen towards the right iliac fossa. The spleen must enlarge two to three times its normal size before it emerges from under the costal margin. A palpable spleen is therefore always abnormal, though it is a common finding in tropical and subtropical countries, on account of the prevalence of malaria and other endemic infections (see p 174).

Left upper abdominal masses may also originate in the kidney, fundus or body of the stomach, splenic flexure of the colon. More uncommon are retroperitoneal sarcomas and masses arising in the tail of the pancreas.

A cyst may be a pseudocyst associated with the tail of the pancreas, a renal cyst or splenic cyst.

Lateral abdominal mass

The lateral abdominal mass is likely to arise from the lower pole of the kidney (malignant or benign renal neoplasm, renal cyst), ureter (hydronephrosis), other retroperitoneal organs (ganglioneuroma, adrenal tumour, soft tissue sarcoma) or colon. The presence of tenderness suggests the presence of a paracolic inflammatory mass, renal abscess, pyonephrosis, psoas abscess or pyomyositis of the lumbar musculature.

Central abdominal mass

The greater curve of the stomach, and with it the transverse colon, usually lies across the mid-abdomen (though is subject to considerable variation in position, and may be higher or lower). Gastric and colonic neoplasms may therefore present as central-abdominal masses. The aorta extends down to the approximate level of the umbilicus, and therefore an aortic aneurysm or enlarged para-aortic nodes can be palpable as a central abdominal, irregular mass. Masses arising from the small intestinal wall (carcinoma, lymphoma) usually cause intestinal obstruction before becoming palpable but *Ascaris* worms, intussusception, mesenteric cysts and mesenteric lymph nodes are other causes of mid-abdominal masses. The involvement of the omentum by metastatic peritoneal malignancy or tuberculosis can result in a large adherent mass through adhesions with adjacent bowel and mesentery.

Lower abdominal mass

Common causes of lateral, lower abdominal masses are those arising from the caecum or appendix (on the right) or sigmoid colon (on the left), ovaries and iliac lymph nodes. Uncommon causes are iliac artery aneurysm, ectopic kidney, psoas abscess, tumours of the iliacus muscle or iliac bone. The hypogastric mass in the male is most commonly an enlarged bladder secondary to bladder outlet obstruction and in the female, an enlarged ovary or uterus. Carcinoma of the bladder may become palpable in both males and females. The horseshoe kidney, in which both kidneys fuse across the midline, is sometimes palpable in the hypogastrium. A sigmoid mass may fall towards the midline. The differential diagnosis of an inflammatory mass in the right iliac fossa includes an appendix mass, ileocaecal tuberculosis, caecal carcinoma, colonic amoebiasis, caecal actinomycosis and in the female, a tubo-ovarian mass.

The distended bladder arises from behind the pubis, is globular, dull to percussion and midline in position. In acute retention of urine, there is **painful** distension of the bladder. In chronic retention of urine, there is **painless** distension of the bladder and the bladder may reach a large size (extending above the umbilicus and resembling a mid-trimester pregnant uterus on inspection and a large cyst on palpation). In chronic retention of urine, the diagnosis of outflow obstruction is sometimes missed because, instead of complaining of difficulty of micturition, the patient has overflow incontinence. The distended bladder is easily diagnosed clinically as it disappears with urinary catheterisation. A cyst-like, lateral lower abdominal mass in the male is likely to be a large bladder diverticulum. The presence of a suprapubic mass persisting after catheterisation may be an advanced bladder neoplasm, often a squamous cell carcinoma, in schistosomiasis-endemic areas.

An ovarian tumour is initially lateral in position but as it enlarges and its mesentery stretches, it falls into the midline. A multilobulated, solid lower abdominal mass in the female is likely to be a uterus enlarged by multiple fibroids. Occasionally long-standing fibroids may be massive and fill almost the whole abdomen. The enlarged, anteverted uterus and the enlarged ovary are made more prominent by a full bladder.

Specific diseases associated with abdominal masses

The specific management of masses due to infections such as amoebiasis, tuberculosis, schistosomiasis and hydatid cysts are discussed in Chapters 3, 6 and 7. In endemic areas the above infections commonly cause abdominal masses. Appendiceal masses are discussed in Chapter 19 and have become increasingly common in urban areas of the tropics where traditional diets have been abandoned. Other causes of abdominal mass that should be considered are discussed below.

Abdominal lymphomas

Burkitt's lymphoma occurs throughout tropical Africa commonly presenting as an abdominal mass with involvement of the kidneys, liver, ovaries or endocrine organs in children. Non-Burkitt's abdominal lymphomas (worldwide) are either primary or secondary to lymphoma elsewhere and may be lymphatic or extralymphatic in site. The two commonest extralymphatic abdominal sites are the stomach and small intestine. HIV infection is associated with an increased incidence of abdominal lymphoma (p 79).

Abdominal cysts

Cysts are classified into true cysts and pseudocysts. True cysts have an epithelial lining and may be developmental, neoplastic or parasitic in origin. Pseudocysts do not have an epithelial lining and are inflammatory or traumatic in origin (Table 10.5). Hydronephrosis, a chronically distended bladder and occasionally, a large diverticulum may mimic a cyst clinically.

Pancreatic pseudocyst (pp 362–3)

Choledochal cyst (Figure 24.10 p 436)

A choledochal cyst results from congenital weakness of the wall of the extrahepatic biliary tract which leads to progressive cystic dilatation of the common bile duct. It can present in childhood or adult life as a right hypochondrial mass, sometimes accompanied by jaundice due to biliary stasis or fever due to biliary infection.

Table 10.5   Abdominal cysts.

	Origin	Site
True cysts		
Development		
Enterogenous	1. Partial intestinal duplication	Para-intestinal
	2. Vitellointestinal duct	Deep to umbilicus
Lymphoepithelial	Lymphatic tissue	Mesentery retroperitoneal
Renal	Congenital	} Retroperitoneal
	Scars of pyelonephritis	
Choledochal	Common bile duct	Right upper abdomen
Urachal	Urachus	Midline, lower abdomen
Neoplastic		
Dermoid		
Cystadenoma		} Most commonly, ovarian;
Cystadenocarcinoma		} also renal, pancreatic
Teratoma		} hepatic
Parasitic		
Hydatid	Echinococcal infection	Liver most commonly
Pseudocysts		
Pancreatic	1. Acute pancreatitis	}
	2. Idiopathic	} Upper abdomen
	3. Trauma	}
Splenic	Liquefied traumatic haematoma	Left upper abdomen
Hepatic	Liquefied traumatic haematoma	Upper abdomen
Urinomas	Traumatised urological	Lateral or lower abdomen
	tract with slow leak urine	
	into soft tissues	

Mesenteric cyst

Mesenteric cysts are of two types, enterogenous and lymphoepithelial. Both are rare. They occur within the leaves of the small bowel mesentery. The lymphoepithelial (lymphatic) cyst is thin walled and has a smooth lining. It can be enucleated without damage to adjacent bowel, because the lymphatic cyst pushes the mesenteric blood vessels aside and a cleavage plane exists between cyst and bowel. The enterogenous (enteric) cyst represents an area of intestinal duplication and has a thick wall lined by intestinal epithelium. The enterogenous cyst shares the same blood supply as the adjacent bowel and is not usually separated by a cleavage plane, so that excision requires removal of adjacent bowel. A special form of enterogenous cyst is that occurring in the remnant of the vitellointestinal duct.

Urachal cyst

A urachal cyst arises in the remnant of the urachus, which forms part of the embryological bladder. The urachal cyst is midline and attached to the posterior surface of the lower abdominal wall.

Renal cysts

Renal cysts resulting from congenital tubular defects or postpyelonephritis scars are common on ultrasound scans but not usually palpable. It is important to exclude these 'simple' renal cysts from cystadenocarcinomas.

Polycystic disease

Polycystic disease presents with multiple abdominal cysts. In the autosomal dominant, adult type, multiple cysts are always present in both kidneys; and additionally in the liver in 40 per cent of cases and occasionally in the pancreas, spleen or lungs. Haemorrhage into a cyst may produce pain. Autosomal recessive disease is less common and usually presents perinatally or in infancy. There is no definitive treatment unless renal transplantation is available. The cysts grow slowly in size until death, which is usually due to renal failure or renal hypertension.

HIV infection

Splenomegaly accompanies persistent generalised lymphadenopathy in about one-fifth of patients. Abdominal tuberculosis and abdominal lymphomas are common in advanced HIV infection, and each may present as solitary or multiple intra-abdominal masses due to retroperitoneal or mesenteric lymphadenopathy, or local involvement of bowel. HIV-associated lymphomas are usually high-grade B-cell, non-Hodgkin's lymphomas (most commonly immunoblastic or so-called Burkitt's-like lymphoma). Intestinal Kaposi's disease occasionally forms the apex of an intussusception. HIV-related intra-abdominal sepsis often complicating gynaecological infection may present with an inflammatory mass or abscess.

Practice point

- *Enlarged intra-abdominal lymph nodes may be palpable in upper mid-abdomen (para-aortic nodes), right upper abdomen (porta hepatis nodes), mid-abdomen (para-aortic or mesenteric nodes) or above one or both inguinal ligaments (iliac nodes).*

Case history 5

A 36-year-old HIV-positive male presented with weight loss and abdominal pain. On examination there were multiple, irregular intra-abdominal masses with enlarged cervical and axillary nodes. Biopsy of a axillary lymph node revealed tuberculous lymphadenitis. The lymphadenopathy and abdominal masses disappeared with anti-tuberculous therapy.

Splenomegaly

Functions of the spleen

The spleen is important in resistance to infection, both bacterial and malarial. The functions of the spleen include:

1. removal of deformed blood cells from the circulation (Howell–Jolly bodies appear in the blood after splenectomy);
2. removal of abnormal particles and antigens from the blood;
3. extramedullary haemopoiesis in the fetus but the potential remains throughout life for the spleen to resume this role e.g. in myelofibrosis;
4. pooling of platelets – normally the spleen contains 30–45 per cent of circulating platelets which may be returned to the circulation in response to stress;
5. immunological function: the spleen contains 25 per cent of the body's T lymphocytes and 15 per cent of its B lymphocytes – antigens removed from the blood are presented to immunocompetent cells which facilitate or make antibodies.

Clinical manifestations

Splenomegaly most commonly complicates infectious disease, particularly in areas endemic for malaria or leishmaniasis where 25–60 per cent of the population may be affected (Table 10.6). The spleen must be two to three times its normal size before it becomes palpable below the left costal margin. Massive splenomegaly is defined as a spleen which is palpable more than half way between the left costal margin and the umbilicus.

Table 10.6 Causes of splenomegaly.

Diffuse enlargement
  Inflammation and infection
    Viral e.g. infectious mononucleosis, HIV and hepatitis
    Bacterial e.g. typhoid, brucellosis and tuberculosis
    Protozoal e.g. malaria and leishmaniasis
  Haematological disorders
    Congenital spherocytosis
    Haemoglobinopathies such as β-thalassaemia
    Acquired haemolytic anaemia
  Venous congestion
    Schistosomal periportal fibrosis
    Cirrhosis of the liver
    Splenic vein thrombosis
  Malignancy
    Leukaemias: hairy cell leukaemia; myelofibrosis (compensatory enlargement); chronic
        lymphatic and prolymphocytic leukaemia; chronic myeloid leukaemia; polycythaemia
    Hodgkin's and non-Hodgkin lymphomas
  Connective tissue diseases
    Felty's syndrome
  Storage disorders
    Gaucher's disease (lipid storage disorder)
    Niemann–Pick disease
    Mucopolysaccharidosis
    Amyloidosis

Focal enlargement
  Splenic cyst
  Splenic abscess
  Arteriovenous malformation
  Splenic trauma with haematoma
  Neoplasm (rare)
    Malignant: lymphoma, haemangiosarcoma
    Benign

A large spleen is uncomfortable and may be acutely painful if it undergoes areas of infarction which provokes peritoneal irritation. Pressure on other intra-abdominal organs may cause discomfort, nausea, bloatedness, constipation or diarrhoea. Most diseases of the spleen cause splenomegaly except for idiopathic thrombocytopenic purpura.

If an infection cannot be identified, screening investigations should include examination of a blood film, blood culture, and blood count, bone marrow aspirate, serum immunoglobulins and abdominal ultrasound. Ultrasound examination allows confirmation of splenomegaly, identifies focal lesions and diagnoses portal hypertension by allowing measurement of the diameter of the portal and splenic veins.

Tropical splenomegaly syndrome

This is a distinct entity in which splenomegaly arises secondary to chronic malaria infection. The splenic enlargement fails to regress after developing immunity to malaria. It is characterised by residence in a malarial area, an IgM level at least two standard deviations above normal for region and response to anti-malarial drugs. The maximum response may take 12–24 months and should be sustained. Splenomegaly which fails to subside or recurrs on antimalarials may be due to some other cause. The spleen may not become impalpable and may enlarge if anti-malarial treatment is stopped. Splenectomy is only indicated if there is diagnostic uncertainty, severe symptoms which do not subside or persistent hypersplenism.

Hypersplenism

Hypersplenism results from overactivity of the spleen so that one or more elements (red cells, white cells or platelets) are deficient in the peripheral blood. Splenectomy is indicated for causes of hypersplenism such as idiopathic thrombocytopenic purpura (the spleen is not enlarged), congenital spherocytosis and primary splenic neutropenia and pancytopenia.

Whenever possible the primary cause of hypersplenism should be treated. Splenectomy should only be considered when hypersplenism persists as indicated by anaemia requiring repeated transfusions, leucopaenia below 1000×10^9 or platelet count below 25×10^9.

Recurrence of hypersplenism after splenectomy may be due to missing an accessory spleen. Howell–Jolly bodies (fragmented nuclear material eccentrically situated in the red cell) appear in the blood after splenectomy. Should they later disappear it suggests there is an accessory spleen which has resumed the functions of the spleen and is removing abnormal cells.

Post-splenectomy sepsis

Splenectomy predisposes to infection, particularly in children. The risk of overwhelming sepsis in adult life is probably around 2 per cent for pneumococcal and other bacterial infections. Pneumococcal vaccine is advisable in splenectomised patients who may also benefit from low dose penicillin therapy for 3–12 months after surgery. Vaccination against *Haemophilus influenzae* type b and *Neisseria meningitidis* may also be considered if these vaccines are available. One study in Papua New Guinea found all splenecomised patients to be infected with malaria within a few years of splenectomy once the patients had lost enthusiasm for malarial prophylaxis. There have also been sporadic case reports of deaths in the tropics due to malaria in splenectomised patients. Other effects of splenectomy include thrombocytosis, which peaks around 7–10 days and subsides within 1–2 months. The risk of postoperative venous thrombosis is increased after splenectomy so that prophylaxis with aspirin is advisable for further major surgery.

Further reading

Adeloye A. Davey's companion to surgery in Africa. Edinburgh: Churchill Livingstone, 1987.

Browse N. An introduction to the symptoms and signs of surgical disease. 2nd ed. London: Edward Arnold, 1991.

Clain A. Hamilton Bailey's demonstrations of physical signs in clinical surgery. Oxford: Butterworth-Heinmann, 1992.

Houston S. Ultrasound: appropriate technology for tropical field work. Trans R Soc Trop Med Hyg 1991;85:321–3.

11

Cancers of the Gastrointestinal Tract

Epidemiology of oesophageal, gastric and colorectal cancer in sub-Saharan Africa

Reports from South Africa, Zimbabwe and Zaire on the incidence of gastrointestinal cancer in Africa indicate that there is a trend towards fewer cancers of poverty and a slow increase in cancers associated with a westernised life-style. In South Africa, the incidence of cancer of the oesophagus, which is the major cancer in black men, is declining while the incidence of colorectal cancer is gradually rising. Unfortunately 90 per cent of cancers are incurable by the time the diagnosis is made.

Cancer registry data in Africa is reasonably accurate with regard to the pattern of disease (Tables 11.1, 11.2 and 11.3). However figures for incidence rates are likely to be inaccurate because of under-reporting. In South Africa studies in both rural and urban areas, suggest that most patients who are severely ill or in pain ultimately seek admission to hospital. However, not all cancers are verified histologically despite the ability of some mission hospitals, to achieve histological confirmation in most patients. Despite under-reporting, the key questions regarding cancer prevention in Africa remain: what can be done to lessen the burden of cancers of poverty? And, what can be done to restrain the rise in the cancers of life-style and prosperity, which accompany urbanisation?

Risk factors

The major risk factors in western populations are diet (35 per cent of cancers); smoking (30 per cent); reproductive and sexual behaviour (7 per cent) and industrial toxic hazards (3 per cent of cancers). In Third World countries other factors are prominent including viruses, parasitic infections, dietary imbalances, chronic inflammation and poverty.

177

Diet

Western diets, high in fat and low in fibre, favour the development of a number of cancers including colorectal cancer. In order to combat cancer and other diseases of life-style it is advised that total energy intake be reduced, fat should supply 25–30 per cent rather than 40 per cent of energy; and dietary fibre should be increased from the present 10–12 g or so to 20–30 g daily, through increases in consumption of cereal products, legumes, vegetables and fruit.

How do these recommendations relate to the diets of African populations? Among those living in much of rural Africa, traditional diets include a variety of foodstuffs, principally cereals and cereal products. Characteristically, the diet is relatively low in energy, with fat providing 10–20 per cent of the energy, but high in fibre-containing foods supplying at least 20–30 g of dietary fibre daily. Intakes of meat and diary produce are low.

In South African black urban dwellers the situation is changing. Energy intake is rising with improvement in socioeconomic conditions. Obesity in black middle-aged women is now more common that among white women. Fat provides 25–30 per cent and more of energy. In everyday nutrition, all blacks avidly wish for much more fat in their diets. Unpublished observations on series of black students at university residences reveal that fat supplies approximately 35–42 per cent energy. As to fibre intake, even in rural populations, intakes are decreasing; indeed, in urban areas, the decrease has fallen to a level lower than that in the white population. The reasons are that maize meal is highly refined with a 70 per cent extraction rate and thus has a low fibre content, consumption of beans has halved, and vegetables and fruit are expensive.

In Western populations, trace elements such as calcium, and antioxidants (vitamin A, β-carotene, vitamin C and vitamin E) have been shown to protect against cancer. Cancers affected by levels of these dietary components include colorectal, stomach, oesophagus, and liver. All African diets have a low calcium content. Intakes of the vitamins mentioned vary regionally, but they are very seldom present in the recommended amounts.

Smoking and alcohol

Smoking is a risk factor for oesophageal cancer. Studies on western populations have indicated a multiplacative effect of alcohol and tobacco on the development of cancer of the oesophagus, with risk increasing more sharply with rising alcohol intake than with rising tobacco consumption. There is also a causal relationship between alcohol consumption and cancer of the rectum. Alcohol consumption is rising in some African countries. Between 1961 and 1981 beer consumption per person over the age of 15 years rose six-fold. Alcohol intakes in The Gambia and Mali are low and may be rising in Zimbabwe and South Africa. In South Africa an unpublished survey indicates that black men would drink more if the money were available.

Infections

It has been suggested that chronic colonic schistosomiasis increases the risk of colorectal cancer but this requires confirmation. Burkitt's lymphoma which may present as an abdominal mass in children or HIV-infected adults is associated with the Epstein–Barr virus. The potential role of *Helicobacter pylori* infection in gastric cancer is outlined in Figure 15.4 (p 278). Recently a Scottish population of chronic carriers of typhoid and paratyphoid were shown to have an increased risk of gallbladder, pancreatic, colorectal and lung cancers. If this finding is confirmed in the tropics a concerted effort to identify and treat carriers will be important for both infection and cancer control.

Poverty and affluence

In the USA, a review suggested that the black population suffers from more cancers because of poverty, not race. However, when adjustment was made for income and education, blacks have a lower cancer rate. In Africa impoverishment is rampant and is even rising. Aid from western countries is diminishing, and in many countries budgets are devoting less to health maintenance, disease prevention and treatment. Hence, a rise in socioeconomic state, sufficient to influence cancer control is very unlikely. In South Africa and for affluent city dwellers elsewhere in the continent, the situation is different in that the cancers associated with poverty may decrease slightly, particularly those arising in the oesophagus, liver and cervix. However the outlook is gloomy with regard to anticipated increases in the cancers of prosperity such as breast, colorectal, lung and prostate. The rates for these cancers might ultimately surpass those of Western populations. It is unlikely that intervention in terms of screening programmes, advice about diet or education concerning the adverse effects of smoking and alcohol will have much effect. Some studies suggest that it is only the cost which restricts the number of cigarettes smoked and amount of alcohol drunk. Health education in schools and through the media may take years to have any influence on the incidence of cancer in Africa.

However, the scale of the problem in the future remains uncertain, and will vary regionally. Other puzzling epidemiological features also discourage prediction. For example, although the dietary fibre intake of South African urban blacks has been progressively falling for several years, the incidence of 'Western' bowel diseases such as appendicitis, diverticular disease, colorectal cancer have risen only slightly. Undoubtedly, in Africa there are other unknown lifestyle factors which affect carcinogenesis.

Major gastrointestinal cancers

The next section which discusses the epidemiological aspects of cancers of the oesophagus, stomach and large bowel is based on work done in Baragwanath hospital, Johannesburg, but it is likely that the results are relevant for other parts of Africa, particularly urban areas.

The population served by Baragwanath Hospital in Johannesburg consists primarily of poor, urbanised blacks. The typical diet in the townships is of low nutritional quality. Fresh fruit and vegetables are expensive and tend to be avoided while vitamin supplements are too costly for most blacks.

Cancer of the oesophagus

Cancer of the oesophagus was an uncommon disease in the South African black population before 1950. Since then a rapid and alarming acceleration in incidence has occurred. It has reached epidemic proportions in some parts of the country and at present is the commonest cancer in black men. Figures from the hospitals in Johannesburg show an increase from 2 per cent of all tumours in men in the 1930s, to 11 per cent in the early 1950s and 28 per cent in the early 1960s. The highest incidence rates that have been reported from Southern Africa are these for the south of the Transkei; 63 per 100 000 for males in 1981 and 65 for females. The 50 per cent survival period of 3–4 months is very short but not much longer in whites in whom it is 6–8 months where earlier diagnosis may account for some of the difference.

Although it occurs in young and old adults, the peak age at diagnosis is 50–55 years. The male:female ratio is 4:1. Patients present with dysphagia, indicating advanced disease. The commonest site is in the middle thoracic oesophagus (50 per cent). The majority of patients show circumferential involvement, manifesting as fungating, ulcerative or infiltrative lesions. Most tumours are moderately differentiated squamous cell carcinomas.

Aetiology

The disease occurs primarily among maize eaters, and is associated to a varying degree with a diet low in micronutrients. It is also associated with excessive cigarette smoking and alcohol consumption. From his studies in Transkei, Van Rensburg concluded that the principle factor in the aetiology was nutritional status. Chronic deficiency of zinc, magnesium, riboflavin, and nicotinic acid together with an adequate energy and protein intake, may promote dysplasia and neoplastic transformation in the oesophageal squamous epithelium. This hypothesis applies equally to alcoholics in New York as it does to Iranians, Chinese, or Africans who all have a high risk of oesophageal cancer. Long-standing deficiencies of a few micronutrients helps explain some epidemiological features such as geographical variation, the recent emergence of the disease in Africa and the role of alcohol abuse.

The risk associated with the consumption of traditional beer may not be restricted to the quantity of alcohol consumed. There is an association with the use of maize for beer making. The traditional alcoholic drink in South African blacks is a beer low in alcohol content (about 3 per cent) made from malted sorghum and a starchy adjunct – sorghum grain or maize corn. In fact maize has been an ingredient of beer since before the turn of the century, but the percentage of maize used in beer has recently increased considerably. A typical recipe given in 1926 contained maize meal – 27.8 per cent, sorghum meal – 37.6 per cent, and sorghum malt – 34.6 per cent. However, by 1964 57 per cent of the content of traditional beer was derived from maize and this use of maize instead of sorghum grain has reduced the thiamine, niacin and riboflavin content of traditional brews. This would have dramatic effects on the vitamin B status of those who consume large quantities of beer and whose low socioeconomic status will result in a generally poor diet that is also largely composed of maize. A recent study from Natal, South Africa, found a high relative risk of oesophageal cancer in those who bought maize daily compared with those who bought it less than once a week. There is no evidence to suggest that carcinogens in home-brewed beer or in home-brewed spirits from other parts of the world are of any importance in the development of cancer of the oesophagus. However, consumption of beer made from maize may be a factor in the development of oesophageal cancer in some parts of Africa, but its carcinogenic potential is due to nutritional deficiencies rather than a direct chemical carcinogen. Direct carcinogens in black South Africans may be derived from tobacco, especially tobacco smoked either in pipes or in hand-rolled cigarettes.

Figures recorded by cancer registries for oesophageal carcinoma elsewhere in sub-Saharan Africa are shown in Table 11.1. The presentation and management of carcinoma of the oesophagus is described in Chapter 12 pp 207–215.

Table 11.1 Oesophageal carcinoma in sub-Saharan Africa.

		Males		Females	
		Number	Per cent	Number	Per cent
Nigeria	1970 – 76	9	1.1	11	1.2
Kenya	1968 – 78	803	9.1	112	1.3
Sudan	1978	16	3.3	21	3.3
Uganda	1971 – 80	33	4.9	28	3.3
Angola	1977 – 80	23	3.2	10	2.1
Gabon	1978 – 84	6	1.1	2	0.4
Malawi	1976 – 80	232	12.8	36	2.8
Tanzania	1981	97	9.5	18	1.4
Zambia	1981 – 83	30	5	9	1.4
Zimbabwe (Bulawayo)	1973 – 77	321	12.8	30	1.8

Per cent is per cent of all cancers. The above figures were obtained from cancer registry data and modified from: Parkin DM. Cancer Occurrence in Developing Countries. IARC Scientific Publications (Lyon) No 75. Oxford: Oxford University Press, 1986.

Gastric cancer

The incidence of gastric carcinoma is high in Colombia, Japan, and Eastern Europe and low in most parts of Africa (Table 11.2), with a 20-fold difference in the incidence of gastric cancer between Miyagi, Japan and Dakar, Senegal. It is also associated with low socioeconomic status. Environmental and cultural factors such as diet, tobacco use, food storage practices, and the composition of the soil and drinking water have all been implicated in the aetiology. More recently, *Helicobacter pylori* infection has been associated with an increased risk for gastric carcinoma (Figure 15.4, p 278).

Gastric cancer in Baragwanath

Gastric carcinoma has been a relatively uncommon diagnosis at Baragwanath Hospital until the last 10 years when there has been a slight increase. This may herald a rise in the incidence of gastric carcinoma in South African urban blacks or merely reflect better diagnostic facilities due to endoscopy. Any conclusions drawn must be guarded because over the last 40 years hospital admission figures were not always accurate, nor were reliable population and death statistics available for Soweto.

Blacks presented at an early age and with advanced disease. Studies in Zimbabwe and Nigeria found the highest incidence of stomach cancer to occur in the sixth or seventh decades. The sex ratio data of our study reflects a trend seen in other developing countries where the incidence was higher in males. The antrum was the main site involved in a third of the patients and late presentation with invasion of the entire stomach occurred in 20 per cent.

Table 11.2   Gastric carcinoma in sub-Saharan Africa.

		Males		Females	
		Number	Per cent	Number	Per cent
Nigeria	1970 – 76	50	6	20	2.2
Kenya	1968 – 78	381	4.3	212	2.4
Sudan	1978	13	2.7	8	1.5
Uganda	1971 – 80	18	2.7	40	1.8
Angola	1977 – 80	71	9.8	22	4.7
Gabon	1978 – 84	6	1.1	10	1.8
Malawi	1976 – 80	38	2.1	7	0.4
Tanzania	1981	17	1.7	19	1.5
Zambia	1981 – 83	30	5	32	4.9
Zimbabwe (Bulawayo)	1973 – 77	113	4.5	43	2.6

Per cent is per cent of all cancers. The above figures were obtained from cancer registry data and modified from: Parkin DM. Cancer Occurrence in Developing Countries. IARC Scientific Publications (Lyon) No 75. Oxford: Oxford University Press, 1986.

The pathology, presentation and management of gastric carcinoma is discussed in Chapter 15 pp 289–90.

Colorectal cancer

Colorectal cancer is the second commonest cancer in many Western countries but remains uncommon in most parts of the tropics. A recent study in Ghana collected 134 cases from two teaching hospitals over 5 years. The number of cases recorded by the cancer registries of various countries in sub-Saharan Africa are listed in Table 11.3. The cites of Hong Kong and Singapore are exceptional in that large numbers of patients with colorectal cancer are seen which suggests that the incidence will increase with development.

Colorectal cancer in Baragwanath

The incidence in South African blacks is one of the lowest in the world, the mortality rate for 1968–71 being 0.8 per 100 000 population compared with the white population of Johannesburg which has a mortality rate of 13 per 100 000 population. During a 12-year period (1957–68) 96 cases of large bowel cancer were diagnosed in our urban Black population of at least one million. During the same period, only six adenomatous polyps were biopsied.

In the South African white population, however, the epidemiology is similar to that in Western countries. In blacks there is not only a low incidence of polyps but also synchronous cancers and diverticular disease are extremely rare. Either the dietary factors are absent, or have not been present for a sufficient length of time to influence the development of polyps or the polyp–

Table 11.3   Colorectal carcinoma in sub-Saharan Africa.

		Males		Females	
		Number	Per cent	Number	Per cent
Nigeria	1970 – 76	29	3.5	27	3
Kenya	1968 – 78	217	2.4	126	1.5
Sudan	1978	22	4.5	19	3.5
Uganda	1971 – 80	34	5	39	4.7
Angola	1977 – 80	25	3.5	10	2.2
Gabon	1978 – 84	11	2.1	16	3
Malawi	1976 – 80	41	2.3	26	1.4
Tanzania	1981	26	2.6	31	2.4
Zambia	1981 – 83	23	3.9	14	2.2
Zimbabwe (Bulawayo)	1973 – 77	54	2.1	30	1.9

Per cent is per cent of all cancers. The above figures were obtained from cancer registry data and modified from: Parkin DM. Cancer Occurrence in Developing Countries. IARC Scientific Publications (Lyon) No 75. Oxford: Oxford University Press, 1986.

cancer sequence. It is also possible that the adenoma–carcinoma progession observed in Western countries may not be relevant to the development of colorectal carcinomas in the tropics.

The pathology, clinical features and management of colorectal carcinoma are described on pp 403–5.

Tumours of the liver

No hepatic tumours, benign or malignant, have a particularly high incidence throughout the tropics. However, two malignant tumours, hepatocellular carcinoma and cholangiocarcinoma, occur very commonly in certain tropical regions. Furthermore, the biological behaviour of these two tumours varies in different parts of the tropics. The characteristics of these two tumours as they are seen in the tropics will be reviewed. Other hepatic tumours do not differ between tropical and non-tropical regions in presentation or response to treatment.

Hepatocellular carcinoma

Epidemiology

Incidence

Neither comprehensive nor consistently accurate information on the incidence of hepatocellular carcinoma is available for tropical countries. Nevertheless, the incidence of the tumour is known to vary considerably in different tropical regions. Hepatocellular carcinoma occurs commonly (age-adjusted rate > 15 per 100 000 of the population per annum) in most countries of the tropical Far East and tropical Africa and has an intermediate incidence (5–15 per 100 000 per annum) in the remainder. The incidence is low (< 5 per 100 000 per annum) in all parts of tropical South America with the exception of Peru, which has an intermediate incidence, as well as in the Middle East and Near East. Given the difficulties that are experienced in recording all cases of hepatocellular carcinoma in rural areas, some of the documented incidences are almost certainly underestimates, perhaps by as much as 50 per cent in some countries.

Mozambique has the highest recorded incidence of hepatocellular carcinoma among tropical countries: Shangaan men have an age adjusted rate of 113 per 100 000 per annum and women of 31 per 100 000 per annum, and the tumour accounts for two-thirds of all malignant disease in men and one-third of that in women. The tumour is also very common in Zimbabwe, the Guanxi Autonomous Region in the People's Republic of China, and Taiwan.

Even in those tropical countries with a high incidence of hepatocellular carcinoma, the tumour may not be uniformly common throughout the country. This phenomenon is well seen in Mozambique, where hepatocellular carcinoma is far more common in the coastal or eastern regions than in the inland or western regions.

Age and gender distribution

The incidence of hepatocellular carcinoma increases progressively with increasing age in all tropical regions, although there is a tendency for it to level off in the oldest age groups. However, in some countries in tropical Africa there is a distinct shift towards the younger age groups. This phenomenon is especially striking in Mozambique, where 50 per cent of Shangaan males with hepatocellular carcinoma are less than 30 years of age and their mean age is 33.4 years.

In all tropical regions men are more susceptible to hepatocellular carcinoma than are women (mean ratio 2.9:1, range 1.4:1 to 5.8:1). However, male predominance is generally more obvious in those tropical countries with a high incidence of the tumour (mean ratio 3.4:1) than in those with a low or intermediate incidence (1.8:1).

Aetiology

The major risk factors for hepatocellular carcinoma in the tropics are chronic hepatitis B virus infection, repeated exposure to the mycotoxin, aflatoxin, and cirrhosis. Chronic hepatitis C virus infection plays a lesser role, being incriminated in only about 20 per cent of the patients. Minor risk factors such as hereditary haemochromatosis, cigarette smoking, oral contraceptive steroids, androgenic anabolic steroids, and α-1-antitrypsin deficiency play an insignificant role in tropical countries.

The high incidences of hepatocellular carcinoma in tropical Africa and the tropical Far East are paralleled by high hepatitis B virus carrier rates, and the great majority of the cancer patients in these regions show serological markers of current infection with this virus. Ninety five per cent of the patients with hepatitis B virus-related hepatocellular carcinomas have integrated sequences of viral DNA in their tumours. The precise way or ways in which hepatitis B virus induces malignant transformation of hepatocytes is uncertain, but both direct and indirect carcinogenic mechanisms are involved.

The warm moist conditions prevailing in the tropics favour contamination of staple crops with the fungus, *Aspergillus flavus*, the main source of aflatoxin. A strongly positive correlation between the incidence of hepatocellular carcinoma and ingestion of aflatoxin has been demonstrated in some tropical countries in Africa and the Far East. More accurate measurements of aflatoxin exposure, based on the detection of aflatoxin metabolites or DNA adducts in urine or serum, are now available but few results have thus far been published from tropical countries. The recent finding of a correlation between heavy exposure to aflatoxin and a specific inactivating point mutation of the third nucleotide of codon 249 of the tumour suppressor gene, p53, in human hepatocellular carcinomas has suggested a way in which the mycotoxin may contribute to hepatocellular carcinogenesis.

Cirrhosis co-exists with hepatocellular carcinoma in many or most tropical patients with this tumour. Although the precise role that cirrhosis plays in tumour formation is uncertain, the increased cell turnover rate in chronic necroinflammatory hepatic disease acts as a promoter of malignant transformation. Cells in mitosis are more susceptible to spontaneous and exogenously-induced mutation, partly because the DNA is temporally single stranded. Moreover, an increased cell turnover rate shortens the time available for DNA repair, making it more likely that changes will be transferred to daughter cells, and provides an opportunity for the selective growth advantage of initiated cells to be exercised. Cirrhosis *per se* is the most important risk factor for hepatocellular carcinoma in tropical South America.

Clinical presentation

The clinical presentation of hepatocellular carcinoma in the tropics differs between regions with high and low or intermediate incidences of the tumour. Black African and Chinese patients usually present when the disease is at an advanced stage. Upper abdominal pain is an almost invariable complaint, and this may be accompanied by weakness, weight loss, and anorexia: the patients may also be aware of an abdominal mass or have generalised abdominal swelling from ascites. Infrequent presentations include tumour rupture with acute haemoperitoneum, obstructive jaundice, bone pain from skeletal metastases, hypoglycaemia, or polycythaemia. The liver is almost invariably enlarged and may be tender: an arterial bruit may be heard over the liver. Ascites may be present and the fluid is often blood-stained. When the patients are first seen, mild or moderate muscle wasting may be present but jaundice is unusual.

In other tropical regions hepatocellular carcinoma often arises as a late complication of known cirrhosis and the symptoms attributable to the tumour may be difficult to differentiate from those of the underlying disease. These patients may present with a sudden change in their hitherto stable condition: they may develop abdominal pain or weight loss, ascites may become troublesome or become blood-stained, the liver may enlarge suddenly, or hepatic failure may supervene.

The usual course in black Africans and Chinese is one of rapid deterioration with progressive wasting, increasing ascites, liver size, and jaundice, and more severe pain. Death generally occurs within 4 months. In other tropical populations the tumour generally runs a somewhat more benign course and prolonged survival may occur.

Diagnosis

Biochemical tests of hepatic function are of little help in the diagnosis of hepatocellular carcinoma. The serum α-fetoprotein concentration may, however, be very useful, especially in black Africans and Chinese patients. About 90 per cent of these patients have a raised serum level, and in approximately 75 per cent the value is diagnostic i.e. above 500 mg/ml. Tropical populations with a low or intermediate incidence of hepatocellular carcinoma are less likely to have a diagnostically raised serum α-fetoprotein concentration. A variety of imaging modalities is currently available to confirm the presence of a mass legion in the liver. Histological confirmation is required for definitive diagnosis.

Treatment

Surgical resection should be undertaken if possible. Unfortunately, this is seldom feasible in tropical populations. Liver transplantation has an unacceptably high recurrence rate and is rarely available in tropical countries. Embolisation may be used to reduce the viable tumour mass. A large number of anti-cancer agents has been tried in the treatment of hepatocellular carcinoma in patients in the tropics, but the predictable response rate has been less than 20 per cent (this is also true of patients in non-tropical areas).

Cholangiocarcinoma

Epidemiology

Incidence

The occurrence of cholangiocarcinoma shows an appreciable geographical variation in tropical regions. The tumour occurs commonly in continental South-East Asia, most notably in north-east Thailand, which has the highest recorded incidence of cholangiocarcinoma in the world – an annual age-adjusted rate of 79 per 100 000 in men and 31 per 100 000 in women. This incidence is 12 times higher than that in other parts of Thailand. In contrast, the incidence of hepatocellular carcinoma is uniform throughout Thailand. In north-east Thailand the majority of cholangiocarcinomas originate from hilar intrahepatic ducts. Other high incidence regions of cholangiocarcinoma are Hong Kong and Guangzhou (Canton) in the People's Republic of China. Elsewhere in tropical South-East Asia, such as in Taiwan and Indonesia, the incidence of cholangiocarcinoma is as low as it is in non-tropical countries.

Age and gender distribution

In those tropical countries in which cholangiocarcinoma occurs commonly, the

tumour presents at a slightly younger age than it does in non-tropical countries: the mean age of patients in north-east Thailand is 55 years compared
with 60 years in non-tropical countries. Men are generally affected slightly
more than are women, although male predominance is less striking than it is
in hepatocellular carcinoma. In north-east Thailand the male:female ratio is
2.2:1.

Aetiology

In South-East Asia the high incidence of cholangiocarcinoma is attributed to
chronic infestation of the biliary tree with the liver flukes, *Clonorchis sinensis*
and *Opistorchis viverrini*. The former are found in Hong Kong and Guangzhou
and the latter is confined mainly to Thailand. In north-east Thailand subjects
with raised serum antibody levels to O. *viverrini* have been shown to have a
relative risk of developing cholangiocarcinoma of 5, and at least two-thirds of
the tumours are attributable to this cause. The liver flukes are confined to the
larger intrahepatic ducts, but the precise way in which they induce malignant
transformation is not known. Neither chronic hepatitis B virus infection nor
exposure to aflatoxin are important risk factors for cholangiocarcinoma.
Minor risk factors – thorium dioxide, α-1-antitrypsin deficiency, long-standing
ulcerative colitis and Crohn's disease, biliary atresia, congenital anomalies of
intrahepatic bile ducts, and intrahepatic cholelithiasis – are as uncommon as
they are in non-tropical countries.

Clinical presentation

Clinically, intrahepatic cholangiocarcinomas are of two types: peripheral
cholangiocarcinomas which arise from small peripherally-situated ducts and
hilar cholangiocarcinomas originating from larger ducts close to the hilum of
the liver. The signs and symptoms of the peripheral type of cholangiocarcinoma
are similar to those of hepatocellular carcinoma. However, the liver tends to be
less enlarged, a bruit is not heard over the tumorous liver, ascites is far less
common, signs of portal hypertension are absent, and fever is less frequent in
patients with cholangiocarcinoma. Hilar cholangiocarcinomas present with
obstructive jaundice.

Diagnosis

Cholangiocarcinomas do not secrete α-fetoprotein. Peripheral cholangiocarcinoma gives a picture similar to hepatocellular carcinoma on hepatic
imaging, and hilar cholangiocarcinomas show the features of biliary
obstruction.

Treatment

The treatment of cholangiocarcinoma in the tropics does not differ from that elsewhere. Surgical resection is seldom possible for peripheral tumours and the results of radiation therapy and chemotherapy are poor. Hilar tumours may, depending upon size and position, be resectable. Palliative surgery involves stenting or dilatation of the tumour to relieve obstructive jaundice.

Tumours of the pancreas

Adenocarcinoma

The incidence of carcinoma of the pancreas in the tropics is unknown due to difficulties with diagnosis and lack of post-mortem data. Figures in sub-Saharan Africa suggest it comprises about 1 per cent of all tumours (Table 11.4). The incidence is higher in South India (Kerala) where chronic (tropical) pancreatitis predisposes to the development of carcinoma.

The tumour most commonly affects the head of the pancreas. Most patients present with painless jaundice and pruritus indicating biliary obstruction or with a palpable mass in the distal pancreas. Upper abdominal pain is an unusual presentation unless there is a large uncomfortable mass.

Biliary and sometimes duodenal bypass are usually the only procedures possible in those who are fit for surgery. A cholecystojejunostomy or hepaticojejunostomy provide palliation of jaundice. A stent can be inserted

Table 11.4   Pancreatic carcinoma in sub-Saharan Africa.

		Males		Females	
		Number	Per cent	Number	Per cent
Nigeria	1970–76	1	1.1	12	1.3
Kenya	1968–78	78	0.9	40	0.5
Uganda	1971–80	5	0.7	1	0.1
Angola	1977–80	11	1.5	4	0.9
Gabon	1978–84	4	0.7		
Malawi	1976–80	1	0.1	2	0.1
Tanzania	1981	1	0.1	1	0.1
Zambia	1981–83	8	1.3	6	0.9
Zimbabwe (Bulawayo)	1973–77	45	1.5	20	1.2

The above figures were obtained from cancer registries and modified from Parkin DM. Cancer occurrence in developing countries. IARC Scientific Publications (Lyon) No 75. Oxford: Oxford University Press, 1986.

endoscopically if endoscopic retrograde cholangiopancreatography (ERCP) is available. A pancreaticoduodenectomy (Whipple's procedure) is a major surgical undertaking indicated only for early tumours in the head or ampullary region which have not yet invaded the portal vein. The management of obstructive jaundice is discussed further in Chapter 13 pp 255–7.

Hormone-secreting tumours of the pancreas

The rare hormone secreting tumours of the pancreas include insulinomas, glucagonomas, VIPomas and gastrinomas.

Insulinoma

Hypersecretion of insulin causes attacks of hypoglycaemia which manifest as drowsiness, confusion, fits and coma. The diagnosis is made by finding a high insulin level and hypoglycaemia after a 72-h fast. The serum C-peptide level is elevated and not suppressed by insulin infusion. Localising the tumour requires angiography, selective venous sampling of the pancreatic vein, computed tomography (CT) scanning or laparotomy.

Gastrinoma

High secretion of gastrin causes peak acid secretion by the chief cells of the stomach and peptic ulceration (Zollinger–Ellison syndrome). The gastrinoma may be part of the multiple endocrine neoplasia syndrome in 25 per cent of cases. Diagnosis depends on demonstrating a high serum gastrin and raised basal acid secretion. Localisation requires arteriography and CT scanning which are effective in only 50 per cent of cases. Proton pump inhibitors or H_2 antagonists may control acidity temporarily but definitive treatment requires surgical excision if the tumour can be located.

VIPoma

Vasoinhibitory peptide (VIP) is the product secreted which results in water diarrhoea of up to 10 litres per day. Potassium losses result in severe hypokalaemia. Dehydration, lethargy and weakness are often present. The diagnosis is suggested by a secretory diarrhoea containing high concentrations of sodium, potassium and bicarbonate. Serum VIP is high. The tumour is unlikely to be localised by arteriography or CT scanning. The treatment involves rehydration, correction of hypokalaemia, control of the diarrhoea with steroid, indomethacin or octreotide and ultimately surgical resection.

Glucagonoma

The tumour arises from the α-cells, is associated with diabetes mellitus and is often malignant. It most often affects females around the age of 50. There may be a characteristic necrolytic migratory erythematous rash involving the perineum. Frequently there is weight loss and anaemia. The diagnosis is made by finding raised fasting serum glucagon levels. Treatment is surgical excision.

Abdominal tumours of childhood

In the past there has been an understandable tendency to regard abdominal tumours of childhood as a somewhat depressing and unimportant area, since the majority are malignant and the overall prognosis has been poor. In the 1990s however, the finding of an abdominal mass in an infant or young child should instil in the clinician an urgency to reach an accurate diagnosis and to embark on treatment – if appropriate – as quickly as possible, since many abdominal tumours of childhood are potentially curable with current treatment regimens.

A wide variety of paediatric malignancies present in the abdomen, but a large proportion is made up of three or four tumours. In endemic areas, Burkitt's lymphoma is important, whereas in all areas Wilms' tumour, and neuroblastoma, occur relatively frequently, and hepatic tumours less commonly. Germ cell tumours should be considered in tumours arising from the pelvis.

Diagnostic approach

History

A thorough history should always be taken, though it has to be admitted that this may not be particularly helpful. Non-specific symptoms of abdominal pain and discomfort may be present and there may be symptoms referable to compression of neighbouring structures. Occasionally, symptoms and signs are referable to tumour type – for example pseudopuberty or virilism would suggest a tumour of the adrenal, germ cell tumour or hepatoblastoma, and profuse watery diarrhoea may suggest a vasoactive intestinal peptide (VIP) secreting neuroblastoma. Wilms' tumour and neuroblastoma both have associations with certain syndromes, such as hemihypertrophy and aniridia for Wilms' and the Beckwith–Weidemann syndrome of organomegaly for both. The majority of abdominal tumours of childhood are, however, first detected incidentally during palpation by the parent, child or clinician.

Examination

The location and characteristics of the mass often point to its organ of origin. Thus a lateral mass which is palpable in the loin as well as anteriorly is highly suggestive of a Wilms' tumour, though neuroblastoma and adrenal tumour would be considered. A mass in the right hypochondrium suggests an hepatic origin, while a mass arising from the pelvis would suggest a germ cell tumour. Midline tumours are more likely to be neuroblastoma or lymphoreticular malignancies. Burkitt's lymphoma may present in any part of the abdomen or pelvis.

Investigation

A full blood count should be routine. The presence of abnormal cells in the film may be suggestive of lymphoreticular malignancy. Urinalysis may reveal microscopic haematuria – present in one-third of children with Wilms' tumour. More specific investigations may help to confirm the diagnosis in some children. Elevated serum α-fetoprotein is found in many liver tumours and in some germ cell tumours – which may also be associated with elevated levels of serum human chorionic gonadotrophin. Elevated serum sex steroids are present in some adrenal tumours.

A plain abdominal X-ray and a chest X-ray should still be considered routine. The former may demonstrate calcification – a common but not unique feature of neuroblastoma – while the chest X-ray may demonstrate evidence of lung or bony metastases and, importantly, the presence of clear lung fields before surgery. Further imaging will depend on the facilities available. Ultrasonography is an excellent diagnositic tool for examination of the abdomen. Intravenous pyelogram may be required if ultrasound is not available, or to confirm an ultrasound diagnosis of Wilms' tumour and to assess the function of the non-affected kidney.

If available, CT scan is the modality of choice for the assessment both of the primary lesion and of metastatic disease. Magnetic resonance imaging (MRI) and nuclear imaging techniques may also be available in sophisticated settings. Occasionally other techniques such as lymphography for staging of lymphoreticular malignancy, may be indicated – but staging laparotomy is more accurate.

Biopsy and histological examination of primary or metastatic tissue is likely to be the most accurate diagnostic technique where possible. Fine needle aspiration biopsy may be sufficient to yield the accurate diagnosis.

Staging of the disease is defined for most tumours of the abdomen and is particularly important in Wilms' tumour and neuroblastoma since it not only determines the treatment used but also gives an indication of prognosis.

Specific tumours of infancy and childhood

Burkitt's lymphoma

Burkitt's lymphoma is the commonest neoplatic disease of children in tropical areas of Africa and Papua New Guinea, and a mass in the abdomen is its second most common presentation – after that of the more well known jaw swelling. Presentation peaks between the ages of 4 and 7 years. The unravelling of its aetiological links with Epstein–Barr virus and malaria is a fascinating story and the tumour continues to give insights into the basis of carcinogenesis. It is now recognised that the translocations of chromosome 8 to chromosome 14 or 22, or the translocation of chromosome 2 to 8 (one of which is present in the majority of cases) result in the over expression of the c-*myc* proto-oncogene.

The original reports of Burkitt's lymphoma indicated that the tumour was highly sensitive to cyclophosphamide and that results with this drug were remarkably good. While early optimism about long-term survival has been tempered by further experience, Burkitt's lymphoma should still be regarded as a potentially curable tumour and children with this condition should be treated as soon as is possible. Chemotherapy remains the treatment of choice. A high fluid intake together with allopurinol, if available, should be given before chemotherapy to reduce the possibility of tumour lysis syndrome. Although cyclophosphamide is the most important agent, best results are achieved with combination therapy using cyclophosphamide, vincristine, methotrexate and Adriamycin.

One regime currently recommended in Papua New Guinea is:

cyclophosphamide	30 mg/kg IV	
vincristine	0.04 mg/kg IV	given every 2 weeks for
methotrexate	0.8 mg/kg IV	at least 4 doses
Adriamycin	0.5 mg/kg IV	

Other regimens use cyclophosphamide, vincristine and oral methotrexate. An antiemetic such as metoclopramide should also be given.

With or without evidence of involvement of the central nervous system four doses of intrathecal methotrexate should be given at weekly intervals (10 mg if below 5 years, 15 mg if above 5 years) in addition to intravenous treatment.

Results from Uganda indicate that with combined chemotherapy, 80 per cent of children can be expected to go into remission. Fifty per cent may relapse – but if this occurs after 3 months the child may respond satisfactorily to further chemotherapy. The relapse rate may be reduced by increasing the number of treatment courses.

Wilms' tumour (Nephroblastoma)

The incidence of Wilms' tumour has been said to be remarkably uniform throughout the world – at around 1 per 15 000 live births. In countries in which Burkitt's lymphoma is not prevalent, Wilms' tumour is the commonest abdominal malignancy of childhood. There are recognised associations of the tumour with aniridia, hemihypertrophy, genitourinary abnormalities, neuro-fibromatosis and the Beckwith–Weidemann syndrome (visceromegaly including macroglossia, omphalocele, mental retardation and hemihypertrophy). Heritable and non-heritable forms of Wilms' tumour conform to the 'two hit' model of the loss of tumour suppressor gene activity, and three such genes have been located to chromosome 11. The mean age of presentation in the western context is 3 ½ years, with bilateral tumours presenting earlier.

In most cases the tumour is discovered 'accidentally' by the parent, child or clinician. While microscopic haematuria occurs in one-third of affected children, macroscopic haematuria is uncommon. Ultrasonography of the kidneys, renal veins and inferior vena cava, or an intravenous pyelogram (IVP) if ultransonography is not available, and a chest X-ray to determine the presence of lung metastases is adequate – and is likely to be all that is available in most settings. Tertiary institutions may have CT scan or MRI facilities.

Staging of the tumour is most important both from the point of view of treatment and prognosis. It can be summarised as follows:

Stage I   Limited to kidney (and completely resected)
Stage II Extends beyond kidney but completely resected
Stage III Residual tumour confined to abdomen (includes spillage)
Stage IV Haematogenous metastases
Stage V   Bilateral renal involvement

Practice point
• *Prognosis depends on staging and histology. Stage I Wilms' tumour is associated with a 90–95 per cent survival with relatively straightforward surgical and medical treatment. Stage II tumours with favourable histology are associated with a greater than 80 per cent survival. Even children with stage III and IV disease may have a relatively good prognosis. Children suspected of having Wilms' tumour deserve an 'emergency' approach to diagnosis and management.*

Surgery, chemotherapy and radiotherapy are all used in the treatment of children with Wilms' tumour. Excision of stage I and II tumours is followed by chemotherapy with vincristine and actinomycin D. More aggressive therapy, with the addition of Adriamycin is used for stage III and IV tumours, together with radiotherapy – which may also be used in some stage II tumours. The management of a child with bilateral tumours is extremely difficult – but chemotherapy is usually given.

One regimen for chemotherapy in stage I and II tumours is:

Actinomycin D   75 µg/kg IV   ⎫   Given either immediately before
Vincristine   0.04 mg/kg IV ⎬   operation or as soon as possible
                                 ⎪   after operation. Repeated after
                                 ⎬   6 weeks and then every 3 months
                                 ⎭   for 15 months.

Adriamycin   0.5 mg/kg is used in stage III and IV disease.

Neuroblastoma

Neuroblastoma can arise in any site containing cells derived from the neural crest. Approximately two-thirds of all neuroblastomas arise in the abdomen, and neuroblastoma is the commonest solid abdominal tumour in infancy. The epidemiology of neuroblastoma and the finding of non-random deletion of chromosome 1 in the majority of tumours support the 'two hit' model of the loss of tumour suppressor gene activity in its aetiology.

Neuroblastoma often presents at a late stage, and as a result the overall prognosis is considerably less optimistic than for Wilms' tumour. Cure may be achieved in the early stages, however, and in addition there is a relatively high rate of spontaneous remission of the tumour in children less than one year old.

Although many children with neuroblastoma present with an asymptomatic abdominal mass, which is usually fixed, may be painful on palpation and which often crosses the midline, extension of the tumour into the spinal cord may cause paraplegia, and bone involvement may present with bone pain and a limp. Other presentations include anaemia and thrombocytopenia – the result of bone marrow infiltration, subcutaneous metastases, proptosis due to retro-orbital metastases, hepatomegaly, and, less commonly, profuse diarrhoea resulting from the production by the tumour of vasoactive intestinal peptide (VIP) and the opsoclonus–myoclonus syndrome of cerebellar ataxia sometimes known as the 'dancing eyes' syndrome. Some neuroblastomas are detected by antenatal ultrasonography.

A plain X-ray of the abdomen to detect calcification, ultrasonography, and a chest X-ray to detect the rare lung metastases and the more common bony metastases may be sufficient to give a high index of suspicion of the diagnosis. If ultrasound is not available an IVP may distinguish a suprarenal from a renal mass. In tertiary institutions CT scan, MRI and nuclear imaging techniques may be employed. The finding of elevated levels of catecholamine metabolites (vanillyl mandelic acid, homovanillic acid and metanephrine) in a 24-h sample of urine confirms the diagnosis of a tumour of neural crest origin. Full or fine needle aspiration biopsy of the tumour, lymph glands or subcutaneous metastasis will yield the definitive diagnosis, while bone marrow examination may reveal bone marrow involvement.

A number of staging systems have been proposed for neuroblastoma – the most widely used is the Evans criteria which can be summarised as follows:

Stage I   Confined to organ or structure of origin
Stage II   Extending beyond the organ, but not across the midline with
             without regional node involvement.
Stage III   Extending across the midline. Regional nodes may or may not be
             involved bilaterally
Stage IV   Remote disease
Stage IVS   As in stage I or II except for remote disease in liver, skin or bone
             marrow.

Surgical resection is the primary treatment for stage I and II tumours. Should surgery be deemed dangerous in view of the position of the tumour the decision to treat children less than 1 year of age with chemotherapy is difficult in view of the relatively high chance of spontaneous remission. Chemotherapy is not generally given after complete removal of stage I tumours but is given to children older than 1 year with stage II tumours. Radiotherapy is not indicated for children less than 1 year old with stage I disease, but is usually considered for children older than 1 year with stage I disease and in all children with stage II disease. With stage III and IV disease surgery is often delayed until chemotherapy has reduced tumour size, and radiotherapy is used for both local and metastatic disease.

Treatment of children with stage IVS disease is somewhat controversial, because of the spontaneous remission rate in those less than 1 year old. A common approach is to limit treatment to surgical removal of the primary tumour if this is feasible.

Cytotoxics used in the management of children with neuroblastoma include vincristine, cyclophosphamide, Adriamycin, cisplatin, VP-16, dacarbazine and nitrogen mustard. It is acknowledged however that some of these agents are very expensive and may not be available in many parts of the world. The decision to use cytotoxics is best accompanied by advice from a tertiary institution if possible.

Hepatic tumours of children

Hepatic tumours are much less common than those already discussed. About one-third are benign – the vascular tumours, haemangioendothelioma and cavernous haemangioma, mesenchymal hamartoma, hepatic adenoma and focal nodular hyperplasia.

Hepatoblastoma

Hepatoblastoma is the most common of the malignant liver tumours of childhood and most frequently presents in the first 2 years of life. The most common presentation is that of a palpable abdominal mass, though with advanced disease there is likely to be weight loss, vomiting and abdominal pain. Hepatoblastoma is one of the tumours that may present with precocious pseudopuberty as a result of human chorionic gonadotrophin production. α-Fetoprotein is elevated in two-thirds of affected children, and serves as a tumour marker. A plain abdominal film will indicate hepatic enlargement with possible compression effects, while ultrasonography will reveal an intrahepatic echogenic mass with indistinct borders. CT scan and MRI should be used if available.

Prognosis is related to the resectability of the tumour and the histological typing. A child with a resectable tumour of fetal histology has a 90 per cent of cure. Chemotherapy is often used after resection, and may sometimes be given in an attempt to render unresectable tumours resectable. Chemotherapeutic agents used include cisplatin, vincristine and 5-flurouracil.

Hepatocellular carcinoma (Hepatoma)

Hepatoma is the most common tumour of adolescents and young adults in the tropics, and is related to the high hepatitis B carrier prevalence. It is rare in the first decade. Abdominal pain fever, anorexia, and malaise are relatively common, and hepatomegaly is almost invariably present. Ultrasonography usually shows multicentric ill-defined echogenic areas within the liver. Serum α-fetoprotein is often elevated.

Where the tumour is detected early and is completely resectable, surgery and postoperative chemotherapy have achieved 50 per cent survival. Unfortunately, however, most affected children have unresectable tumours and the prognosis is dismal.

Other abdominal tumours of childhood

Non-Hodgkin's lymphoma

In contrast to lymphoblastic lymphoma which characteristically presents above the diaphragm, non-differentiated lymphomas often appear to arise in the abdomen, and may present with abdominal pain, nausea, vomiting, change in bowel habit and weight loss. The peak incidence of non-Hodgkin's lymphoma is 7–10 years. Prognosis depends on staging and on histology, which also determines the chemotherapeutic agents employed. Surgery other than biopsy has little role in the curative management of this condition.

Hodgkin's lymphoma

Hodgkin's disease is rare before the age of 10 years, and abdominal presentation is relatively uncommon. As in non-Hodgkin's lymphoma, surgery has little part to play in the management of Hodgkin's disease other than in the form of diagnostic biopsy and, in some cases, staging procedures. Treatment is with chemotherapy and radiotherapy.

Germ cell tumours

Germ cell tumours are rare but are the most frequently diagnosed malignant tumours of the ovary and testis in children. They may also occur extragonadally. The diagnosis should be considered in any abdominal tumour arising from the pelvis. The germ cell tumours characteristically produce the tumour markers, α-fetoprotein and human chorionic gonadotrophin. CT scan and MRI are the imaging modalities of choice, but ultrasonography is extremely useful where these are not available. Staging and cell type are prognostic indicators. Surgery is important in the management of children with germ cell tumours, and complete excision of the primary tumour should be performed if possible. Both chemotherapy and radiotherapy are important components of therapy.

Virilising adrenal tumours

These rare tumours may present in boys or girls. The pathological distinction between adenoma and carcinoma is often difficult and all such tumours should be treated with surgical removal.

Rhabdomyosarcoma

This soft tissue tumour, consisting of primitive mesenchymal cells may rarely present in the abdomen, more commonly affecting the head and neck, genitourinary tract and extremities. Treatment is with a combination of surgery, radiotherapy and chemotherapy.

Advanced malignant disease of the abdomen

It is a sad fact that many children with malignant tumours presenting in the abdomen do so at an advanced stage. For such children the decision to attempt treatment or not should be carefully and humanely made, taking into account the type of tumour, its staging (where relevant), the availability of treatment modalities, and the parents' wishes after they have been informed as fully as possible. It is not the clinician's function to treat every child as if they have a curable condition. Neither should malignant disease be regarded by clinicians as a medical challenge without due thought to the comfort of the child and parents. Surgery, chemotherapy and radiotherapy are all likely to be extremely unpleasant experiences for the child. The clinician's main role may be in helping the child by the provision of adequate analgesia and sedation if required, and by attention to the mundanities of bowel and bladder function and feeding, and in being available to help the parents in discussing the child's condition and preparing them for the likely outcome. Particularly, but not only, in the tropical world, clinicians must accept the fact that many parents may wish to make use of alternative medicines, and, once they realise that the child will die, will wish to take the child home to do so among the family and in familiar surroundings. Religious and cultural beliefs must always be respected.

Conclusion

The majority of abdominal tumours of childhood are malignant. However, because of the very good prognosis for Wilms' tumour and early stage neuroblastoma using surgical excision and chemotherapy, the presentation of a child with an abdominal tumour should be regarded almost as an emergency. Every effort should be made to reach a firm diagnosis as quickly as possible so that appropriate treatment can be instituted within the shortest possible time. Where treatment is unlikely to be effective however, the role of the clinician is to help the child and the family through the last part of the child's life.

Further reading

Epidemiology

Ajao OG. Gastric carcinoma in a tropical African population. S Afr Med J 1982;54: 70–5.

Bordeaux L, Renard F, Gigase PL, Nukolo-Ndjolo, Maldague P, De Muynck A. L'incidence des cancers a l'hopital de Katana, Kivu, Est-Zaire, de 1983 a 1986. Ann Soc Belg Med Trop 1988;68:141–56.

Caygill CPJ, Hill MJ, Braddick M, Sharp JCM. Cancer mortality in chronic typhoid and paratyphoid carriers. Lancet 1994;343:83–4.

Day NE. The geographic pathology of cancer of the oesophagus. Br Med Bull 1984;40:329

Gwavava NJT, Gelfand M. Prevalence and pathology of gastric carcinoma in Zimbabwe. Cent Afr J Med 1983;29:158–63.

Koshland DE. Cancer research: prevention and therapy. Science 1991;254:1089.

McWhorter et al. Schatzkin AG, Brown CC. Contribution of socioeconomic status to black/white differences in cancer incidence. Cancer 1989;63(5):982–7.

Modan B. Diet and cancer; causal relation or just wishful thinking? Lancet 1992;340: 162–3.

Muir CS, Sasco AJ. Prospects for cancer control in the 1990s. Ann Rev Public Health 1990;11:143–63.

Naader SB, Archampong EQ. Cancer of the colon and rectum in Ghana: a 5-year prospective study. Br J Surg 1994;81:456–9.

Pantanowitz D. Modern surgery in Africa. Baragwanath experience. Johannesburg: Southern Book Publishers, 1988.

Parkin DM. Cancer occurrence in developing countries. IARC Scientific Publications (Lyon) No 75. Oxford: Oxford University Press, 1986.

Pollack ES, Nomura AMY, Heibrun K, Stemmerman GN, Green SB. Prospective study of alcohol consumption and cancer. N Engl J Med 1984;310:617–21.

Segal I, Cooke SAR, Hamilton DG, Outtim L. Polyps and colorectal cancer in South African Blacks. Gut 1981;22:653–7.

Segal I, Reinach SG, De Beer M. Factors associated with oesophageal cancer in Soweto, South Africa. Br J Cancer 1986;58:681–6.

Tomatia L, Aitio A, Day NE. Cancer: Causes, occurrence and control. IARC Scientific Publications, No. 100. Lyon: International Agency for Research on Cancer, 1990.

Van Rensburg SJ. Epidemiological and dietary evidence for specific nutritional predisposition to oesophageal cancer. J Natl Cancer Inst 1981;61:243–51.

Walker ARP, Burkitt DP. Colonic cancer-hypothesis of causation, dietary prophylaxis, and future research. Am J Dig Dis 1976;21:910–17.

Walker ARP, Walker BF, Funani S, Segal I. Survival of black patients with gastric cancer in Soweto, Johannesburg, South Africa. Trop Gastroenterol 1989;10:102–5.

Walker ARP, Walker BF, Segal I. Cancer patterns in three African populations compared with the US Black population. Eur J Cancer Prev 1993;2:313–320.

Tumours of the liver

Kew MC. The development of hepatocellular cancer in humans. Cancer Surv 1986;5: 719–39.

Kew MC. Hepatic tumours. In Zakim D, Boyer TD, editors. Hepatology. A textbook of liver disease. 2nd ed. Philadelphia: Saunders, 1990:1206–39.

Okuda K, Ishak KG, editors. Neoplasms of the liver. Tokyo: Springer Verlag, 1987.

Parkin DM, Srivatankul P, Khlat M, *et al.* Liver cell cancer in Thailand. 1. A case-control study of cholangiocarcinoma. Int J Cancer 1991;48:323–8.

Abdominal tumours of childhood

Caty MG, Shamberger RC. Abdominal tumours in infancy and childhood. Pediatr Clin North Am 1993;40(6):1253–71.

Fletcher BF, Pratt CB. Evaluation of the child with a suspected malignant solic tumour. Pediatr Clin North Am 1991;38(2):223–45.

Olweny CLM. Neoplastic diseases. In: Stanfield P, *et al.*, editors. Diseases of children in the subtropics and tropics. London: Edward Arnold, 1991:873–87.

12

Dysphagia

Oesophagus: anatomy and physiology

The oesophagus is approximately 25 cm in length with the gastroesophageal junction usually located at 40 cm from the incisor teeth. The term upper oesophageal sphincter (UES) describes a zone of resting high pressure 2–4 cm in length that exists between the pharynx and oesophagus which excludes air from the oesophagus and oesophageal contents from the pharynx. This sphincteric segment comprises the cricopharyngeus muscle, the muscles of the hypopharynx and proximal oesophagus. The fan shaped cricopharyngeus muscle is anatomically distinct from the inferior pharyngeal constrictor muscle above and the circular muscle of the oesophagus below. The swallowing reflex includes sensory input via the V, X and XI cranial nerves and motor activity transmitted via the V, VI, IX, X and XII cranial nerves.

Primary peristaltic waves traverse the entire length of the oesophagus whereas secondary peristalsis involves clearance of the distal oesophagus of refluxed gastric contents. This secondary peristalsis may be impaired by the inflammatory changes of oesophagitis leading to delayed oesophageal emptying of refluxate. Oesophageal inflammation in reflux oesophagitis could cause or contribute to a reduction of lower oesophageal sphincter pressure (LOSP) and diminished oesophageal peristaltic propagation and amplitude. Once established, a vicious circle could be created, whereby LOS hypotension and oesophageal motor dysfunction lead to increasingly severe oesophagitis which, in turn, further impairs LOSP and motor function.

A high pressure zone (HPZ) at the gastro-oesophageal (GO) junction is believed to be the manometric manifestation of an intrinsic physiological sphincter as no anatomical sphincter has ever been convincingly demonstrated. In recent years the LOS, 2–5 cm in length, has been regarded as the single most important determinant in the prevention of GO reflux (GOR). The amplitude of the LOS-HPZ and the length of the abdominal oesophagus determine gastro-oesphageal competence and are related to a mechanical valvular function.

201

Clinical assessment

Despite the limited symptomatology of diseases of the oesophagus, it is possible to make a current diagnosis on the basis of a clinical history, which considers the subjective symptoms in terms of onset, duration, intensity, rhythmicity or their various combinations (Table 12.1, Figure 12.1). Patients with difficulty in swallowing (dysphagia) usually present in the outpatient clinic. An accurate history is important in patients with oesophageal disease as diagnostic physical signs are often lacking – except in cachectic patients with

Table 12.1 Oesophageal disorders.

Dysphagia

Oesophagus: anatomy and physiology

Clinical assessment

Presenting problem
   Difficulty with swallowing (dysphagia)
   Painful swallowing (odynophagia)
   Bleeding
   Perforation
   Pulmonary aspiration
   Hoarseness
   Weight loss

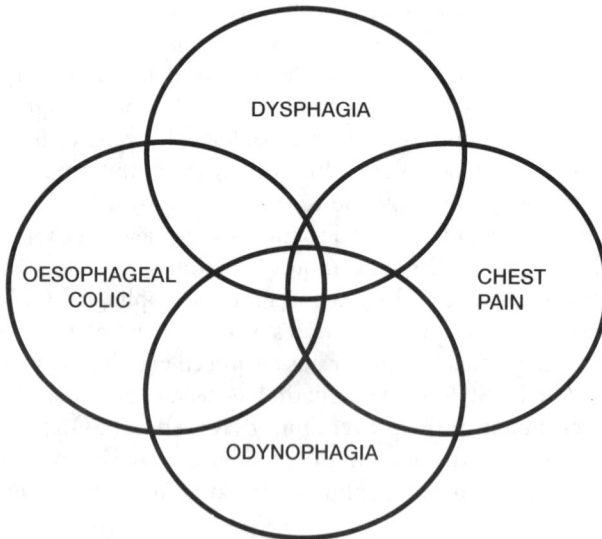

Figure 12.1 Oesophageal symptoms.

disseminated malignant disease. Heartburn and regurgitation are the hall-marks of GOR disease in adults and often precede dysphagia secondary to reflux stricture by many years. About 20 per cent of patients presenting with dysphagia due to a benign peptic (reflux) stricture have not had symptoms severe enough to seek advice from a medical practitioner previously. In other words, some patients have 'silent' reflux, which may be producing oesophagitis and subsequent oesophageal narrowing, but do not have a history of trouble-some heartburn or regurgitation. As the developmental origin of the oesopha-gus and heart are related it is not uncommon for oesophageal symptoms to mimic those of ischaemic heart disease. Atypical oesophageal pain may e.g. be felt across the chest, be brought on by exercise, relieved by rest and radiate into the neck/jaws, back or inner aspect of the left arm. It may be very difficult to distinguish between an oesophageal or a cardiac origin for chest pain, and this may be compounded by co-existence of both conditions, particularly in west-ern societies. Spasm of oesophageal muscle may give rise to 'oesophageal colic' which may be a feature of motility disorders.

Often patients who have dysphagia for solids can still tolerate a liquid diet. Usually more than 50 per cent of the oesophageal circumference is involved by tumour before difficulty in swallowing solid food occurs. This generally means that a majority of patients presenting with dysphagia due to malignancy have advanced disease with extra-oesophageal invasion. Dysphagia for liquids implies gross luminal narrowing with perhaps only a pinhole passageway to the stomach or even complete obstruction. A food bolus which becomes impacted above a stricture may cause acute complete obstruction. Painful swallowing, odynophagia, may occur with malignant disease but is more common following iatrogenic or spontaneous perforation of the oesopha-gus. Pain during swallowing may be due to lesions of the mucosa and are then of a burning quality, or may be of muscular origin in which case, they are of a cramping nature. Odynophagia is often provoked by sour, spicy, very hot or very cold food or beverages. A submucosal haematoma following muscle injury may make swallowing painful while a full thickness oesphageal tear (usually left posterolateral) arising spontaneously following an episode of retching or vomiting (Boerhaave's syndrome) produces acute epigastric/chest pain and, perhaps, features of surgical emphysema and peritonitis.

Gastro-oesophageal reflux is uncommon in Africa and Asia and this may be attributable to high basal LOS pressure which has been documented in asymptomatic Hong Kong Chinese. Barrett's oesophagus which predisposes to the development of oesophageal dysphagia and adenocarcinoma is now re-garded as being secondary to reflux damage to the oesophagus. The longer the history of dysphagia the more likely it is that weight loss will be a prominent feature. Hoarseness may indicate direct involvement of the recurrent laryngeal nerve with tumour and is generally regarded as a contraindication for an open surgical procedure in a patient with incurable disease. Also important in this regard is third nerve palsy giving rise to Horner's syndrome with ipsilateral loss of facial sweating, a pin point pupil and lagging of the eyelid on that side (ptosis). This is seen occasionally in patients with extensive oesophageal cancer involving the superior mediastinum. The development of a tracheo-oesopha-geal fistula secondary to oesophageal cancer may cause a severe coughing episode when swallowed fluids pass directly from oesophagus to tracheo-bronchial tree.

Bleeding is usually chronic in patients with mucosal lesions although oesophageal varices may give rise to catastrophic acute haemorrhage. Dysphagia is not a feature of oesophageal varices unless injection sclerotherapy has produced severe ulceration with perforation or stricture formation. Haemate-mesis and/or melaena may also occur with a Barrett's ulcer in the oesophagus but this is encountered almost exclusively in western societies.

Perforation may be secondary to tumour growth or ingestion of a foreign body, drugs or corrosives. It may also be the consequence of instrumental examination of the oesophagus and be iatrogenic in nature. Pulmonary aspira-tion with sometimes repeated episodes of chest infection may be secondary to regurgitation of food or fluid in the obstructed oesophagus with spillover into the lungs, or of infection secondary to contamination via a tracheo-oesophageal fistula. Such a fistula may cause vigorous coughing if patients swallow liquids which pass into the trachea and major airways. Spillover to the larynx and trachea is more likely if the recurrent laryngeal nerve is involved with tumour giving rise to vocal cord paralysis.

In addition to careful history-taking it is important to undertake a thor-ough physical examination. Emphasis is placed on the detection of anaemia, jaundice, stigmata of chronic liver disease, Horner's syndrome, pleural effusion or other respiratory signs, hepatomegaly, and the presence or absence of an upper abdominal mass or ascites.

In the absence of obvious features of disseminated disease dysphagia requires special investigations to enable a diagnosis to be confirmed. In many hospitals in developing countries only barium swallow and rigid oesophagoscopy may be available. Oesophageal manometry, pH monitoring and nuclear medi-cine studies of oesophageal function are employed in developed countries to evaluate GOR disease and other motility disorders.

Dysphagia requires urgent investigation and treatment (Figure 12.2), of-ten palliative for malignant disease, but which will enable a return to swallow-ing and social interaction at meal times.

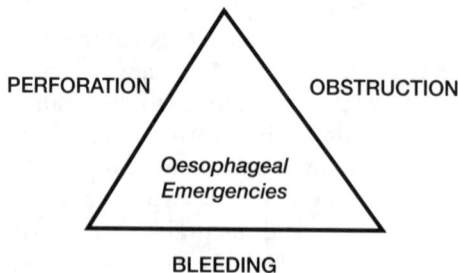

PERFORATION   OBSTRUCTION

Oesophageal
Emergencies

BLEEDING

Figure 12.2 Oesophageal emergencies.

Investigation and diagnosis

A diagnosis of benign or malignant disease may be apparent on consideration of the clinical history. When the presence of a stricture is suspected then investigation, including histological examination of biopsy specimens if such services are available, is essential to determine the cause of oesophageal narrowing. Fine needle aspiration biopsy of a 'lump' in the neck is often helpful for diagnosis of metastatic disease in lymph nodes. The nature of an enlarged left supraclavicular lymph gland, hard in consistency, and extending behind the medial clavicle may be elucidated by needle biopsy. In the developed countries cytology of fine needle aspirates and paraffin section of resected specimens are usually readily available. A barium swallow examination may reveal the length, size and site of any stricturing (Figure 12.3). Angulation of the narrow area is generally regarded as indicating disease with advanced local

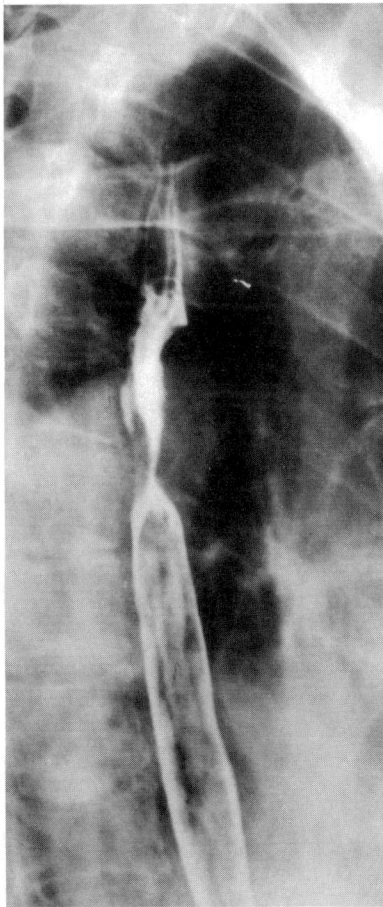

Figure 12.3 Oesophageal carcinoma evident with stricturing high in the middle third of the oesophagus.

spread for which surgery is considered inadvisable. A contrast study also enables the relationship to the clavicles of a tumour in the proximal third of the oesophagus. This may be of help in determining the operative approach to be employed – either a two-phase or three-phase procedure (with anastomosis in the neck). In developed countries modern imaging methods of endoscopic ultrasound (EUS), computed tomography (CT) will also provide useful information regarding staging of malignant disease. EUS is claimed to be more accurate than CT scanning for staging purposes. Ultrasound or CT examination of the liver may not be available to detect metastatic disease but gross irregular hard hepatomegaly on clinical examination is consistent with the presence of secondary deposits.

Oesophagoscopy

This may be therapeutic as it enables a foreign body or impacted food bolus to be identified and removed. Fibreoptic endoscopy under local anaesthesia and intravenous sedation, e.g. Diazemule (10 mg), is sufficient for the management of a majority of impacted coins, fish bones, etc. in the oropharynx, laryngopharynx or oesophagus. When this is not available, and particularly for large bones, then rigid oesophagoscopy, ideally with the wide-channelled Negus oesophagoscope, is necessary. Rigid endoscopy (Figure 12.4) is more traumatic and requires general anaesthesia. The advantage of the fibreoptic scope is that

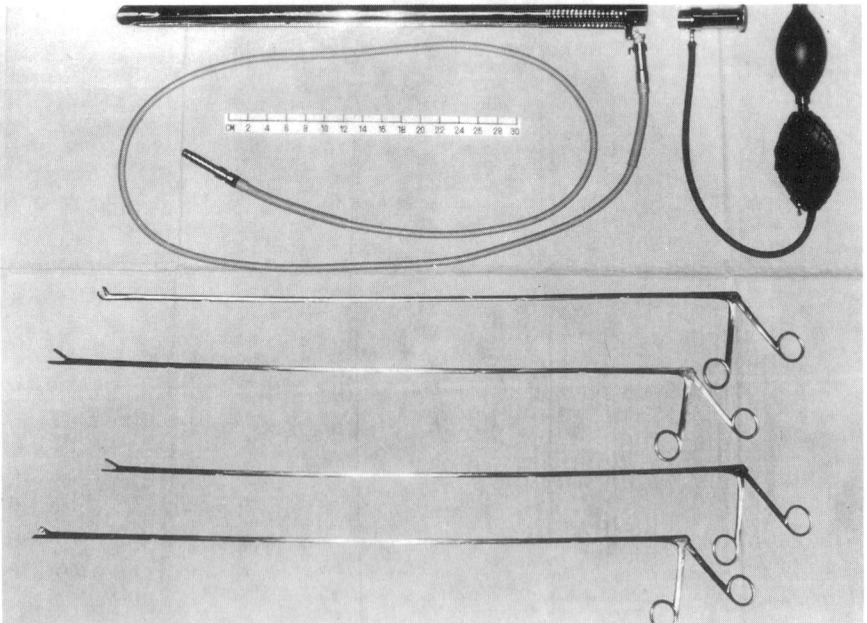

Figure 12.4 Rigid wide channelled Negus oesophagoscope.

it is particularly valuable for insertion of a guidewire to negotiate tight strictures. The wider rigid scope permits clearance of retained debris when the oesophagus is obstructed and permits the use of large biopsy forceps (Figure 12.5). Removal of impacted foreign bodies is most successful if the procedure is undertaken within 12–24 h of the onset of symptoms. The longer the delay in carrying out oesophagoscopy the lower is the success rate in identifying and removing a swallowed fish bone, which is usually to be found impacted in the hypopharynx, valleculae or piriform fossa.

Oesophagoscopy may also be diagnostic enabling inspection of the mucosal lining of the oesophagus and identification of inflammatory changes, (erythema, friability, ulceration) as well as disorders, such as varices and infective conditions e.g. the white patchy appearance of moniliasis. A stricture may be inspected and the proximal margin biopsied. Alternatively, if dilatation of the stricture is performed then biopsies or brushings can be made for cytological studies from within the mid portion of the stricture. If fibreoptic endoscopy is available then dilatation of the stricture over a guide wire will permit subsequent inspection of the distal oesophagus, stomach and duodenum.

Specific disorders

Pathological processes that involve the oesophagus include circulatory, neuromuscular disorders and neoplastic disease (Table 12.2). Oesophageal

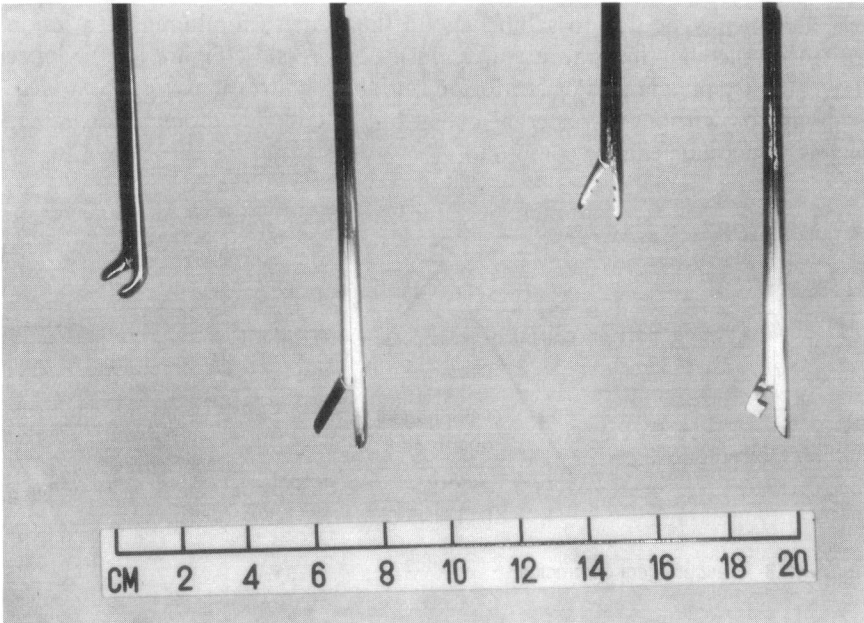

Figure 12.5 Range of biopsy forceps for use with rigid scope.

Table 12.2   Specific disorders causing dysphagia.

Goitre
Oesophageal tumours
  Benign
  Malignant (squamous or adenocarcinoma)
Infection
  Tuberculosis
  Chagas' disease
  Moniliasis
  Viral infections
    Herpes simplex, CMV, AIDS
Ingestion
  Foreign body
  Drugs
  Corrosives
Trauma
  Spontaneous tear/rupture
  Iatrogenic perforation
Irradiation
Motility disorders
  Pharyngeal/upper oesophageal sphincter dysfunction
  Gastro-oesophageal reflux
  Achalasia
  Diffuse oesophageal spasm

---

obstruction may be due to a blockage in the lumen (intraluminal), a lesion growing in the wall (intramural) or extrinsic compression (Figure 12.6). Goitre may cause dysphagia and/or stridor and nodular goitres may assume a large size, with or without retrosternal extension, in endemic mountainous areas where iodine deficiency is common.

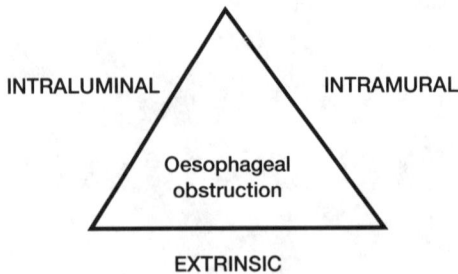

Figure 12.6   Oesophageal obstruction.

Benign oesophageal tumours

These are sometimes incidental findings but can give rise to dysphagia if very large. Epithelial (papilloma, adenoma) and mesenchymal lesions (lipoma, leiomyoma) have been described. In practice, a leiomyoma is the most common which appears as an extramucosal lesion although mucosal ulceration can occur. These tumours arise from the oesophageal muscle wall and can be treated, if less than 2 cm in size, by myotomy and ennucleation at thoracotomy or thoracoscopy with suture closure of the defect. Lesions greater than 5–6 cm in size and those with a mitotic count greater than five per high power field on microscopy are regarded as being malignant in nature.

Carcinoma of the oesophagus and cardia of the stomach

Carcinoma of the oesophagus is common particularly in China, and areas of South-East Asia, (e.g. Hong Kong, Thailand and Japan), parts of Africa (e.g. Transkei, Western Kenya) and Iran. The aetiology of the disease is believed to be multifactorial with presentation late in its course being characteristic. Early lesions have been detected in China by balloon cytological screen but this is not generally believed to be cost effective, even in areas with a high incidence. Endoscopic dye spray techniques with e.g. Lugol's iodine or Toluidine blue will detect early lesions which may be otherwise difficult to visualise endoscopically. Frank malignant change in Barrett's oesophagus secondary to GOR disease may be obviated by the detection of dysplastic lesions on endoscopic surveillance with biopsies every 6 months. The presence of severe dysplasia suggests that overt malignancy is likely and a case can be made for oesophageal resection in fit patients in whom surgery is deemed justifiable. It is of interest that anti-reflux procedures to correct GOR are not usually successful in reversing the extent of involvement of the oesophagus with Barrett's columnar lined epithelium. Dyplastic change in Barrett's oesophagus may lead to the development of an adenocarcinoma. Achalasia, Chagas' disease, and corrosive ingestion may each give rise to malignant change, usually in the form of squamous cell carcinomas.

Squamous cell carcinoma of the distal oesophagus has a better prognosis than adenocarcinoma of the cardia, squamous lesions responding better to treatment with chemotherapy and/or irradiation. The management of this condition depends upon the nature and extent of the disease and the fitness of the patient for surgical intervention. The majority of patients in the tropics present with incurable and irresectable disease (Figure 12.7). The site and size of the lesion is helpful in determining treatment. Malignant strictures longer than 7 cm or with gross angulation on contrast study are unlikely to be curable or resectable. Such patients are best treated by some form of palliation which enables them to spend their remaining months out of hospital with their ability to swallow restored (Figure 12.8). There is little or no place for bypass procedures in patients with advanced unresectable disease as these may carry

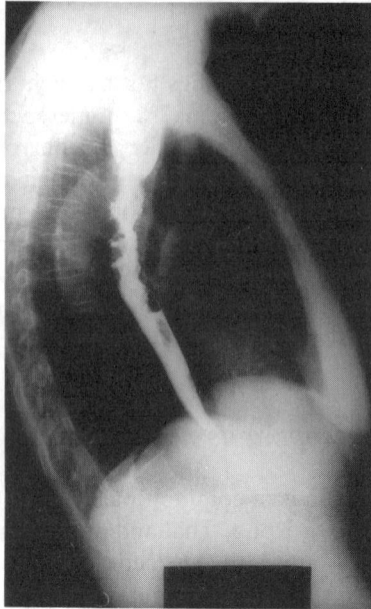

Figure 12.7 Advanced middle third carcinoma only suitable for palliative therapy.

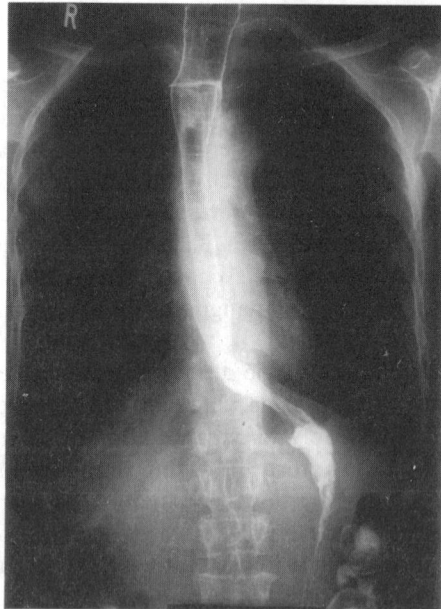

Figure 12.8 A 56-year-old man with advanced middle third squamous carcinoma of the oesophagus. A Livingstone tube has been inserted by pulsion intubation using a rigid oesophagoscope. The patient was able to swallow minced food within a few hours of the procedure and was discharged the following day.

a high morbidity similar to that for resection. Bypass procedures involve extensive open surgery without any proven survival benefit compared with intubation. Those patients with shorter, resectable lesions who are fit for surgery may not often be cured but are certainly best palliated by resection if the surgical skill and facilities for good perioperative care are available. Until 1980 the hospital mortality for oesophageal resection was almost 30 per cent world-wide, but in specialised units the operative mortality should be below 10 per cent and often below 5 per cent if cases are well selected. The 5-year survival for resected cases is low, less than 30 per cent, but it is hoped that more effective chemotherapy will improve this in the future.

Surgical approaches for resection of oesophageal cancer

Lower third lesions
  • Left thoraco-abdominal (Sweet)
  • Laparotomy and right thoracotomy (Lewis–Tanner)
Middle third
  • Laparotomy and right thoracotomy (Lewis–Tanner)
  • Three phase oesophagectomy (McKeown, Ong)
  • Transhiatal resection (Orringer)
Proximal third
  • Transhiatal resection (Orringer)
  • Three phase oesophagectomy (McKeown, Ong)
  • Pharyngo-laryngo-oesophagectomy (PLO)

Thoracoscopic resection using newly introduced techniques of minimally invasive surgery may be possible for lesions at any of these sites, in conjunction with laparotomy and anastomosis in the neck.

The aims of treatment are to (1) restore swallowing; (2) obtain resection margins of sufficient length, usually 10 cm for oesophageal lesions, to make local anastomotic recurrence unlikely and (3) to undertake a radical resection when cure is considered possible, this dissection to include regional lymph glands which may be involved by metastatic disease. Although Japanese surgeons have advocated bilateral block dissection of neck glands for lesions in the proximal third of the oesophagus, this is not accepted practice in most other parts of the world.

There are few indications for PLO as this will lead to sacrifice of the patient's larynx. The loss of speech is usually not justifiable for patients who often have disease at an incurable stage at presentation. Radiotherapy, if available, is a better option for very proximal lesions in the oesophagus. Laryngectomy will require the creation of an end stoma and its continued care. In addition, in western societies, speech therapists are available to help patients develop 'speech' from regurgitated air from the stomach.

A transhiatal resection involves cervical and abdominal dissection only with the omission of thoracotomy, these may be undertaken synchronously.

This procedure is suitable for lesions in the distal third of the oesophagus but is not recommended for tumours involving the oesophagus above the level of the carina, which may be damaged during the blunt dissection required for such proximal lesions. There has been some debate as to whether the Lewis–Tanner procedure, with an abdominal gastric mobilisation followed by right thoractomy, is superior to the transhiatal approach as regards long-term survival. To date no clear survival advantage of either approach has been convincingly demonstrated.

Continuity of the gastrointestinal tract may be restored using stomach small bowel or colon. An oesophagogastric anastomosis is generally most often employed. The route for recontruction may be subcutaneous, retrosternal orthotopic, i.e. via the posterior mediastinum in the previous oesophageal bed. The orthotopic route is preferred by most surgeons but it carries the disadvantage that local recurrence or residual mediastinal disease may involve the restored food conduit. If the risk of mediastinal recurrence is considered high then a retrosternal route is preferable, subcutaneous placement is unsightly and more likely to be associated with ischaemic necrosis of the conduit postoperatively.

A three-phase oesophagectomy involves an abdominal incision for gastric mobilisation, thoracotomy for mobilisation of the oesophagus and the tumour followed by cervical anastomosis. It is generally advisable to perform right thoractomy in the first instance to ensure that the tumour is indeed resectable. The patient may then be turned from the left lateral to the supine position. In this way the abdominal and cervical phases may be performed synchronously by two teams of surgeons. It is important, however, to try and ensure, laparoscopically if this is available, that there is no evidence of intrabdominal metastatic disease before embarking on thoractomy which is in most instances not appropriate if the disease is considered incurable.

It is now recognised that combination chemotherapy (particularly including cisplatin in the regimen) and irradiation can give excellent results in patients with squamous cell lesions, and there are increasing trends for preoperative chemoirradiation (neoadjuvant therapy) or for definitive treatment using chemoirradiation with the avoidance of surgery altogether. In the developing world where radiotherapy services may not be available then chemotherapy alone with oesophageal dilatation (Figure 12.9) and tube intubation (Figure 12.10) may give good palliation. Pulsion tube intubation may be performed at oesophagoscopy or retrograde insertion of a Celestin or Mousseau–Barbin tube via a gastrotomy may enable solids to be ingested.

Whenever oesophageal dilatation needs to be performed for a tight benign stricture which has previously proved difficult to dilate or for malignant disease then it is advisable to administer parenteral antibiotic therapy e.g. using a cephalosporin or chloramphenicol administered intravenously combined with metronidazole administered by suppository or intravenously 1 hour before instrumentation. If the dilatation is difficult and oesophageal perforation occurs then the consequences of mediastinitis are reduced, with a greater chance of survival, if antibiotics have been given prophylactically. Gastrostomy

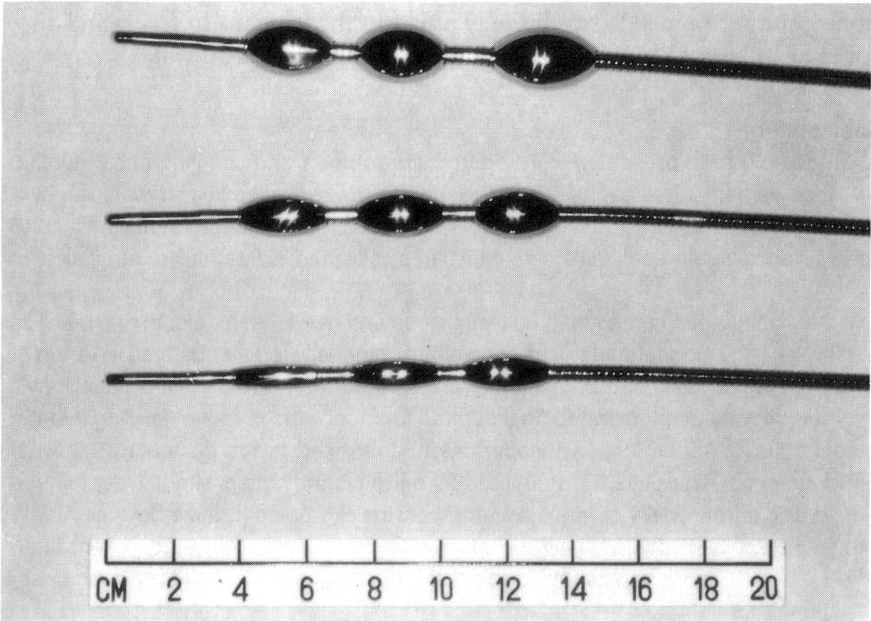

Figure 12.9 Tridil dilators with three graduated metal olives to each flexible rod.

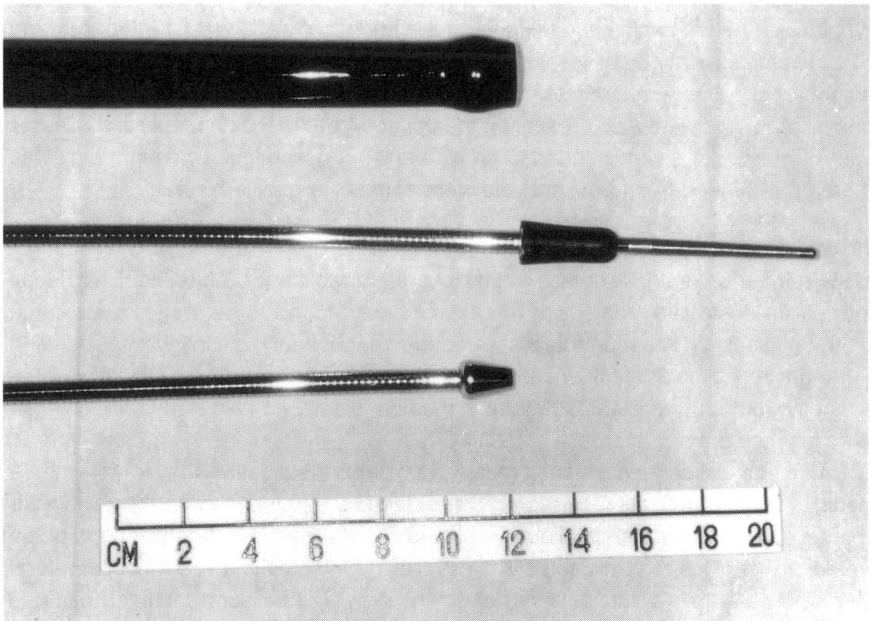

Figure 12.10 Nottingham introducer and rammer for placement of 'Atkinson' silicone tube.

alone is not recommended as this only prolongs the patient's suffering and does not give a reasonable quality of life as swallowing is not possible.

Case history 1
A 60-year-old man presented with regurgitation of food and vomiting for 3 months. Two months earlier he developed total dysphagia and was given liquid medicine by a traditional healer which enabled him to swallow food for a further month. He came to hospital once again complaining of difficulty swallowing solids and regurgitation of food.

On examination he had marked weight loss and had a haemoglobin of 6 g/dl. His chest X-ray was normal and upper endoscopy demonstrated an obstructing lesion at 35–40 cm in his oesophagus which proved to be an adenocarcinoma on histology.

Barium meal demonstrated an ulcerated tumour of the cardia extending into the oesophagus. At laparotomy an inoperable tumour fixed to the posterior abdominal wall was found. The patient was treated by palliative intubation with a Celestin tube placed at gastroscopy. He was discharged on the 5th postoperative day with a life-expectancy of 3–4 months. Had the tumour been resectable and the patient fitter, resection of the proximal stomach and distal oesophagus would have provided better palliation.

Case history 2
A 40-year-old father of three, recently widowed, presented to his GP with upper abdominal pain and dysphagia. This persisted despite anti-ulcer therapy for 3 months. Eventually he went to his base hospital where endoscopy showed a tumour growing in his oesophagus at 40 cm. He was prepared for thoracolaparotomy as he was fit for major surgery. Sadly at laparotomy he was found to have two liver metastases and tumour seedlings were also present on the upper border of the pancreas in the lesser sac. A Celestin tube was inserted to provide relief of dysphagia. Chemotherapy was offered but refused by the patient who went home to organise his affairs.

Case history 3
A 55-year-old patient presented with dysphagia for solids for 3 months. Endoscopy showed an obstructing tumour at 36 cm which was found to be a squamous carcinoma on histology. A barium meal showed the tumour was 4 cm in length, extending to the gastro-oesoophageal junction but not involving the stomach. Palliative resection of the tumour which was adherent to the right pleura was achieved through a left thoracolaparotomy incision.

A gastro-oesophageal anastomosis was performed below the aortic arch. A feeding jejunostomy was inserted but when feeding commenced on the third post-operative day, the patient developed a chylous fistula from the abdominal end of the thoracic duct. This was treated by 7 days of gastrointestinal rest and parenteral feeding. The patient's fistula closed spontaneously and he soon resumed diet and was discharged on the 17th postoperative day. His life expectancy is probably 1–2 years. Had a curative resection been attempted the entire thoracic oesophagus would have been excised to achieve a 10-cm proximal clearance of tumour and the stomach would then have been anastomised to the cervical oesophagus.

Case history 4
A 65-year-old Indian was admitted with dysphagia for 8 months. Recently he had begun to cough every time he swallowed. A barium swallow demonstrated a oesophago-airway fistula and a tumour of the middle third of the oesophagus. This was treated by intubation of the tumour using a Procter–Livingstone tube inserted over a gum elastic bougie at rigid oesophagoscopy. Postoperative barium swallow confirmed the fistula was sealed and the patient was able to swallow minced foods. He was discharged home swallowing on the first postoperative day. His life expectancy was only 4–6 weeks, but at least his ability to swallow was restored.

Oesophageal tuberculosis

Oesophageal tuberculosis is the rarest form of gastrointestinal tuberculous disease. It is usually associated with acute pulmonary disease but occasionally is secondary to mediastinal tuberculosis, without overt pulmonary disease. Presenting features include dysphagia, chest pain, cough and sometimes haematemesis, upper endoscopy and biopsy is helpful for diagnosis. There have been over 50 reports of oesophageal tuberculosis but in only nine patients was isolated oesophageal involvement alone identified. The diagnosis is made when endoscopy reveals an ulcer crater filled with cheesy caseating material. Confirmation may be obtained by demonstrating caseating granulomas in biopsies of miliary nodules or by the direct identification of *Mycobacterium tuberculosis* on histology or culture of biopsies. Most of the well established principles of treatment for pulmonary tuberculosis are also applicable to intestinal tuberculosis. Ideally, drug susceptibility studies are required. If the patient has received anti-tuberculous treatment previously or if the patient is from an endemic area (e.g. South-East Asia) it must be assumed that the bacillus will be resistant to isoniazid (INAH).

Case history 5
A 28-year-old male presented with dysphagia for solids. Endoscopy revealed an unusual ulcer at 37 cm which seemed to be clear with undermined edges. The barium swallow (Figure 12.11) had the appearance of a sinus tract or diverticulum emerging from the ulcer. Biopsy showed tuberculosis. The patient's symptoms completely resolved after 6 weeks of anti-tuberculous chemotherapy.

Chagas' disease (American trypanosomiasis)

Megaoesophagus is particularly frequent in the American continent, and is endemic in certain areas of Brazil, affecting all races equally, with a male:female ratio of 2:1, a majority of patients coming from rural areas. Progression from acute to chronic disease may take several decades, determinants being unknown, a 1 per cent incidence of megacolon or megaoesophagus has been

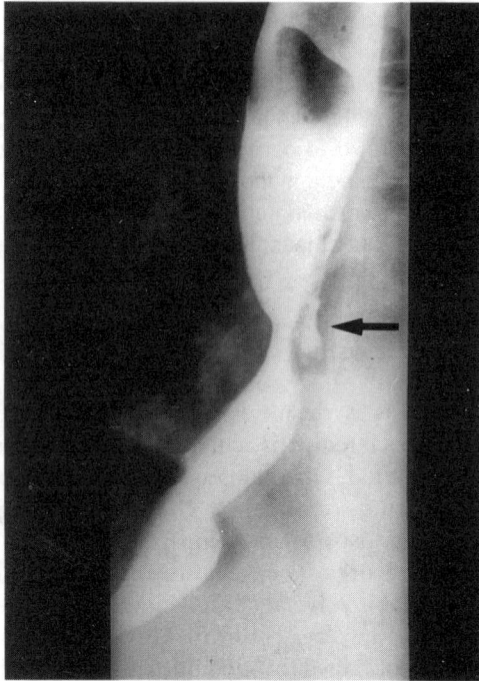

Figure 12.11   Tuberculous ulcer of the oesophagus in a 28-year-old male.

reported in 15 000 autopsies from an endemic area. Chronic Chagas' disease may give rise to dilated congestive cardiomyopathy and/or the 'mega syndrome' that usually involve the digestive tract and rarely the ureter or bronchi. Chagasic patients with megaoesophagus have less than 95 per cent of the normal number of ganglia. There is a decrease in Auerbachs' and Meissner's plexus neurons in the gut, preganglionic lesions also occur with a reduction in dorsal cells of the motor nucleus of the vagus.

Initially, thickening of the muscularis mucosa and muscularis propria followed by dilatation of the gut with thickened muscle layers and finally dilatation with thinning of the muscle layers is observed. Muscle thickening seems to compensate for lack of neuronal control. Both the smooth and skeletal muscle of the oesophagus thicken with most of the increase occurring in the inner circular layer rather than the outer longitudinal muscle layer. Circular muscle contracts to overcome obstruction whereas the function of longitudinal muscle is receptive relaxation. A megaoesophagus can hold up to 2 litres of fluid and the thickened mucosa may have erosions or oesophagitis due to stagnation. Presenting symptoms include dysphagia, regurgitation, odynophagia, eructation, fullness, cough and weight loss. If dilatation of the Chagasic megaoesophagus is very great, dysphagia may be absent, the oesophagus acting only as a reservoir. Regurgitation is found in about two-thirds of cases and occurs in the initial stages during or immediately after eating, and in advanced disease with great dilatation, many hours after the meal, commencing at night. Odynophagia is present in about half the patients, especially when the organ is not markedly dilated. There is a report of megaoesophagus in a neonate born with congenital disease. Radiologically, according to the diameter of the oesophagus, on barium swallow examination, four grades have been described: (1) < 4 cm, (2) 4–7 cm, (3) 7–10 cm and (4) > 10 cm. Contrast fluoroscopy shows irregular and non-propulsive contractions of the oesophagus or, in advanced disease, absence of motility and failure of opening of the terminal portion. The thoracic oesophagus appears dilated, sometimes tortuous, with a smooth fusiform and beak-like narrowing at the lower extremity. In manometric studies of symptomatic patients with oesophageal dilatation, the LOS rarely relaxes with swallowing, oesophageal body abnormality can occur independently of LOS dysfunction.

Treatment of megaoesophagus is either surgical myotomy or dilation of the LOS, pneumatic bag dilatation being regarded as superior to standard bougienage. A 10 per cent incidence of squamous cell carcinoma of the oesophagus has been reported, the diagnosis of malignant change in the Chagasic megaoesophagus often being made late in its course. Nifedipine and isosorbide dinitrite have been shown to reduce LOSP in patients with Chagas' disease and may be useful for therapy.

Infections

Involvement of the oesophageal mucosa may occur in a number of conditions such as measles and herpes simplex. Oesophagitis due to herpes simplex or *Candida albicans* is usually encountered in immunocompromised patients, or those with malignant disease or diabetes. Thus, it is that with an increasing incidence of AIDS these two disorders are encountered more frequently (pp 74–5).

Moniliasis

Moniliasis with candidiasis-induced oesophageal strictures is observed occasionally following antibiotic therapy and has been reported to give rise to dysphagia. Often, however, oesophageal involvement is asymptomatic. Endoscopically, erythema and friability may be evident alone, although the formation of patchy or confluent pseudomembranes is more typical. Oesophagobronchial fistulae have been reported.

Herpes simplex

In herpes simplex infection, the earliest lesion to develop is a vesicle which ruptures to form an ulcer. This may have a discreet punched out appearance with a slightly raised yellow granular border in the distal two-thirds of the oesophagus. Large confluent ulcers may be observed. It is the finding of a characteristic vesicle which establishes the diagnosis but appearances may actually be less specific and more variable than previously suggested.

AIDS

Aphthous ulcers in the pharynx and oesophagus are described in AIDS, cytomegalovirus (CMV) also gives rise to oesophageal ulceration and odynophagia. It is estimated that two-thirds of oesophageal ulcers in AIDS are idiopathic. The latter responds to corticosteroid therapy and at times resolves spontaneously whereas CMV ulcers require ganciclovir.

Idiopathic oesophageal ulceration may be > 2.5 cm in diameter and 0.5 cm in depth. Ulcers usually occur in the distal oesophagus, penetration into the mediastinum and fistula formation crossing the gastro-oesophageal junction may occur. Fistulisation is not a feature of CMV ulcers.

Prompt diagnosis is crucial. These giant ulcers are much larger, perhaps 12 × 9 cm, than peptic or drug induced (including zidovudine) oesophageal ulcers and do not respond to antipeptic therapy or drug withdrawal. Contrast radiology is of diagnostic value, findings being more clearly defined by endoscopy.

Foreign body ingestion

Blunt or round foreign bodies such as coins tend to lodge in the oesophagus. If the patient is able to lateralise symptoms, then it is useful to perform endoscopy in the lateral position with the symptomatic side uppermost so that saliva does not pool on the side suspected to have the foreign body. Coins may be extracted by special forceps which grip the rim, though the hold is sometimes tenuous. Keys or other objects may also be removed on simultaneous withdrawal of the scope and forceps. Other useful devices include stone extraction baskets, a variety of grasping forceps – rubber-clad, rat-toothed, alligator jaws and three-pronged (Figure 12.12). It is helpful to try out the retrieval device on a similar or identical object on the endoscopy trolley before attempting the procedure in the patient.

If the foreign body to be retrieved is pointed and/or sharp, the oesophagus may be damaged on its removal. This risk may be lessened by ensuring that the long axis of the foreign body is in the line of the long axis of the oesophagus and by turning the object so that the sharpest position is furtherest away during its retrieval. For large sharp objects, an overtube may be used into which the scope and foreign body can be withdrawn.

Foreign bodies which pass into the stomach will normally progress through the gastrointestinal tract without problem. Even sharp objects like safety pins and pieces of metal are unlikely to perforate the bowel. Foreign bodies in the

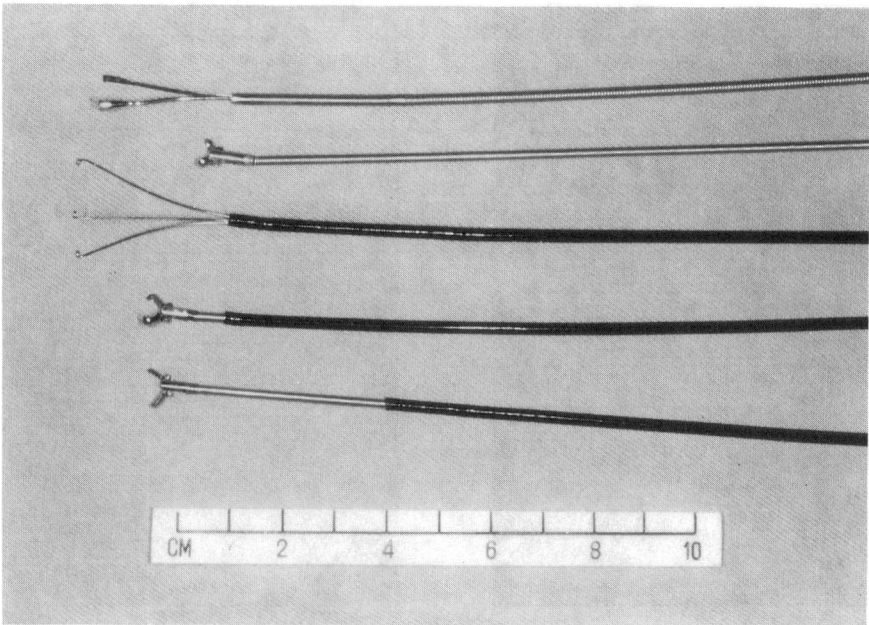

Figure 12.12 Range of biopsy forceps for use with flexible scope.

stomach should be observed though not necessarily in hospital, particularly if it is a blunt object like a coin (Figure 12.13 a and b). The rare development of abdominal pain and tenderness with signs of peritonism or failure to progress after 1–2 weeks would be indications to intervene. Some foreign bodies in the stomach might be retrieved with an endoscope if special grasping instruments are available (Figure 12.12), but usually in the tropics intervention will involve gastrotomy.

Drug ingestion

Oesophagitis following drug ingestion can occur when passage of medication is held up by oesophageal motility disorders or a stricture. It is important to take liquids when ingesting tablets to avoid such oesophageal damage. Over 250 cases of drug-related oesophageal inflammation have been reported in the literature and more than 25 drugs have been implicated. These include aspirin, tetracycline, clindamycin, ferrous sulphate, ascorbic acid, potassium chloride and quinidine. Most often only transient retrosternal pain and dysphagia occurs but fatal complications such as perforation to the mediastinum or haemorrhage have occurred. Endoscopically focal oedema, erythrema or ulceration may be seen and late stricture formation can also develop.

The first report of a drug related oesophageal injury occurred in a patient with achalasia, treated with aspirin, who developed an oesophageal fistula.

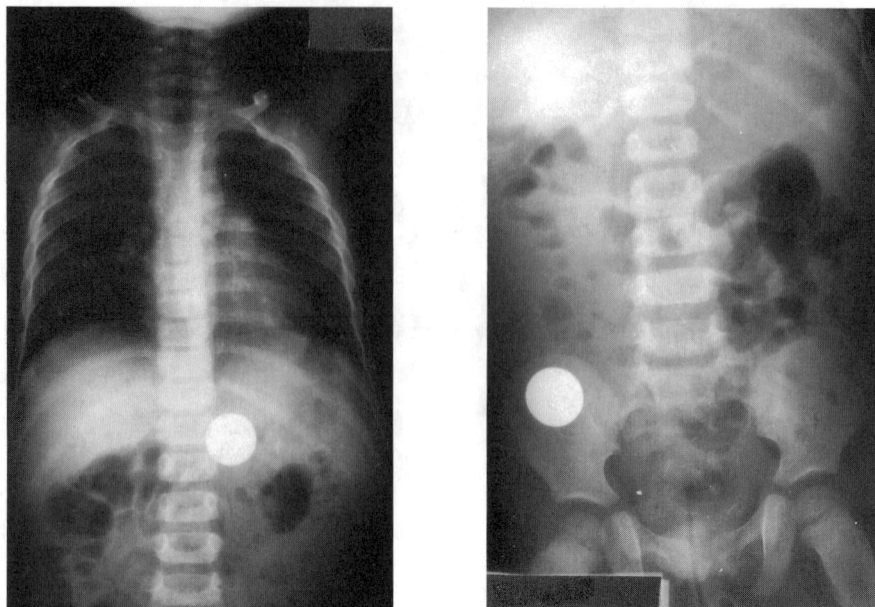

Figure 12.13 *Left* A swallowed coin in a child's stomach. *Right* Follow up X-ray 2 days later showing progression of the coin to the ileum or caecum. The coin was passed in the stool on the third day.

Non-steroidal antiflammatory drugs are now regarded as the most important aetiological agents of drug-induced oesophagitis and benign strictures. Their usage is best avoided if possible in patients with known oesophageal disease.

Corrosive ingestion

This may be secondary to ingestion of dilute hydrochloric or sulphuric acid, or alkali (Figure 12.14). Oesophageal injury can occur even in the absence of oropharyngeal involvement. Early endoscopy is essential to determine the location and extent of damage whenever corrosive injury is suspected. In view of the risk of subsequent stricture formation endoscopy should be performed even in the complete absence of symptoms and signs on presentation following ingestion. The larynx may also have been damaged interfering with the arytenoids and ability to close the glottis during swallowing. Some reports suggest that the endoscope should not be passed beyond the start of the first mucosal lesion, although there is a strong case for a more complete examination unless full-thickness damage is encountered. Swelling and erythema of mucosal folds may occur with the development of ulceration, fibrinous excudate and extensive loss of mucosa. There may be evidence of mucosal gangrene (brown or black discolouration) as a sign of impending perforation.

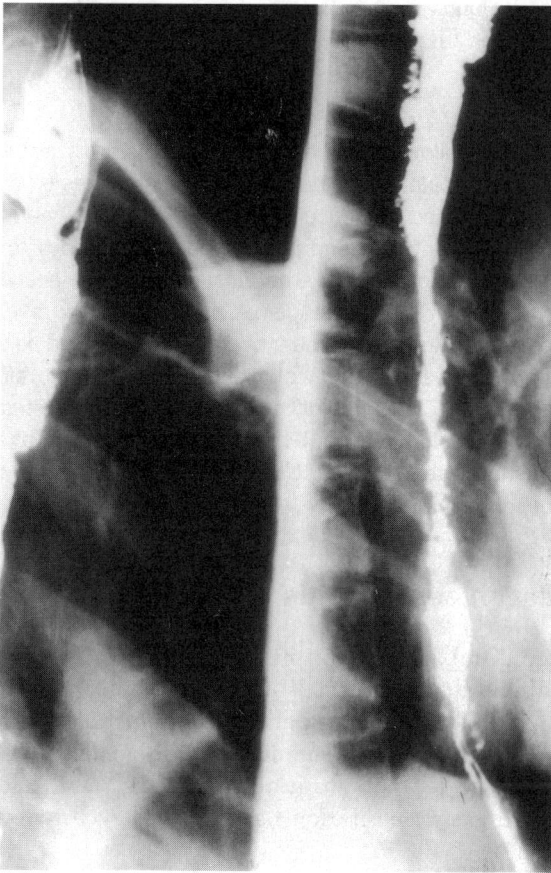

Figure 12.14 Extensive oesophageal stricture formation following caustic soda ingestion 2 months earlier.

The early development of stenosis can be assessed at the end of the first week, and at 2 weeks, oesophageal dilatation can be performed. Some surgeons recommend dilatation only when stricturing occurs causing dysphagia but there is some evidence that in children early bougienage commencing within 24 h of ingestion can prevent stricture development. Bougienage may be easy, when the stricture responds to repeated dilatation or it may be undilatable without force which threatens to rupture the oesophagus. In an intermediate group, dilatation is difficult but possible and a trial of dilatation appears justified before considering open surgery. Oesophagectomy may be necessary in patients with persistent dysphagia or recurrence despite frequent dilatation. Occasionally, following acid ingestion, gastric involvement with vomiting will be the predominant feature at follow-up.

In the long term, the oesophagus damaged by corrosive injury may undergo malignant change. This may not be evident until late in the course of the disease as dysphagia may be attributed incorrectly to recurrent stricturing due to benign fibrotic narrowing.

Case history 6
A 22-year-old male swallowed acid after a dispute with his girlfriend. He came to hospital after 2 days complaining of retrosternal pain and was unable to swallow any liquid. Endoscopy revealed a diffusely inflamed oesophageal mucosa. He was treated empirically with antacids and had a weekly endoscopy to try and maintain oesophageal patency. Unfortunately he absconded from hospital and returned 2 months later with complete dysphagia. A barium swallow revealed two sites of stricture. These were dilated on a number of occasions over the next 3 years. He was offered oesophageal resection and colonic replacement but refused such major surgery. On some occasions it was difficult to dilate the lower stricture using a rigid bougie and a rigid oesophagoscope. Fibreoptic dilatation was not available. On two occasions the stricture had to be dilated by performing a gastrotomy and inserting the dilator up the oesophagus from below.

Acute irradiation oesophagitis

Following deep X-ray therapy in the chest, endoscopy may reveal mucosal erythema, friability and superficial ulceration. Oesophageal stricturing may occur with extreme fibrosis. In the patient who undergoes postoperative radiotherapy for residual mediastinal tumour after oesophagectomy, there is a risk of radiation damage to the substitute organ, e.g. fatal haemorrhage from radiation induced gastric ulceration has been observed following the Lewis–Tanner procedure.

Achalasia/diffuse oesophageal spasm

Disturbances of motility in the upper oesophagus, which possesses striated muscle, are rare, and lesions responsible are located in the brain stem or medulla. Abnormalities in the body of the oesophagus (DOS) or cardia (achalasia) are more common.

In achalasia dysphagia for liquids and solids is evident. Symptoms worsen with the passage of time and active prandial or postprandial regurgitation, often mistaken for vomiting, occurs in almost all patients. Retention of large quantities of food in the oesophagus may lead to regurgitation or pulmonary aspiration during recumbency. About a third of patients complain of coughing spells at night.

Endoscopic appearances are usually normal in DOS whereas in achalasia, it is common to find erythema and erosions due to stagnation of food debris, biopsy changes are non-specific. The diagnosis of achalasia may be suspected clinically in a young adult with dysphagia and confirmed by barium swallow examination with evidence of dilatation of the oesophagus throughout its length with absent peristalsis. The head of the barium column may have a characteristic bird's beak appearance (Figure 12.15). Manometric studies may show abnormal findings but it can be difficult to manipulate the catheter into the stomach for assessment of the lower oesophageal sphincter, unless fibreoptic endoscopy is available for its placement. Manometric criteria for diagnosis of achalasia and aperistalisis in the body of the oesophagus and defective relaxation of the LOS. In cases of 'vigorous achalasia' the amplitude of contractions is high, the pressure waves are repetitive and spontaneous contractions occur. Grossly abnormal LOS function may be diagnostic. Treatment in fit patients is by Heller's myotomy, a 2-cm myotomy being sufficient with attention paid to ensuring that this crosses the cardia and extends just into the stomach. Pneumatic bag dilatation is best reserved for the elderly and those considered unfit for open surgery, and this may need to be repeated. The bag may be insufflated to 300 mmHg for 3 min under general anaesthesia, but it noteworthy that

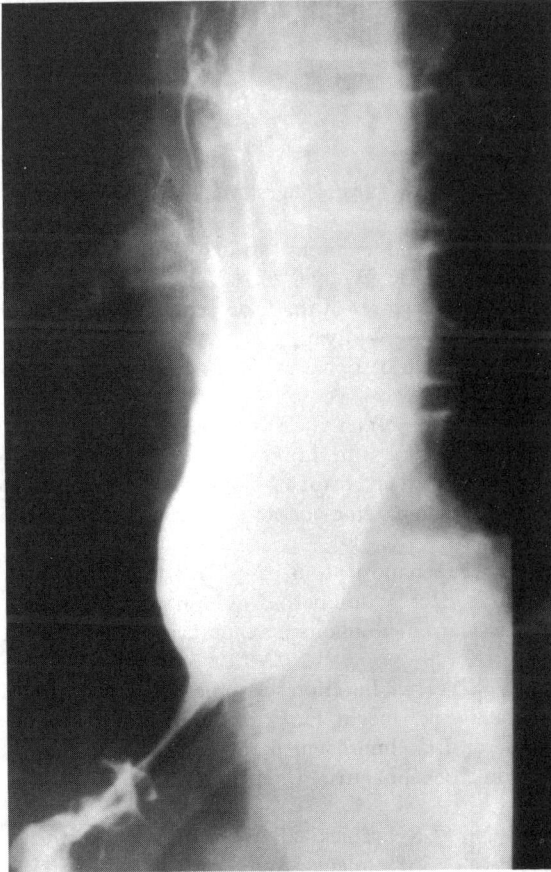

Figure 12.15 Achalasia with bird's beak appearance.

occasionally complete perforation of the distended oesophagus can occur requiring immediate surgical repair.

Diffuse oesophagus spasm may give rise to chest pain, and/or dysphagia in the absence of demonstrable pathology and abnormal non-peristaltic contractions. Most patients have normal LOS function. However, manometry may reveal simultaneous contractions, contractions of high amplitude and duration, repetitive waves of abnormal distal propagation.

Pneumatic bag dilatation and myotomy, long and extending to the aortic arch, have each been advocated as treatment for diffuse spasm. The results of bag dilatation are less favourable in diffuse spasm than in achalasia and long myotomy is preferred for diffuse spasm.

Case history 7
A 30-year-old Zambian nurse complained of difficulty in swallowing for 2 years. Endoscopy was normal. A barium meal showed a 'rat-tail' appearance at the lower end of the oesophagus indicating achlasia. She was treated by a Hellers' cardiomyotomy performed at open operation and her dysphagia was completely relieved.

Further reading

Adam JS, Birik HG. Pediatric caustic ingestion. Ann Otol Rhinol Laryngol 1982;91: 656–8.

Anon. Oesophageal reflux and its myths [leading article]. B M J 1979;1:3–4.

Branicki FJ, Fok PJ, Choi TK, Wong J. Benign oesophageal disease: diagnostic and therapeutic endoscopy. Diseases of the Esophagus 1988;1(2):87–102.

Branicki FJ, Lam DKH, Tse CW, Evans DF, Tang APK, Atkinson M, Hardcastle JD. Why is symptomatic gastro-oesophageal reflux a rarity in Chinese? Surg Res Comm 1990;7(2–3):119–26.

DeMeester TR, Johnson LF, Joseph GJ, Toscano MS, Hall AW, Skinner DB. Patterns of gastro-oesophageal reflux in health and disease. Ann Surg 1976;184:459–70.

Demling L, Ester K, Koch H *et al*. Histopathology of esophageal diseases. In: Endoscopy and biopsy of the esophagus, stomach and duodenum. Philadelphia: W B Saunders Co. 1982;21–84.

Dow CJ. Oesophageal tuberculosis: four cases. Gut 1981;22:234–6.

Frager D, Kotler DP, Baer J. Idiopathic oesophageal ulceration in the acquired immunodeficiency syndrome: radiologic reappraisal in 10 patients. Abdom Imaging 1994;19:2–5.

Lai ECS, Choi TK, Fok M *et al*. Injection sclerotherapy of oesophageal varices with the free-hand technique: experience in Hong Kong. Br J Surg 1986;73:193–5.

Marshall JB, Gerhardt DC. Improvement in oesophageal motor dysfunction with treatment of reflux oesophagitis: a repeat of two cases. Am J Gastroenterol 1982;77(6):351–4.

Ngan JHK, Fok PJ, Lai ECS, Branicki FJ, Wong J. A prospective study on fish bone ingestion: experience of 358 patients. Ann Surg 1990;211(4):459–62.

Raizman R, Rezende J, Neva F. A clinical trial of pre and post treatment manometry comparing pneumatic dilation with bouginage for treatment of Chagas' megaoesophagus. Am J Gastroenterol 1980;76:405-9.

Tanowitz HB, Simon D, Gumprecht JP, Weiss LM, Wittner M. Gastrointestinal manifestations of Chagas' disease. In: Rustgi VK, editor. Gastrointestinal infections in the tropics. Basel: Karger, 1990:56-75.

Vinayek R. Tuberculosis of the gastrointestinal tract. In: Rustgi VK, editor. Gastrointestinal infections in the tropics. Basel: Karger, 1990:19-34.

Wilkins EW, Ridley MG, Pozniak AC. Benign strictures of the oesophagus. Role of non-steroidal anti-inflammatory drugs. Gut 1984;25:478-80.

Wong J, Branicki FJ. In: Delarue NC, Wilkins EW Jr, Wong J editors, International trends in general-thoracic surgery. Vol. 4 Oesophageal cancer. St Louis: CV Mosby 1988;36-44.

13

Jaundice

Jaundice is the yellow discolouration of sclerae, mucous membranes and skin caused by accumulation of bilirubin. The other causes of yellow hyper-pigmentation such as hypercarotenaemia, mepacrine therapy and melanosis do not involve the sclerae. Jaundice is probably the most characteristic feature of liver disease. The jaundiced patient remains a major clinical challenge despite considerable advances in the understanding of bilirubin metabolism and sophisticated improvements in technical investigation.

Jaundice is detectable when serum bilirubin level is greater than 30–60 µmol per litre (3 mg per 100 ml). Jaundice results if there is excessive production or defective elimination of bilirubin. Jaundice is subdivided into haemolytic (lemon-yellow), hepatocellular (orange-yellow) and cholestatic (greenish-yellow) jaundice.

In the Western World alcohol is the major cause of liver disease, while in the tropics and subtropics the hepatitis B virus is the single most important factor.

Bilirubin metabolism

Bilirubin is largely produced from the reticuloendothelial system where haemo-globin from effete red cells is broken down to haem, then to bilirubin. A small amount of bilirubin (up to 15 per cent) is derived from the catabolism of other haem-containing proteins, such as myoglobin cytochromes and catalases. Normally 250–300 mg of bilirubin are produced daily.

The bilirubin is lipophilic and is carried in the plasma tightly bound to albumin. This bilirubin is unconjugated and water-insoluble. The bilirubin then dissociates from albumin and is taken by the hepatic cell membrane and transported to the endoplasmic reticulum by cytoplasmic proteins, where it is conjugated with glucuronic acid and excreted as a diglucuronide into bile. The enzyme uridine diphosphoglucuronyl transferase catalyses the formation of bilirubin diglucuronide.

The conjugated bilirubin is water-soluble and is actively secreted into the bile canaliculi and excreted into the intestine with the bile. In the terminal ileum bacterial enzymes hydrolyse the molecule releasing free bilirubin which is then reduced to urobilinogen. Some of this is excreted in the stools as stercobilinogen while the rest is absorbed in the terminal ileum, passes to the liver and is re-excreted into bile. Urobilinogen bound to albumin enters the circulation and is excreted in the urine.

Causes of jaundice

These can be broadly divided into the following categories:

Excessive production of bilirubin

Excessive production of bilirubin occurs in the haemolytic anaemias. It also occurs in thalassaemia and pernicious anaemia which are associated with a marked degree of ineffective erythropoiesis and intramedullary destruction of red cell precursors.

Reduced uptake of bilirubin

A defective uptake of bilirubin to the hepatocyte is the explanation for the unconjugated hyperbilirubinaemia associated with **Gilbert's syndrome**, severe congestive heart failure and portocaval shunts.

Reduced hepatic conjugation of bilirubin

Reduced hepatic conjugation of bilirubin is probably the cause of neonatal jaundice. It also occurs in the **Crigler–Najjar syndrome** where it results from a specific deficiency of glucuronyl transferase.

Reduced excretion of conjugated bilirubin

Very rarely this is a result of a congenital defect of hepatic excretion in the **Dubin–Johnson** and **Rotor's syndromes**. Usually it is a consequence of hepatocellular injury as in viral hepatitis; inflammatory, granulomatous or extrahepatic bile duct obstruction.

Clinical assessment

When faced with a jaundiced patient one should look for features of chronic liver disease such as parotid gland enlargement, gynaecomastia, palmar erythema, loss of body hair, testicular atrophy, leuconychia, Dupuytren's contracture, bruises and spider naevi. Features of portal hypertension such as dilated veins on the abdominal wall, splenomegaly and ascites should also be looked for. In cirrhosis the liver may be small or enlarged. An irregular hard liver with or without a bruit suggests liver malignancy.

Urine examination is a quick method of differentiating between unconjugated and conjugated hyperbilirubinaemia. If bilirubin is absent in the urine, splenomegaly, anaemia, reticulocytosis and a family history of anaemia suggest a haemolytic cause of the jaundice. If bilirubin is present in the urine, the common causes are hepatitis and obstruction of the biliary system. A history of travel, exposure to toxins, viral hepatitis, drugs and a recent anaesthetic should be obtained. When the typical features of hepatitis are absent, jaundice with bilirubinaemia accompanied by pale stools and pruritus suggests cholestasis due to an intrahepatic or extrahepatic cause. Severe abdominal pain of abrupt onset preceding jaundice by a couple of days suggests gallstone obstruction. Rigors in association with dark urine due to bilirubinuria suggests mechanical biliary obstruction with ascending cholangitis. Painless cholestatic jaundice with a palpable gallbladder and absent urinary urobilinogen usually indicates a neoplastic cause (Courvoisier's law).

Liver function tests: the ratio between the serum aspartate aminotransferase (AST) (or alanine aminotransferase (ALT)) and alkaline phosphatase helps to distinguish between hepatitic (high ratio) and cholestatic (low ratio) types of jaundice. The determination of conjugated and unconjugated serum bilirubin is of considerable value in confirming a diagnosis of pre-hepatic jaundice in cases of isolated hyperbilirubinaemia. In cases where the prothrombin time is prolonged, the prothrombin time rapidly corrects on vitamin K therapy in cholestasis but remains abnormal in severe hepatitis or chronic liver disease.

Ultrasound is an important tool in the investigation of the jaundiced patient. The aim is largely to determine whether or not there is intrahepatic obstruction. If the ducts are dilated, then it is usual to proceed to endoscopic retrograde cholangiopancreatography (ERCP) or percutaneous transhepatic cholangiography (PTC) to define the morphology of the ducts and identify the site of obstruction before surgery or interventional radiology. If the ducts are of normal calibre, then other tests including liver biopsy are more appropriate.

Specific disorders

Unconjugated hyperbilirubinaemia

There are two major groups namely, congenital hyperbilirubinaemias (non-haemolytic) and haemolytic anaemia.

Congenital hyperbilirubinaemias

These result from defects in bilirubin uptake or conjugation. The commonest of these is Gilbert's syndrome. The others – Crigler–Najjar, Dubin–Johnson and Rotor's syndromes – are rare (Table 13.1).

Gilbert's syndrome is usually asymptomatic and is usually detected as incidental finding of slightly raised bilirubin. It is of no functional significance but is often the cause of much diagnostic confusion with other diagnoses such

Table 13.1 Congenital hyperbilirubinaemias.

	Inheritance	Age at presentation	Prognosis	Defect	Liver history
Unconjugated bilirubin					
Gilbert's syndrome	Autosomal dominant	Young adults but variable	Excellent	↓ Bilirubin uptake ↓ Glucuronyl transferase ↓ Red cell survival	Normal
Crigler–Najjar syndrome					
Type I	Autosomal recessive	Neonate	Fatal (due to kernicterus)	No glucuronyl transferase	Normal
Type II	Autosomal dominant	Neonate	Survive to adult life	Glucuronyl transferase	Normal
Conjugated bilirubin					
Dubin–Johnson syndrome	Autosomal	Any	Good	Bilirubin excretion	Melanin deposition
Rotor's syndrome	?Autosomal dominant	Variable (usually childhood)	Good	↓ Bilirubin uptake ↓ Storage of bilirubin	Normal

as 'recurrent hepatitis' often being made. The cause is probably the defective uptake of bilirubin by the hepatocytes and secondary deficiency of hepatic glucuronyl transferase, although many cases also have a minor decrease in red cell survival which could increase the bilirubin load. The finding of unconjugated hyperbilirubinaemia, rising further after a 48-h fast, and a normal reticulocytic count without other liver abnormalities is highly suggestive of this diagnosis. No specific treatment is necessary.

Haemolytic jaundice

The increased breakdown of red cells leads to an increase in the production of bilirubin. The resulting jaundice is usually mild as normal liver function can easily handle the increased bilirubin derived from excessive haemolysis.

The bilirubin is unconjugated and water-insoluble and therefore does not pass into the urine ('alcholuric' jaundice). Urinary urobilinogen is increased. Investigations show features of haemolysis. The level of unconjugated bilirubin is increased but serum transferases, alkaline phosphatase and albumin are normal.

Acute hepatitis

Acute liver damage can be attributed to a large number of causes (Table 13.2). Viral causes constitute an important cause of acute hepatitis. The other important causes include drugs and alcohol.

Table 13.2 Causes of acute hepatitis.

Viral infections
  A, B (D), C, E
  Epstein–Barr Virus
  Cytomegalovirus
  Yellow fever virus
  HIV
  Others – rare

Alcohol

Drugs
  Halothane
  Paracetamol

Poisons
  Amanita phalloides (mushrooms)
  Aflatoxin
  Carbon tetrachloride

Non-viral infections
  Toxoplasma gondii
  Leptospira icterohaemorrhagiae
  Coxiella burneti ('Q' fever)

Viral hepatitis

The different viral causes of hepatitis are shown in Table 13.3. Although the general features of hepatitis are similar, there are major differences in the epidemiology and prognosis of the various hepatotrophic viruses. Identification of the responsible agent by serological tests is therefore highly recommended.

The clinical features of the major hepatotrophic viruses are summarised in Table 13.4.

Hepatitis A virus (HAV)

This is an RNA virus. Serologically the diagnosis of an acute infection is made by the finding of specific IgM-anti-HAV antibodies which are present in the serum for about 80 days after the acute illness.

Table 13.3 Viral causes of hepatitis.

Virus	Features
Hepatotrophic	
Hepatitis A virus (HAV)	RNA virus, 27 nm; faecal/oral transmission
Hepatitis B virus (HBV)	DNA virus, 42 nm; blood and sexual transmission
Hepatitis Delta virus (HDV)	RNA virus with HBsAg coat, 36 nm; blood transmission; needs HBV
Hepatitis C virus (HCV)	RNA virus, 30–60 nm; blood and sexual transmission
Hepatitis E virus (HEV)	?RNA/DNA virus, 27 nm; faecal/oral transmission
Other viruses causing hepatitis	
Epstein–Barr Virus (EBV)	DNA herpes-type virus; close contact/aerosol transmission
Cytomegalovirus (CMV)	DNA herpes-types virus; blood and close contact transmission
Herpes simplex and H. zoster	Rarely involves liver; causes severe liver damage especially in HIV patients
Lassa fever, Ebola virus and Marburg virus	Rare diseases; may cause severe damage

Table 13.4 Clinical features of viral hepatitis.

Type	Incubation period	Clinical features	Outcome	Vaccines
A	4 weeks	Mild often subclinical	No chronic disease	Available
B	12 weeks	Variable severity	Neonatal 90% carriers Adult 1–10% carriers	Available and in national programmes
E	6 weeks	High mortality in pregnancy	No chronic disease	None
C	8 weeks	Mild often subclinical	20–40% progress to chronic disease	None

The hepatitis A virus (HAV) is excreted in the faeces of infected persons for about 2 weeks before the onset of the illness and for up to 7 days after. The disease is maximally infectious just before the onset of the jaundice.

The pre-icteric or prodromal phase lasts up to 2 weeks. The patient feels unwell with nausea, vomiting, diarrhoea, anorexia (plus a distaste for cigarettes), headache and malaise. Fever is usually mild and there may be upper abdominal discomfort.

The patient becomes jaundiced after 1–2 weeks and the symptoms often improve. The appetite improves and the patient feels better. As the jaundice deepens the urine becomes dark and the stools pale owing to intrahepatic cholestasis. The liver is moderately enlarged and the spleen is palpable in about 10 per cent of patients. Thereafter the jaundice lessens and in the majority of cases the illness is over within 3–6 weeks. Relapses may occur. Occasionally the disease can be quite severe with fulminant hepatitis and death. The sequence of events after exposure to the hepatitis A virus is shown in Table 13.5.

Hepatitis B virus (HBV)

This is a member of the HepaDNA viruses. The Dane particle is the whole virus and consists of an inner core formed by the liver cell nucleus and an outer coat (HBsAg) product by multiplication of the cytoplasm. The liver core contains double-stranded DNA, DNA polymerase, the core antigen (HBcAg) and the 'e' antigen (HBeAg) (Figure 13.1). The 'e' antigen is also found in excess in the serum as a non-particulate soluble antigen. Thus when HBsAg and HBeAg are found together in the serum, this signifies active viral replication in the liver and HBeAg is commonly used as a marker of infectivity.

Each of these antigens can elicit a corresponding response (anti-HBs, anti-HBc and anti-HBe). In an acute hepatitis B infection the appearance of the antigens and antibodies follows a well defined pattern (Figure 13.2).

The main route of HBV infection is by parenteral inoculation. The virus has a world-wide distribution. Chronic carriers are especially prevalent in sub-Saharan Africa, the Far East, Alaska and the Amazon Basin in Latin America with carrier rates sometimes reaching 30 per cent of the population. In these

Table 13.5 Sequence of events after exposure to hepatitis A virus.

Weeks	1	2	3	4	5	6	7	8
Bilirubin	−	−	−	+	+	−	−	−
AST	−	−	+	+	−	−	−	−
Anti-HAV (IgM)	−	−	±	+	+	±	−	−
Anti-HAV (IgG)	−	−	−	−	±	+	+	+
Clinical	Incubation		Malaise Anorexia		Jaundice		Recovery	

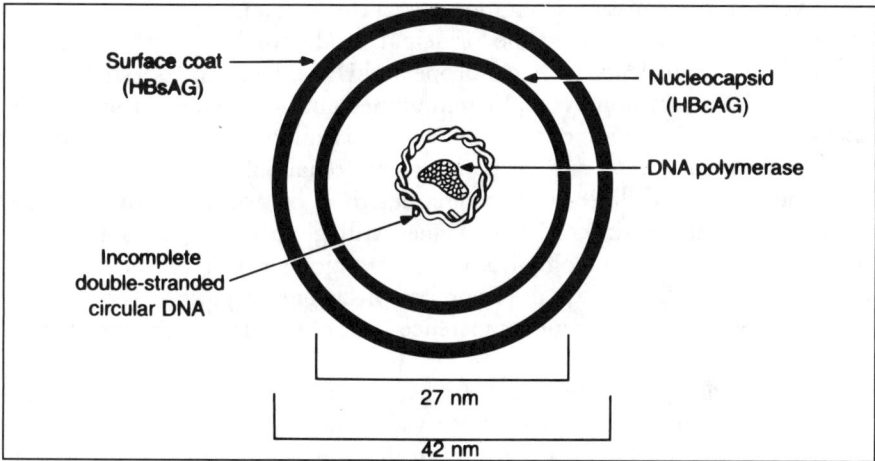

Figure 13.1 The structure of hepatitis B virus.

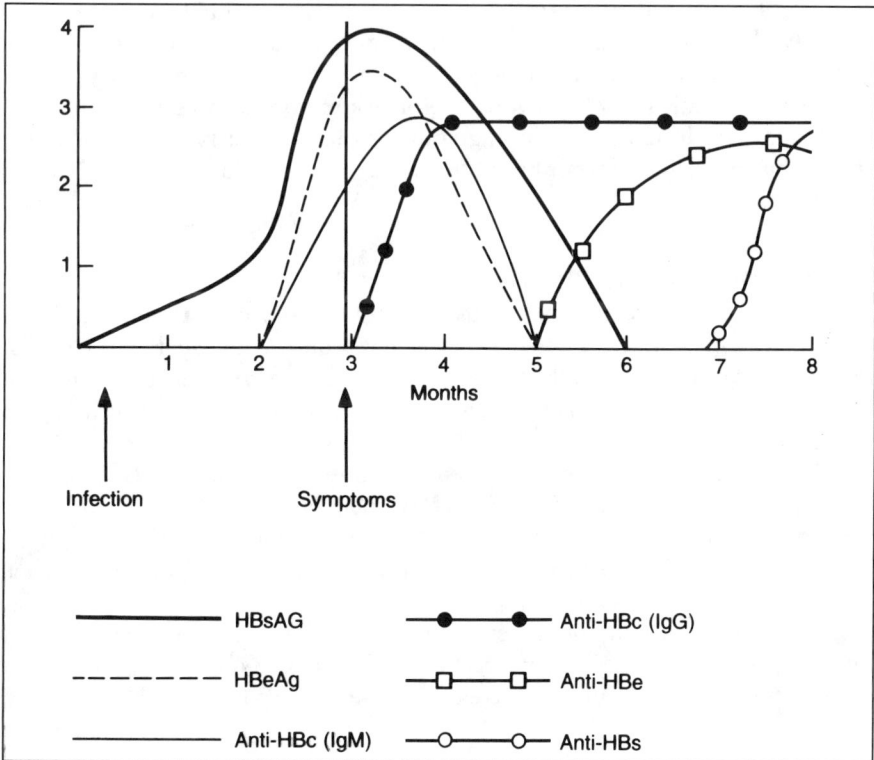

Figure 13.2 Serological changes in hepatitis B infection.

areas vertical transmission from mothers to children and horizontal spread in early childhood seem to be the principal modes of infection. In areas of relatively low prevalence such as Europe and USA, the main reservoirs for the virus are the urban homosexual communities and intravenous drug abusers. The carrier state is commoner in infancy and childhood and in people with immunodeficiency states such as patients with renal failure, HIV infection etc.

The prodromal illness may be characterised by arthralgia, urticaria and occasionally a 'serum sickness' type of illness with glomerulonephritis. Fulminant hepatic failure is a rare complication. The major worry is progression to a chronic carrier state or the development of chronic hepatitis. The outcome depends the age and immunocompetence of the patient and the virulence of the virus.

There is no specific treatment. Active immunisation with either a plasma-derived vaccine or a recombinant yeast vaccine is now widely available. Three (0, 1, 6 months) injections are given intramuscularly into the deltoid muscle. The vaccine is highly immunogenic and effective. Boosters may be required after 5 years. The vaccine should ideally be integrated into the Expanded Programme of Immunization (EPI) alongside the other EPI vaccines and many countries have already done so. The other groups that should be vaccinated are the individuals with a special risk of developing hepatitis B such as all health staff and spouses of HBsAg carriers.

Prevention also involves avoidance of risk factors such as shared needles, prostitutes etc. In many developing countries blood and blood products are still a hazard and efforts should be made to introduce universal blood screening.

Hepatitis Delta virus (HDV)

The Delta virus is a small RNA virus with a genome which does not code for its own protein coat. It is a defective virus that requires the hepatitis B virus for its propagation. Serologically Delta infection can be detected by testing for anti-Delta antibodies in serum. These appear early in the course of infection and may not persist.

Like HBV it is spread by the parenteral route or sexual contact. There are two forms of infection: co-infection, where there is a dual infection with HBV and HDV, and super-infection where HDV infects an existing HBsAg carrier. It is endemic in countries around the Mediterranean basin, Northern Europe and USA particularly among drug abusers.

Co-infection usually produces an acute hepatitis similar to that produced by HBV infection alone. Super-infection of an HBsAg carrier can produce a severe acute hepatitis and in some cases fulminant hepatic failure.

Hepatitis C virus (HCV)

This form is due to an RNA virus (HCV) and is responsible for the majority of post-transfusion hepatitis in all countries where blood is screened for hepatitis B. It is also seen in intravenous drug abusers and homosexuals.

An acute hepatitis occurs although it is less severe than that due to hepatitis A or B. Rarely fulminant hepatic failure occurs. Progression to chronic liver disease is common. Fifty per cent of patients go on to develop chronic liver disease and cirrhosis occurs in 20 per cent of these. A chronic carrier state also occurs. HCV antibodies can be detected in the serum and in some countries, blood donors are screened for this virus.

Hepatitis E virus (HEV)

Hepatitis E causes the epidemic form of non-A, non-B hepatitis and is thought to be water-borne. It produces an illness similar to that of hepatitis A and it does not go on to chronic liver disease. There is a mortality of 1–2 per cent but this rises to nearly 10 per cent in pregnant women.

Drug induced jaundice

Many drugs impair liver function and drugs should always be considered in the differential diagnosis of jaundice. There are two main types of adverse reaction: **dose-dependent** or **predictable** and **dose-independent** or **idiosyncratic**.

The type of damage produced by various drugs is shown in Table 13.6. Some of the common causes of drug induced jaundice are discussed in further detail.

Paracetamol

Paracetamol produces a severe hepatitis if taken in overdose (more than 10 g or 20 tablets). Liver damage is due to the formation of highly reactive metabolites. Paracetamol is converted to a toxic metabolite, N-acetyl-*p*-benzoquinonimine, which is normally rapidly conjugated with reduced glutathione. After a large overdose, glutathione is depleted and the reactive intermediate binds covalently to liver-cell membranes causing necrosis. Compounds acting as -SH donors can prevent this process. The most effective and non-toxic of these is N-acetyl cysteine.

Halothane

Halothane is a commonly used anaesthetic agent which very rarely produces a hepatitis in patients having repeated exposure. It is an example of an unpredictable (idiosyncratic) hepatotoxic agent. An unexplained fever occurs approximately 10 days after the anaesthetic and is followed by jaundice. Progression to fulminant hepatic failure is common.

Steroids

Cholestasis is caused by natural and synthetic oestrogens as well as methyltestosterone. The cholestatic effect is dose-related. Histologically, there is centrilobular cholestasis without obvious evidence of hepatocellular damage.

Phenothiazines

Phenothiazines, e.g. chlorpromazine, can produce an cholestatic picture. About

Table 13.6 Drugs causing liver damage.

Type of reaction	Drug
Hepatocellular damage	
Dose-dependent	Paracetamol
	Salicylates
	Tetracycline
Dose-independent	*Anti-depressants:*
	Tricyclic antidepressants
	Monoamine-oxidase inhibitors
	Anti-convulsants:
	Phenytoin
	Carbamazepine
	Phenobarbitone
	Sodium valproate
	Anti-tuberculous drugs:
	Isoniazid
	Rifampicin
	Pyrazinamide
	Para-aminosalicylic (PAS)
	Anti-inflammatory drugs:
	Non-steroidals
	Anaesthetics:
	Halothane
	Antibiotics:
	Penicillin
	Sulphonamides
	Anti-fungal:
	Ketoconazole
	Cardiovascular drugs:
	Amiodarone
	Methyldopa
Cholestasis	
Pure cholestasis	Oral contraceptives
	Synthetic anabolic steroids
Cholestatic hepatitis	*Hypoglycaemic drugs:*
	Chlorpropamide
	Glibenclamide
	Anti-thyroid drugs:
	Carbimazole
	Anti-psychotic drugs:
	Chlorpromazine
	Antibiotics:
	Erythromycin

Fatty change	Tetracycline
Hepatic fibrosis	Methotrexate
	Amiodarone
Chronic active hepatitis	Methyldopa
	Nitrofurantoin
	Sulphonamides
Granulomatous reaction	Allopurinol
	Methotrexate
	Hydralazine
	Chlorpropamide
Liver tumours and	Oral contraceptives
peliosis hepatitis	Synthetic androgens

1–2 per cent of patients taking chlorpromazine develop a severe cholestasis, usually within 4 weeks of starting the drug. This usually persists for weeks after the drug has been stopped. Typically it is associated with fever and eosinophilia.

Anti-tuberculous therapy
Rifampicin produces a hepatitis, usually within 3 weeks of starting the drug. Pyrazinamide produces abnormal liver function tests and, rarely, liver cell necrosis. Isoniazid produces elevated aminotransferases in 10–20 per cent of patients. Hepatic necrosis with jaundice occurs in a smaller percentage.

Fulminant hepatic failure

This is a rare but often life-threatening syndrome due to acute hepatitis from any cause. Encephalopathy is the commonest and most obvious complication. Some of the potential causes of this include release of toxins from damaged liver, failure to detoxify metabolites, and alterations in cerebral neurotransmitters due to amino acid imbalances. Renal failure due to endotoxaemia or septicemia may occur and has a grave prognosis.

Clinical features
Fulminant hepatic failure develops within 8 weeks for the onset of illness, with no previous history of liver disease. Examination shows a jaundiced patient with the physical signs of hepatic encephalopathy. The mental state varies from slight drowsiness to unresponsive coma (Table 13.7). Convulsions may occur. Ascites and oedema may be present. A small liver is usually found. Terminally hypotension, renal failure, cardiac arrthymia and respiratory arrest occur.

Table 13.7   Grades of coma in liver failure.

Grade	Clinical features
1	Slowness of mentation; mild confusion; untidiness; slurred speech; alternating euphoria and depression
2	Accentuation of grade I; drowsy; inappropriate behaviour
3	Marked confusion; drowsy but rousable; incoherent speech
4	Unrousable; may or may not respond to noxious stimuli

Treatment

There is no specific treatment. Patients should be managed in the intensive care unit. Cerebral oedema is the major cause of death and 20 per cent mannitol infusions are useful in reducing raised intracranial pressure. Dexamethasone is of no value. Coagulation disorders are also common and fresh frozen plasma is the usual treatment for the clotting disturbance. Hypoglycaemia, hypokalaemia and hypocalcaemia should be anticipated and corrected with 10 per cent dextrose infusion and calcium. Erosive oesophagitis and gastritis leading to gastrointestinal haemorrhage may occur and prophylatic H_2-receptor antagonists should be given. When faced with a jaundiced patient one should look for features of chronic liver disease such as parotid gland enlargement, gynaecomastia, palmar erythema, loss of body hair, testicular atrophy, leuconychia, Dupuytren's contracture, bruises and spider naevi. Features of portal hypertension such as dilated veins on the abdominal wall, splenomegaly and ascites should also be looked for. In cirrhosis the liver may be small or enlarged. An irregular hard liver with or without a bruit suggests liver malignancy. Charcoal haemoperfusion has been used but its value has not been proved. Rarely a suitable donor may become available and liver transplantation then becomes another treatment option. However even with the most skilled intensive care support, the mortality of fulminant hepatic failure is over 80 per cent in those who develop grade IV encephalopathy.

Acute alcoholic hepatitis

Acute alcoholic hepatitis is an acute illness associated with alcohol abuse, in which deep jaundice, abdominal pain, fever, marked polymorphonuclear leucocytosis and an elevated prothrombin time are the principal features. Cutaneous stigmata of chromic liver disease are common, even in the absence of cirrhosis. Cholestasis is prominent and mimicks extrahepatic obstruction. The mortality of this condition is high (30–60 per cent).

Histology shows Mallory's hyaline in hepatocytes in, or near to, areas of spotty inflammatory response consisting largely of polymorphonuclear leucocytes. There may or may not be associated cirrhosis.

Trials of specific drug treatments have been disappointing. Abstinence from alcohol remains the most effective therapy.

Chronic active hepatitis

Chronic active hepatitis is a syndrome consisting of several diseases with similar histological appearances on liver biopsy (Table 13.8). By definition the hepatitis should have lasted at least 6 months and the diagnosis is confirmed on liver biopsy. The portal tracts contain chronic inflammatory cells. The cells extend beyond the limiting plate of periportal hepatocytes with 'piecemeal necrosis' of liver cells in this part of the lobule. Fibrosis septa linking portal tracts to each other and to central veins are usually present. The process may lead to the development of cirrhosis.

Autoimmune chronic active hepatitis

Autoimmune chronic active hepatitis is considered to be one of the organ-specific autoimmune diseases. Women are affected more than men and there is an association with other autoimmune diseases.

Humoral disturbances are associated with a hypergammaglobulinaemia (mainly IgG) and nuclear smooth muscle and liver/kidney microsomal antibodies are found in the serum. Suppressor T-cell function is impaired and this may play a part in the pathogenesis.

The majority of patients present with an illness indistinguishable from acute hepatitis. Alternatively the onset may be insidious. Some patients are

Table 13.8 Causes of chronic active hepatitis.

Viral
Hepatitis B ± delta virus
Hepatitis C
Other viruses

Autoimmune

Drugs
Isoniazid
Methyldopa
Nitrofurantoin

Hereditary
Wilson's disease
α-1-antitrypsin deficiency

Others
Ulcerative colitis
Alcohol

asymptomatic for many years and the signs of chronic liver disease are discovered on routine examination. Jaundice may be present in those with an initial acute hepatitis. Biochemical evidence of continued liver cell necrosis is present in these patients. Multisystem involvement is common. In advanced cases, the complications of cirrhosis occur.

Prednisolone 30 mg daily is given for 2 weeks followed by a maintenance dose of 10–15 mg/daily. Azathioprine in a dose of 1–2 mg/kg is a useful adjunct to steroid therapy and may allow a lower dose of steroid to be used.

Chronic hepatitis B infection

Hepatitis B virus is the commonest cause of chronic active hepatitis on a worldwide basis. Many patients are asymptomatic. When symptoms occur, these are often mild and non-specific. Some progress from an acute HBV infection. There is a striking male predominance. The incidence of multisystem disease is lower than that found in the autoimmune variety. The liver function tests usually show a relatively mild hepatic picture. Fifty per cent present with established cirrhosis.

Ideally patients with chronic active hepatitis and asymptomatic carriers who have HBcAg and HBV-DNA in the serum should be treated. All patients with progressive liver disease should be treated but decompensated cirrhosis is a contraindication. The aim of treatment is not to inhibit HBV replication.

Many antiviral agents have been tried but interferon seems to be the most successful. Even so, the response rate is disappointingly low (10–30 per cent) with untreated patients seroconverting at a rate of 15 per cent per year. Other anti-viral agents such as adenine arabinoside and acyclovir have also been tried. Corticosteroids are of no benefit and may be harmful.

Chronic hepatitis C infection

Chronic active hepatitis can occur following HCV infection. HCV antibodies can be measured. Recombinant interferon produces chemical and histological improvement but relapse occurs following cessation of therapy.

Chronic Delta virus infection

The diagnosis of chronic active hepatitis due to HDV is made by finding histological changes of chronic active hepatitis and anti-Delta antibodies in the serum or demonstrating Delta antigen in the nuclei of liver cells using immunofluroscence. Progression to cirrhosis occurs very rapidly and the prognosis is poor. The mechanism of tissue damage is unknown. No specific treatment has been shown to be effective.

Drug-induced chronic active hepatitis

This is usually due to idiosyncratic reactions to drugs. The disease responds to withdrawal of the drug. The drugs most commonly implicated are isoniazid, methyldopa and nitrofurantoin. The clinically picture is similar to that of autoimmune chronic active hepatitis.

Jaundice in pregnancy

There are two causes of jaundice that are peculiar to pregnancy.

Cholestasis of pregnancy

This occurs in the last trimester of pregnancy and is characterised by pruritus with or without jaundice. It also affects women taking the oral contraceptive thus suggesting that it is due to high oestrogen levels. The itching can be very troublesome but usually responds to cholestyramine. The symptoms disappear after birth but cholestasis tends to recur with subsequent pregnancies.

Acute fatty liver of pregnancy

Acute fatty liver of pregnancy presents in the last trimester of pregnancy with a prodromal illness which is similar to acute viral hepatitis and which starts about a week before the jaundice appears. Histology shows widespread centrilobular, microversicular fatty change in hepatocytes. The cause is unknown but similar changes are rarely seen following tetracycline therapy. Liver enzymes are grossly elevated and prothrombin time is markedly elevated. Maternal and fetal mortality is high and urgent delivery is recommended.

Cirrhosis

Cirrhosis is a major clinical problem in the tropics. It results from necrosis of liver cells followed by fibrosis and nodule formation.

    The liver architecture is distorted. There is disturbance of liver function and liver blood flow resulting in liver dysfunction and portal hypertension. Cirrhosis in the tropics is closely linked to hepatocellular carcinoma.

Aetiology

The causes of cirrhosis are shown in Table 13.9. Cirrhosis in the tropics affects relatively young people. The male to female ratio is 3:1. The most important causative agents are the hepatitis viruses although alcohol also plays a significant role in some of the countries.

    There is no evidence that malnutrition is a predisposing factor to liver cirrhosis. Nor is there evidence that parasitic disease plays a role. Although schistosomiasis leads to pipe-stem fibrosis and portal hypertension, it does not produce a true cirrhosis. Other possible causative factors such as dietary toxins

Table 13.9 Causes of cirrhosis.

1. **Infections** Hepatitis B Hepatitis C ?Other Non-A, non-B	6. **Metabolic** Haemochromatosis Porphyria Wilson's disease α-1-antitrypsin deficiency Galactosaemia Tyrosinosis Abetalipoproteinaemia
2. **Alcohol**	
3. **Autoimmune** Chronic active hepatitis Primary biliary cirrhosis	7. **Drugs** Methotrexate Isoniazid Methyldopa
4. **Biliary obstruction** Gallstones Strictures Sclerosing cholangitis Biliary atresia Mucoviscidosis	8. **Miscellaneous** Indian childhood cirrhosis Sarcoidosis Neonatal hepatitis syndrome Intestinal by-pass
5. **Vascular** Chronic right heart failure Budd–Chiari syndrome Veno–occlusive disease Hereditary telangiectasia	9. **Idiopathic (cryptogenic)**

and mycotoxins have been considered but there is no clear evidence linking these to cirrhosis in the tropics.

Pathology

Histologically two types of liver cirrhosis have been described.

1. **Macronodular cirrhosis** in which nodules are of variable size and normal lobules may be seen in the larger nodules. This type is often seen following hepatitis B infection.
2. **Micronodular cirrhosis** in which regenerating nodules are usually less than 3 mm in size and are surrounded by fibrous septa and the condition uniformly involves all lobes. This type is often caused by alcohol.

A mixed picture of both micronodular and macronodular cirrhosis is sometimes seen and this is not surprising since some of the patients have a number of underlying causes such as alcohol and hepatitis B infection. It should be emphasised however that the aetiological cause cannot necessarily be inferred from the pathological picture.

Clinical presentation

Many of the patients in the tropics present late with **decompensated cirrhosis**.

The features to look for are jaundice, ascites with or without peripheral oedema, evidence of portosystemic encephalopathy and evidence of collateral vein circulation around the umbilicus. Cutaneous stigmata of liver disease should be looked for although some of these such as spider naevi may be difficult to detect in black or brown skins.

Practice point
- *Poor prognostic indicators in cirrhosis include:*
  - *Persistent jaundice*
  - *Ascites*
  - *Haemorrhage from varices, particularly with poor liver function*
  - *Neuropsychiatric complications with progressive liver failure*
  - *Small liver*
  - *Persistent hypotension*
  - *Continued alcohol abuse in alcoholic liver cirrhosis*
  - *Failure to respond to therapy*

Investigations

1. **Serum electrolytes.** A low sodium level indicates severe liver disease because of dilution secondary to free water clearance or to excess diuretic therapy.
2. **Haematology.** The prothrombin time is prolonged commensurate to the severity of liver disease.
3. **Serum α-feto-protein** is a useful screening test for a hepatoma.
4. Viral markers, serum antoantibodies, immunoglobulins, copper, α-1-antitrypsin, iron, total iron binding capacity (TIBC) and ferritin should be done to determine the underlying cause of cirrhosis.
5. **Liver biopsy** is necessary to confirm the type and severity of liver disease.
6. **Imaging.** Ultrasound is extremely useful in determining the extent of changes in liver. Fatty change and fibrosis produce a diffuse increased echogenicity. The patency of the portal and hepatic veins can also be assessed. Hepatomas can be detected. Other radiological imaging techniques such as barium studies, scintiscanning and computed tomography (CT) scan all have a role in the investigation of liver disease in specialised centres.
7. **Endoscopy** is performed particularly if oesophageal varices are suspected.

Practice point
- *Poor prognostic indicators in cirrhosis – laboratory tests:*
  - *Low albumin (< 25 g/l)*
  - *Low serum sodium (< 120 mmol/l)*
  - *Prolonged prothrombin time*

Management

Management is that of complications seen in decompensated cirrhosis. There is no treatment that will reverse the cirrhotic changes. Progression may however be altered by correcting the underlying cause e.g. stopping alcohol. Patients with compensated cirrhosis should lead a normal life and no particular diet is helpful.

Prognosis

This is extremely variable and is dependent on the aetiology and severity of cirrhosis. The poor prognostic indicators have already been mentioned. In general the 5-year survival rate in the best centres is approximately 50 per cent, but this also depends on the stage at which the diagnosis is made. The majority of patients in the tropics present with Child's grade C (Table 13.10) and consequently the prognosis of these patients is extremely poor.

Types of cirrhosis of special tropical interest

Indian childhood cirrhosis

This type of cirrhosis presents in childhood (usually between 1 and 3 years of age) and is found mainly in Southern India, Calcutta and Punjab. The disease is known to run in families. Possible aetiological causes that have been studied include malnutrition, viral hepatitis, autoimmunity, dietary aflatoxins, zinc deficiency and a disorder of tryptophan metabolism. What is clear however is that there is an excess of copper in the hepatocytes of these patients and it has been suggested that this may be the cause of the cirrhosis.

It normally starts with vague mild symptoms. The disease may run an acute or subacute course. In the subacute type there is a gradual onset of jaundice and cirrhosis with the development of features of hypertension is a feature.

Histologically there is a progressive fibrosis with little or no evidence of regeneration. Fibrosis extends periportally and progresses to a true cirrhosis. Malignant change is rare. There is at present no known treatment other than liver transplantation.

Veno-occlusive disease

This condition was first reported in the West Indies. Other reports have come from the Middle East, India, Afghanistan and South Africa.

Patients present with acute hepatomegaly and ascites. Approximately 20 per cent of the patients die in the acute stage, 30 per cent go on to develop chronic liver disease with portal hypertension and 50 per cent recover completely. The differential diagnosis includes Budd–Chiari syndrome and secondary thrombosis of the hepatic veins due to tumours or sepsis.

Histology shows subendothelial oedema, intimal overgrowth of connective tissue and narrowing and occlusion of the lumen. This is followed by centrizonal congestion, necrosis of hepatocytes and fibrosis – changes similar to those of cardiac cirrhosis. Thrombosis of larger hepatic veins may also occur.

Table 13.10   Child's classification of severity of liver cirrhosis.

Feature	Points scored for increasing abnormalities		
	1	2	3
Encephalopathy (grade)	None	1 and 2	3 and 4
Ascites	None	Mild	Moderate/severe
Plasma bilirubin (mmol/l)	< 25	25–40	> 40
Plasma albumin (g/l)	> 35	28–35	< 28
Prothrombin time (seconds prolonged)	1–4	4–6	> 6

Total score: 5–6   = grade A
7–9   = grade B
10–15 = grade C

The disease is caused by 'bush-teas' containing pyrolidine-containing alkaloids such as *Senecio*, *Crotalaria* and *Heliotropium*.

Iron overload (African siderosis)
This condition has been described in South Africa, Zimbabwe, Uganda, Tanzania, Zambia and Ghana. Men are affected much more often than women. The cause of the iron accumulation in the liver is probably due to an increased dietary intake of iron through the drinking of traditional beer brewed in iron containers. A possible defect resulting in an excess iron absorption rate has also been postulated.

Histologically iron is present in the hepatocytes, Kupffer cells and portal tracts with or without liver cirrhosis.

Pericellular cirrhosis
Pericellular cirrhosis is a diffuse interstitial cirrhosis of unknown aetiology found in adult Mexicans. An association with tuberculosis has been postulated but not proven. Similar lesions may occur in congenital syphilis but a true cirrhosis is uncommon. Histologically the individual hepatocytes are surrounded by cellular fibrous tissue and chronic inflammatory cells. Features of cirrhosis are present.

Porphyria
The disease has marked geographical variation. The disease has been described in many countries particularly South Africa, Ethiopia, Kenya, Turkey and Sweden.

There are four main types of porphyria:

1. **Porphyria variegata** – inherited as a Mendelian dominant gene and common in South Africa.
2. **Acute intermittent porphyria** – inherited as a Mendelian dominant gene, common in Sweden.
3. **Porphyria cutanea tarda** – often familial and common in Ethiopia.
4. An **acquired** type – common in Turkey and also with a familial basis.

Many patients with porphyria are chronic alcoholics. Fibrous changes in the liver and cirrhosis of the liver occur in the first three types of porphyria. In addition haemosiderosis is present. Hepatic pathology does not occur in the acquired type.

Sickle cell disease (SS)

Impaired liver function tests and hepatomegaly are common in sickle cell disease. The picture may be indistinguishable from that chronic hepatitis.

In a 'sickle cell crisis', the hepatic sinusoids are filled with sickled red blood cells. The blood flow is often obstructed by engorged necrosis with fibrosis, cirrhosis is common. Haemosiderosis may be prominent. Gallstones may occur.

β-thalassaemia major

Mild hepatomegaly is often present. Other features include anaemia and reticuloendothelial and parenchymal haemosiderosis. Cirrhosis may complicate the disease.

Hepatocellular carcinoma and other hepatic malignancies

Jaundice may develop as a result of primary or secondary liver cancers or due to obstruction to the biliary ducts due to carcinoma of the pancreas or ampulla of Vater. Carcinoma of the liver is discussed in Chapter 11. Obstructive jaundice due to carcinoma of the pancreas is discussed later in this chapter and in Chapter 11.

Specific management problems in patients with liver disease

Pruritus

Pruritus is one of the most distressing symptoms experienced by jaundiced patients. Its exact cause remains unclear. One possible aetiology is increased bile salts which either effect the cutaneous nerve endings or stimulate the hepatocytes to produce a pruritogen. Another mechanism may be raised levels of endogenous opiates (metenkephalins).

General measures which may relieve mild symptoms include antihistamines, warm baths, skin emollients or phenobarbital. Severe pruritus will require specific treatment but no agent is either well understood or always effective. The different therapies available listed are in Table 13.11 but no agent is well understood, always effective or free from side effects.

Ascites

Ascites is a term used to describe the accumulation of free fluid inside the peritoneal cavity. The common causes are listed in Table 13.12.

Clinical features

The abdominal swelling associated with ascites may accumulate slowly over many weeks or rapidly. The presence of fluid is confirmed by demonstrating shifting dullness. Abdominal discomfort is common but if this is severe, spontaneous bacterial peritonitis should be suspected. A pleural effusion may be present and this is usually on the right side. Peripheral oedema may also be present.

Pathophysiology

Ascites due to cirrhosis and portal hypertension is associated with impairment of the renal handling of sodium which may be related to peripheral arterial

Table 13.11 Different therapies for pruritus.

Treatment	Dose	Mode of action	Comments
Cholestyramine	4 g 1–3 times daily	Non-absorbable anion exchange resin	May be poor compliance
Rifampicin	10 mg/kg day	Lowers hepatocyte bile salt concentration	Monitor LFT's for hepatitis Hypersensitivity reactions
Ursodeoxycholic acid	600 mg t.d.s. oral	Modifies bile salt composition	Slow onset Safe in pregnancy
Propofol	1.5 mg IV twice	Probably opiate antagonist in spinal roots	Still being evaluated Sub-hypnotic doses
Naloxone	0.2 µg/kg per min infusion for 1–2 days	Opiate antagonist	Oral nalmefene may become available Still experimental
Phototherapy	UV-B for 10 days	Increased bile salt turnover or alters skin sensitivity	Premature ageing Skin carcinogenesis
Plasmapheresis	2–3 treatments for 4 hours	Removal of bile salts	Expensive Time consuming

Obstructive jaundice which often causes pruritus is best managed by surgical or endoscopic relief of the obstruction whenever possible.

Table 13.12 Common causes of ascites.

Portal hypertension	Malignancy
Cirrhosis	Hepatocellular carcinoma
Hepatitis	Cholangiocarcinoma
Schistosomal portal fibrosis	Peritoneal metastases (esp. ovarian cancer)
Portal vein block	Carcinoma of pancreas with obstructive jaundice
	Lymphomas
Cardiac failure	
Congestive heart failure	**Infections**
Constructive pericarditis	Tuberculosis
	Filariasis
Hepatic venous obstruction	Schistosomiasis
Budd–Chiari syndrome	
Veno-occlusive disease	**Miscellaneous**
	Pancreatitis
Hypoproteinaemia	Chylous ascites
Nephrotic syndrome	Hypothyroidism (myxoedema)
Malnutrition	Bile ascites
Protein losing enteropathy	Ovarian disease – Meigs' syndrome/stroma ovarii

vasodilation and reduced effective plasma volume. This stimulates the renin angiotensin system (through reduced renal blood flow), the sympathetic system (through the baroreceptors) and antidiuretic hormones. Despite increased endogenous natriuretic peptides (from the atrium and brain) and intra-renal vasodilators, there is sodium and water retention with little sodium excretion in urine. In patients with ascites, urine sodium excretion rarely exceeds 5 mmol/24 h.

Practice point
- *A diagnostic paracentesis of 10–20 ml should be performed*
  The fluid should be clear or straw coloured and any cloudiness should lead to a suspicion of spontaneous bacterial peritonitis. Bacterial culture may be negative but if the polymorph count is above $500 \times 10^9/l$ broadspectrum antibiotics should be started.

Management

Ascites in patients with liver disease does not usually require immediate therapy unless severe. The aim is to reduce sodium intake and increase renal sodium excretion. The maximum rate at which ascites can be mobilised is 500–700 ml/24 h.

1. **Dietary sodium restriction** should always be part of the management. The sodium intake is restricted to 22 mmol/day.
2. **Best rest** alone, probably by improving renal perfusion, may lead to a diuresis in a small number of patients.
3. **Diuretic therapy** should lead to a loss of 300–900 g/daily of body weight.

The serum and urinary electrolytes, hydration, urea and creatinine should be monitored. Side effects include a rise in urea and creatinine levels, hypokalaemia, metabolic alkalosis and precipitation of encephalopathy.

4. **Paracentesis** involving removal of ascites has been reintroduced as a means of rapid therapy to reduce hospital stay. The main complication is hypovolaemia which can be prevented or treated by the administration of albumin to maintain plasma volume. In practice up to 20 litres can be removed over 3 h. This should always be followed by 40 g of salt-poor albumin given over half an hour, 3 h after paracentesis.

5. **Le Veen peritoneovenous shunt.** The introduction of a catheter from the peritoneal cavity (subcutaneously) into the internal jugular vein, incorporating a one-way valve, allows passage of ascites directly into the circulation. Complications include Gram-negative septicaemia, disseminated intravascular coagulation and fibrinolysis. It should be reserved for patients with resistant ascites.

Other causes of ascites

Specific treatment is available for some forms of ascites. For example surgery may be indicated for constrictive pericarditis, ovarian tumours and biliary ascites. Thyroxine is needed for myxoedema and appropriate chemotherapy for infective causes.

The management of malignant ascites is an important clinical problem particularly when it does not respond to conventional systemic chemotherapy. Repeated paracentesis may be needed to control the abdominal discomfort and breathlessness. Occasionally intra-abdominal injection of chromic phosphate (^{32}P) colloidal suspension gives good results. Alternatively immunotherapy with intraperitoneal injection of OK–432 (a penicillin heat-treated lyophilised powder of a *Streptococcus pyogenes* strain) can be used and is reported to give good results in about 60 per cent of patients.

Hepatorenal syndrome

Renal failure may complicate severe liver disease, particularly in patients with ascites, and is characterised by a low sodium excretion with a residual capacity to concentrate urine (i.e. tubular function is intact). As in ascites there is a low peripheral vascular resistance and a low arterial pressure that leads to increased secretion of the vasoconstrictors noradrenaline, angiotensin and vasopressin. There is a functional renal failure due to active vasoconstriction of the renal arteries.

Initially the vasoconstriction causes postglomerular constriction with little or no impact upon the preglomerular arterioles, thus maintaining perfusion pressure. Later constriction of the preglomerular arterioles also occurs causing a reduction of renal blood flow and the characteristics of the hepatorenal syndrome.

Endotoxin absorption in the portal venous blood from Gram-negative bacilli in the gastrointestinal tract may also play a role. In cirrhosis there is diminished phagocytosis of this endotoxin by the Kupffer cells and extensive portosystemic channels exist resulting in endotoxin appearing in the systemic circulation where it may cause renal vasoconstriction and fibrin deposition in the renal microvasculature.

This condition occurs in the deeply jaundiced patient who often has ascites and must be distinguished from pre-renal failure which is often precipitated by diuretic therapy.

Hepatorenal syndrome should, if possible, be avoided by maintaining renal perfusion and preventing endotoxaemia. Once it occurs the prognosis is poor.

Hepatic encephalopathy

Development of this complication of cirrhosis is a sign of severe liver failure and is associated with a poor prognosis. A treatable precipitating factor is usually present and its identification and correction are important clinical objectives. This condition occurs with cirrhosis as well as in acute fulminant liver failure.

Pathophysiology

The two most important ingredients in this condition are a reduction in liver cell mass and diversion of portal blood past the liver via the portosystemic circulation whether through 'spontaneous' shunts or following portocaval shunt operations. This leads to a disturbance of cerebral function but the precise mechanisms are not known.

Many 'toxic' substances have been suggested as causative factors. These include ammonia, mercaptans, amines and indoles. All have been shown to cause encephalopathy in experimental animals. Increased serum levels of aromatic amino acids and decreased levels of branch chain amino acids have led to the theory that the encephalopathy is due to an alteration in the balance of cerebral neurotransmitters.

Clinical features

An acute onset often has a precipitating factor (see Table 13.13). The patient becomes increasingly drowsy and comatose.

Chronically, there is a disorder of personalty, mood and intellect with a reversal of the normal sleep rhythm. These changes may be fluctuating and a history from a relative should be obtained. The patient is often irritable, confused and disorientated. The speech is slurred. Convulsions and coma occur as the encephalopathy becomes more marked. Hyperventilation and pyrexia may occur.

Table 13.13 Factors precipitating encephalopathy.

Gastrointestinal haemorrhage
Blood acts a protein load and hypotension impairs liver functions.

Fluid and electrolyte imbalance
Hyponatraemia and hypokalaemia usually resulting from diuretic use, paracentesis and vomiting.

Dietary indiscretion
High-protein meal
Alcohol abuse

Reduced colonic motility
Constipation

Intercurrent infections
Chest
Urinary tract
Spontaneous bacterial peritonitis
Septicaemia

Drugs
Sedatives
Diuretics
Surgery
Portosystemic shunt operations

Other important signs include foetor hepaticus (a sweet smell to the breath) and a coarse flapping tremor (asterixis). There is a constructional apraxia and the patient cannot write or draw, for example, a five-pointed star.

The diagnosis is clinical and routine liver biochemistry merely confirms the presence of liver disease. Additional investigations if available include an electroencephalogram (EEG) which shows a decrease of the normal alpha waves (8–13 Hz) to delta waves (1.5–3 Hz), visual evoked responses and increased blood ammonia levels.

Management

Management consists of restricting protein intake and decontaminating the bowel.

Immediate management

1. Identify and remove the possible precipitating cause e.g. sedative drugs.
2. Give purgatives and enemas to clear the bowel of nitrogenous substances. Lactulose (10–30 ml) three times daily is an osmotic purgative that reduces colonic pH and limits ammonia absorption.
3. Institute a protein-free diet, with adequate calories, given if necessary via a nasogastric tube.

4. Oral neomycin 1 g hourly orally can be used if lactulose alone fails. Neomycin can also be given in retention enemas. It is mainly unabsorbed but in the long term can produce deafness.
5. Diuretic therapy should be stopped.
6. Any electrolyte imbalance should be corrected.
7. Give intravenous fluids – 10 per cent dextrose is recommended.
8. Treat any infection.

Long-term management
1. Increase protein in the diet to the limit that can be tolerated (20–50 g) as the encephalopathy improves.
2. Avoid constipation.
3. Give lactulose 10–30 ml three times daily.
4. Avoid precipitating factors e.g. narcotic drugs and loop diuretics.

Course and prognosis

Acute encephalopathy, often seen after fulminant hepatic failure, has a very poor prognosis as the disease itself has a very high mortality. In cirrhosis, encephalopathy is variable and the prognosis is that of the underlying disease.

Portal hypertension

Portal hypertension is mainly due to resistance to blood flow although increased flow in such conditions such as tropical splenomegaly syndrome can also produce portal hypertension. Portal hypertension can be classified according to the site of obstruction:

1. **Prehepatic** due to blockage of the portal vein;
2. **Intrahepatic** due to distortion of the liver architecture which can be pre-sinusoidal e.g. in schistosomiasis or post-sinusoidal e.g. cirrhosis;
3. **Posthepatic** due venous blockage outside the liver.

The normal pressure within the portal vein is 5–8 mmHg. As the pressure rises above 10–12 mmHg the compliant venous system dilates and collaterals within the system develop. These collaterals occur at the gastro-oesophageal junction, the rectum, the left renal vein, the diaphragm, the retroperitoneum and the anterior abdominal wall via the umbilical vein. The collaterals at the gastro-oesophageal junction (varices) are superficial and tend to rupture whereas the other portosystemic anastomoses rarely give rise to any symptoms. The causes of portal hypertension are shown in Table 13.14.

Clinical features

Patients with portal hypertension are often asymptomatic and the only clinical evidence of portal hypertension is splenomegaly. Presenting features are:

Table 13.14 Causes of portal hypertension.

Prehepatic
  Portal vein thrombosis

Intrahepatic
  Cirrhosis
  Hepatitis
  Schistosomiasis
  Non-cirrhotic idiopathic portal hypertension
  Granulomata
  Partial nodular transformation
  Congenital hepatic fibrosis

Posthepatic
  Budd–Chiari syndrome
  Veno-occlusive disease
  Constrictive pericarditis

1. Haematemesis/melaena from the rupture of varices (discussed below on pp 259–62);
2. Ascites (discussed above p 247);
3. Encephalopathy (discussed above p 250).

Management of variceal haemorrhage

Approximately 30 per cent of patients with gastro-oesophageal varices will bleed from them. Bleeding is likely to occur with large varices, high pressure and more severe liver disease.

Initial management
1. Assess **general condition** and check **vital signs**.
2. Insert **intravenous line** and obtain blood for grouping and cross matching haemoglobin, urea and electrolytes, prothrombin time and liver function tests.
3. Restore **blood volume** with plasma expanders or blood transfusion if necessary.
4. **Endoscopy** should be performed to confirm diagnosis and exclude bleeding from other sites e.g. gastric erosions/ulceration.
5. **Injection sclerotherapy**. The varices should be injected with a sclerosing agent which arrests bleeding by producing vessel thrombosis. This can be achieved in most cases except when major bleeding occurs.

Other specific measures
1. **Vasoconstrictor therapy** may be used to control bleeding in an emergency. Particularly if endoscopy or sclerotherapy is delayed. The vasoconstrictor agents restrict portal flow by splanchnic arterial constriction.

- *Vasopressin* – 20 units per hour intravenous infusion should be administered. In patients with ischaemic heart disease it is important to give nitrates either by patch, sublingually or intravenously to reduce cardiac complications of vasopressin. The patient will complain of abdominal colic, evacuate his bowels and have facial pallor due to generalised vasoconstriction.
  - *Ocreotide* – a somatostatin analogue (250 mg bolus followed by an infusion of 250 mg per hour) will also produce splanchnic vasoconstriction without any significant systemic vascular effect or complications. If available it is safer and as effective as vasopressin.
2. **Balloon tamponade** is used mainly to control bleeding if vasoconstriction therapy has failed. The tube should be left in place for 12–48 h and then removed before definite therapy e.g. sclerotherapy.
3. **Emergency surgery** is used when sclerotherapy has failed to control bleeding particularly if the bleeding is from gastric fundal varices. Oesophageal transection and ligation of the feeding vessels to the bleeding varices is the most common surgical technique and discussed on p 262.
4. **Measures to prevent encephalopathy** Hepatic encephalopathy can be precipitated by a large bleed (since blood contains protein).
   The management of hepatic encephalopathy is described above (page 250).

Prevention of recurrent variceal bleeding

Following an episode of variceal bleeding, the risk of recurrence is 60–80 per cent over a 2-year period with an approximate mortality of 20–30 per cent per episode. It is therefore necessary to try and stop re-bleeding and the following measures are available:

1. **Long-term injection sclerotherapy.** The use of repeated courses of injection sclerotherapy at weekly intervals leads to obliteration of the varices. Follow-up sclerotherapy should be performed at intervals to keep varices ablated.
2. **Beta-adrenoreceptor blockage.** Oral propranolol in a dose sufficient to reduce the resting pulse by 25 per cent has been shown to reduce portal pressure by a decrease in cardiac output and also by the blockade of B_2 receptors in splanchnic arteries, leaving an unopposed vasoconstrictor effect. This has been shown to decrease the frequency of re-bleeding in patients with well-compensated liver disease including schistosomiasis and cirrhosis. The usual dose of propranolol is 40–120 mg twice daily.
3. **Surgical procedures.** Surgical shunts are associated with a low risk of re-bleeding but the major problem is hepatic encephalopathy. Operative mortality is low with Child's grade A (0–5 per cent) but encephalopathy still occurs. Child's grade C has a very poor prognosis. The shunts performed today are usually an end-to-side portacaval anastomosis or a selective distal splenorenal shunt (Warren shunt). Selection of patients for shunts should only be done in specialist centres where other alternative methods of treatment may be tried first.

The prevention of the first variceal haemorrhage has been attempted by medical and surgical therapy. At the present time, no prophylactic measures have been shown to reduce mortality. However β-adrenoreceptor blockade has been shown to reduce the frequency of the first haemorrhage and should be prescribed.

Obstructive jaundice

Clincal features

In obstructive jaundice the sclerae are usually deeply icteric, the urine dark (due to bilirubinuria) and the stools pale (due to absence of bile pigment). The patient is itchy and there are often visible scratch marks. Painful jaundice suggests bile duct stones. Gradual onset of painless jaundice with weight loss is characteristic of carcinoma of the head of the pancreas or the periampullary region. The gallbladder is palpable if the site of obstruction is distal to the confluence of common hepatic and cystic ducts (Courvoisier's sign). A palpable gallbladder implies the obstruction can at least be bypassed if not resected. Carcinoma of the gallbladder may also cause a palpable mass.

Investigations
Obstructive jaundice is confirmed biochemically by markedly raised bilirubin, markedly raised alkaline phosphatase and some (but not marked) elevation of transaminases. In complete obstructive jaundice urobilinogen is absent from the urine and bilirubin is increased in the urine.

The most important investigation is an ultrasound scan. This will demonstrate which parts of the biliary tree are dilated and visualise the gallbladder, bile ducts, and head of the pancreas. Further definition must be achieved by cholangiogram. The two non-operative routes available are a retrograde cholangiogram using a side viewing endoscope (ERCP) or an antegrade cholangiogram performed by percutaneous cannulation of a dilated intrahepatic duct with a fine needle (PTC). Endoscopic assessment is preferred as it allows biopsy of any ampullary tumour or sphincterotomy and removal of common duct stones or *Ascaris lumbricoides*. Where cholangitis has complicated bile duct stones a nasobiliary drain may be inserted (pp 348–50). Intravenous cholangiography is contraindicated in the presence of jaundice because the liver cannot excrete the contrast into the obstructed bile ducts. If no further investigation is possible an operative cholangiogram can be be performed during a diagnostic laparotomy.

Management

Try to define the cause of obstructive jaundice (Table 13.15). The next stage is to relieve the jaundice preferably before any definitive surgery. Invasive procedures and open surgery in obstructive jaundice present three specific problems:

Table 13.15   Some causes of obstructive jaundice in the tropics.

Intraluminal
  Common bile duct stones
  Intrahepatic stones
  Ascaris lumbricoides
  Cholangitis
  Ruptured hydatid cyst

Mural
  Cholangiocarcinoma
  Sclerosing cholangitis
  Stricture
    Iatrogenic
    Post-inflammatory
  Ampullary tumour

Extramural
  Carcinoma head of pancreas
  Chronic pancreatitis and psuedocyst
  Hepatoma
  Carcinoma stomach or duodenum
  Lymph nodes in the porta hepatis
  Inflammation adjacent to bile duct as in acute cholecystitis
  Subhepatic collection of fluid (e.g. pus, bile)
  Hydatid cyst

---

1. **Bleeding tendency.** Patients with obstructive jaundice may have a clotting deficiency due to inadequate absorption of vitamin K which is responsible for liver synthesis of coagulation factors prothrombin, V, VII and IX. Always give 10 mg vitamin K_1 daily for at least 3 days to patients with obstructive jaundice and check their clotting time. In district hospitals unable to do coagulation profiles the time taken for blood to clot in a plain glass tube can be measured (normal = 5–7 min). Fresh frozen plasma or whole blood contains the missing clotting factors and can be given if a patient is bleeding. It is unwise to perform invasive procedures if the clotting time is greater than one and half times normal.

2. **Risk of hepatorenal failure.** Renal failure in obstructive jaundice is partly linked to endotoxaemia secondary to poor Kupffer cell filtration of endotoxins in the portal circulation coming from the bowel. To minimise the risk of renal failure 3 days of oral bile salts (cholic or chenodeoxycholic acid) appear to make the intestinal flora less prone to cause endotoxaemia. Dehydration should be avoided so that renal perfusion is maximal. Before surgery check creatinine, urea and electrolytes, insert an intravenous line to cover the period of fasting and monitor the urine output postoperatively with an indwelling catheter. A central venous pressure line may be indicated. A urine output of less than 30–50 ml/h in an adult is an indication for a fluid challenge and/or mannitol as guided by the central venous pressure if the patient is not already in established renal failure or fluid overloaded.

3. **Sepsis.** Obstruction to bile flow predisposes to secondary infection which may in turn be complicated by cholangitis, septicaemia or liver abscess. Since any invasive procedure may be complicated by septicaemia, use of antibiotic prophylaxis is indicated. A broad-spectrum cephalosporin is better than aminoglycosides because of the latter's nephrotoxic effects. In the absence of cephalosporins chloramphenicol can be used but this is not as effective, particularly where drug resistance is common.

Relief of the jaundice

1. **Endoscopic palliation.** Jaundiced patients benefit from the least invasive method of relieving their jaundice, particularly if it is longstanding. Procedures include endoscopic nasobiliary drainage for cholangitis, sphincterotomy and stone removal (pp 348–51) or stenting for malignant or other strictures of the bile duct. Stenting may spare patients with advanced cholangiocarcinoma open surgery. Where ERCP is not available an access jejunostomy may allow further bile duct dilatation and stenting after open surgery.

2. **Palliative surgery.** In carcinoma of the head of the pancreas the tumour is rarely resectable. Life expectancy is usually only a few months or a little longer in cholangiocarcinoma. If stenting is impossible then a bypass cholecystojejunostomy can be performed using the dilated gallbladder. The jejunum can also be directly anastomosed to the hepatic ducts if the site of obstruction is proximal to the cystic duct. Hepaticojejunostomy is the operation of choice for strictures of the common bile duct caused by malignancy, dying ascaris worms, bile duct calculi or iatrogenic damage during cholecystectomy. Adding a gastrojejunostomy to the bypass may prevent subsequent duodenal obstruction by tumour invasion of the duodenum. If possible a biopsy should be taken at the time of the procedure, providing this can be done without complication. Occasionally obstructive jaundice may be due to fibrosis from chronic pancreatitis rather than malignancy.

3. **Definitive surgery.** A pancreaticoduodenectomy (Whipple's procedure) offers the best chance of cure although the tumour has usually spread even in resectable cases. The surgical challenge is to remove the tumour from the portal vein and restore gastrointestinal continuity.

Practice points

- *A palpable gallbladder in the presence of jaundice suggests obstruction and that the obstruction can be relieved surgically.*
- *Patients with obstructive jaundice are prone to bleeding, renal failure and sepsis.*

Further reading

Gentilini P, Laffi G. Pathophysiology and treatment of ascites and the hepatorenal syndrome. Baillière's Clin Gastroenterol 1992;6(3):581–607.

Khandelwal M, Malet PF. Pruritus associated with cholestasis – a review of pathogenesis and management. Dig Dis Sci 1994;39:1–8.

Pauly MP, Ruebner BH. Hepatic fibrosis and cirrhosis in tropical countries (including portal hypertension). Baillière's Clin Gastroenterol 1987;1:273–95.

Schiff L. Diseases of the liver. 6th ed. Philadelphia: Lippincott, 1987.

Sherlock S. Diseases of the liver and biliary system. 8th ed. Oxford: Blackwell Scientific, 1989.

Wright R, Millward-Sadler GH, Alberti KGMM, Kavian S. Liver and biliary disease 2nd edn. London: Baillière Tindall, 1985.

Obstructive jaundice

Al-Hadeedi SY *et al*. Carcinoma of the gallbladder: a diagnostic challenge. J R Coll Surg Edinb 1991;36:174.

Barker EM, Winkler M. Permanent access hepaticojejunostomy. Br J Surg 1984;71: 188–91.

Cahill CJ. Prevention of postoperative renal failure in patients with obstructive jaundice – the role of bile salts. Br J Surg 1983;70:590–5.

14

Gastrointestinal Bleeding

Patients with gastrointestinal haemorrhage in tropical countries are difficult to manage – they present late, blood for transfusion is scarce, sophisticated facilities for investigation and treatment are not available and most of the publications on this subject have originated from Western countries where the causes of bleeding are very different. However, if managed in a rational manner by a dedicated and knowledgeable team of physicians and surgeons, then even under the difficult circumstances of the tropics these patients can be saved and the results of treatment will approach those obtained in Western countries.

The principles of management are first to resuscitate the patient, to attempt a quick identification of the cause of bleeding and finally to take steps to stop it. Although these principles are similar for patients with bleeding originating from anywhere in the gastrointestinal tract, the details of their application vary depending on whether he or she has upper gastrointestinal haemorrhage (haemorrhage from a source proximal to the duodenojejunal flexure) or lower gastrointestinal haemorrhage (from a source in the remaining small bowel and colon). The management of each will be discussed separately.

Upper gastrointestinal haemorrhage

This type of haemorrhage manifests as either the vomiting of blood (haematemesis) or the passage of black, tarry stools (melaena). Most large hospitals admit 100–200 patients every year and our own 1400 bedded general hospital admits 220 annually. There are generally more admissions in winter than in summer.

Aetiology

The three main causes of upper gastrointestinal bleeding, accounting for 90 per cent of cases world-wide, are peptic ulcers, portal hypertension and erosive mucosal disease. However the proportions of these conditions vary from country to country (Table 14.1). In the USA the relative frequency of bleeding from peptic ulcer varies from 40 to 50 per cent, portal hypertension constitutes 10–15 per cent and erosive mucosal disease 25–40 per cent. In the UK although the proportion of patients bleeding from peptic ulcer is similar variceal bleeding is much less common constituting less than 5 per cent of all episodes. In India variceal bleeds are by far the largest group constituting 52 per cent of the total; 36 per cent have peptic ulcers and 9 per cent bleed from gastric erosions. The remaining causes of bleeding in the patients include oesophagitis, cancer of the oesophagus and stomach, gastric leiomyoma and the Mallory–Weiss syndrome. In up to 10 per cent no cause for bleeding will be found.

Age and sex

Patients with upper gastrointestinal haemorrhage in tropical countries are younger (mean age 40 years) than those reported from Western countries (mean age 55 years) and there is a slightly greater preponderance of males over females (3:1) than in the West.

Management

After dealing with more than 2300 patients with upper gastrointestinal haemorrhage (UGIH) over the last 19 years we have now evolved a simple stepwise approach to their management.

Step I: Resuscitation

If, on admission, a patient has a systolic blood pressure of less than 100 mmHg and a pulse rate of greater than 100 per minute the first action should be to

Table 14.1 Causes of upper gastrointestinal haemorrhage in different countries.

Country	Varices (%)	Ulcer (%)	EMD (%)	Others (%)
India	52	36	9	3
Zimbabwe	27	40	12	21
USA	15	51	28	4
UK	2	49	12	32

EMD, erosive mucosal disease; ulcer, gastric and duodenal ulcer restore his blood volume. Start by inserting two good and reliable intravenous lines using wide-bore needles inserted into each antecubital vein at the elbow and running in 2 litres of normal saline as quickly as possible. This should be followed by an infusion of colloids such as plasma, Hemaccel (Hoechst, Germany) or Dextran (Pharmacia, Sweden) because they remain longer in the intravascular compartment. However it should be remembered that colloids are more viscous and less easily infused than crystalloids and Dextran interferes with blood cross-matching. A 10-ml sample of blood should therefore be drawn before infusing Dextran.

After raising the blood pressure to above 100 mmHg we pass a large (16 Fr) Levin tube into the stomach, aspirate its contents, and wash it with ice-cold saline and antacids every 2 h. If bleeding persists we instil a solution of noradrenaline (8 mg in 100 ml saline) through the nasogastric tube into the stomach every 30 min for 4 h. If a patient has had hypotension a urinary catheter should be inserted and the hourly urinary output maintained above 30 ml. This is a simple and fairly reliable way of assessing the adequacy of tissue perfusion and of fluid replacement. We have not found that the insertion of a central venous pressure line to be very useful because our nurses seem to be hesitant to manipulate the complicated fluid system and long intravenous catheters are a potent source of serious infection.

The hourly urine output, visual estimation of the jugular venous pressure and auscultation of the lung bases for crepitations usually provide enough information on the state of hydration. When the patient is haemodynamically stable we go on to the next step which is to try and make a diagnosis.

Step II: Diagnosis

Placing a hand on the abdomen and feeling for an enlarged spleen will provide the diagnosis in up to half our patients. If the spleen is palpable the patient is very likely to be bleeding from oesophageal varices. Although there are many other causes of splenomegaly in tropical countries, such as chronic malaria and kala-azar, we found that 98 per cent of our patients with upper gastrointestinal haemorrhage who had palpable spleens were bleeding from varices. Associated bleeding lesions other than varices, present in up to 50 per cent of patients with alcoholic cirrhosis in the USA, are very rare in India. When the spleen is not enlarged the patient is probably bleeding from a peptic ulcer or erosive mucosal disease. A young patient with no history of indigestion, who has had only moderate bleeding and has a haemoglobin level of greater than 10 g/100 ml on admission and who has been taking antipyretics or analgesics, is likely to have erosive mucosal disease. A middle-aged patient with a history of dyspepsia lasting longer than a month who has a haemoglobin level of less than 10 g/100 ml is more likely to be bleeding from a peptic ulcer.

Step III: Control of bleeding

The third step is to stop the bleeding. In up to 70 per cent it will stop spontaneously and it is important to identify these patients who can be managed at home (low-risk group). The others will need admission to hospital for subsequent care (high-risk group).

Low-risk group

These are patients with non-variceal bleeding who are below 40 years of age, have melaena rather than haematemesis and do not need resuscitation when first seen i.e. have a blood pressure of greater than 100 mmHg and a pulse rate of less than 100/min. These patients can be managed at home with bed rest, ice-cold antacid sips every 2 h and then mobilised after 3 days. After a week a barium meal or endoscopy should be done to confirm the diagnosis and appropriate treatment started. A few of the patients in the low-risk group will continue to bleed or have a recurrence of bleeding after it has stopped initially. These should be moved to the high-risk group.

High-risk group

This also includes patients with variceal haemorrhage, those above 40 years of age, those who have had a haematemesis and those who have had an episode of hypotension (BP < 100 mmHg). These patients should be admitted.

Hospital treatment

In the 30 per cent of patients who continue to bleed in hospital, it may be useful, though not essential, to do a fibreoptic endoscopy to confirm the diagnosis of the cause of the bleeding and attempt to control it by local injection of sclerosant. If this facility is not available or if it fails to control haemorrhage then further management depends on the diagnosis.

Variceal haemorrhage

A Sengstaken–Blakemore double ballooned tube should be passed into the stomach and the gastric balloon inflated with 200 ml of air. When mild traction is placed on the tube (using tape at the nose) haemorrhage from varices is controlled in most instances. If it is not, the oesophageal balloon is inflated to a pressure of 30 mmHg (measured against a sphygmomanometer). The tube is kept in position for 48 h when, if bleeding recurs, surgery becomes necessary. The best procedure when little help is available is to open the abdomen through an upper midline incision, perform high gastrotomy and underrun the bleeding varices with 10 silk sutures. Both gastric as well as oesophageal varices can be dealt with in this way the latter being gradually pulled into view using a continuous interlocking stitch and progressing from below upwards. The mortality rate after emergency surgery for bleeding varices in patients without cirrhosis is 10 per cent whereas in those with cirrhosis it is in the region of 70 per cent.

Peptic ulcer

We operate on a patient with peptic ulcer if the bleeding is continuing even after 4 units of blood transfusion, if there is rebleeding in hospital and if blood of that particular group is in short supply. For a gastric ulcer probably the best operation is a partial gastrectomy with a gastroduodenal anastomosis but in a high-risk patient is it probably better to excise the ulcer locally and do a vagotomy and gastrojejunostomy. For a small ulcer in the duodenal bulb it is sufficient to underrun the bleeding artery with two or three strong silk sutures inserted deep into the ulcer bed and follow this with a pyloropasty and a truncal vagotomy. For ulcers larger than 2 cm or those which are situated in the postbulbar region we prefer a more radical procedure such as vagotomy and antrectomy with a gastrojejunal anastomosis. With a smaller operation the incidence of recurrent bleeding is high. The mortality rate for bleeding peptic ulcer is about 10–15 per cent and my feeling is that this rate is increasing because not only is there a longer delay before operation but also because ulcers which bleed do so in spite of H_2 blocker treatment and are probably more virulent.

Erosive mucosal disease

A truncal vagotomy and antrectomy is probably the most effective procedure – it lowers acid secretion, reduces the area of stomach from which bleeding is occurring and the vagotomy improves mucosal blood flow. The mortality rate averages 30 per cent not because of the upper gastrointestinal haemorrhage (UGIH) but because bleeding mucosal erosions which need operation usually occur in patients who have other serious illness – such as major operations or multiple trauma.

Operation without preoperative localisation

The surgeon should open the abdomen through an upper midline incision and then look for evidence of portal hypertension, i.e. for an enlarged spleen (which may not have been detected by abdominal palpation), the characteristic salmon pink appearance of the peritoneum and distended tortuous veins over the omentum and bowel. If there is no portal hypertension the wall of the stomach and duodenum should be carefully inspected and palpated by dividing the gastrocolic omentum and using a Kocher manoeuvre. If no lesion is found, the interior of these structures should be inspected through a gastrotomy near the pylorus. If in some cases still no lesion is found, the liver, gallbladder and bile ducts (haemobilia) and the pancreas (haemosuccus pancreaticus) should be examined.

There remains the occasional patient in whom the cause of bleeding remains obscure. We have encountered four such patients recently in whom we performed a 'blind' truncal vagotomy and antrectomy. In three the bleeding stopped. The fourth, a girl of 13, rebled and we subsequently did a total gastrectomy but she bled yet again and died. Even after a careful post-mortem examination no cause for bleeding was found.

Prognosis

The effectiveness of management of patients with upper gastrointestinal haemorrhage cannot be determined only by the operative mortality rates (because if only good risk patients are operated upon the rate will be low) but also by what proportion of patients admitted leave hospital alive. The mortality is higher when the patients are older and also if the predominant cause of bleeding is portal hypertension. The overall mortality rates of upper gastrointestinal haemorrhage (UGIH) range between 10 and 15 per cent and there has been little change in these figures in Western countries despite the advent there of more accurate diagnostic methods like flexible fibreoptic endoscopy and angiography as well as non-surgical endoscopic methods of control like local sclerosant injection, electrocautery, laser photocoagulation and selective vessel embolisation. These methods are too expensive and sophisticated for most hospitals in the tropics and I believe their use delays operation and may be contributing to the rising mortality from upper gastrointestinal haemorrhage (UGIH) reported by some Western centres.

Author's experience

In the Gastrointestinal Surgery Department of the All-India Institute of Medical Sciences we have records of 2300 patients with UGIH admitted between 1976 and 1993. The mean age of our patients was 43 years and males outnumbered females by a ratio of 3.2:1. The causes of bleeding were as follows:

Portal hypertension	51 per cent
Duodenal ulcer	24 per cent
Gastric ulcer	4 per cent
Erosive mucosal disease	9 per cent
Other causes	12 per cent

In 73 per cent, bleeding was controlled by initial conservative management. Of the remainder 15 per cent died in hospital without operation because they bled so massively that they could not be taken to the operating theatre, because they were in deep coma from liver failure, or because the relatives refused operation. Overall 27 per cent underwent operation of whom 22 per cent died (i.e. 6 per cent of those who presented initially with bleeding). Thus 83 per cent of our patients left hospital alive. Our mortality rates are higher than the best Western figures because although our patients are young, a larger proportion of them have portal hypertension and there is often difficulty in getting blood for transfusion which delays our operative procedures.

Lower gastrointestinal haemorrhage

Patients with lower gastrointestinal haemorrhage are seen about one-tenth as frequently as those with upper gastrointestinal haemorrhage. They present with haematochezia (red, maroon or brownish-black stools) rather than haematemesis and melaena. However they are more difficult to manage even in Western countries, because the source of bleeding is not easily identified. (The small gut below the duodenojejunal flexure is inaccessible to fibreoptic endoscopy and colonoscopy is unrewarding in the presence of blood which obscures the field and cannot be easily removed.)

Aetiology

The causes of lower gastrointestinal haemorrhage (LGIH) (Table 14.2) are very different in India from those in the West. In the West the aetiology has changed; the main cause in the 1920s was colonic carcinoma, in the 1940s diverticular disease, and now it is angiodysplasia (a predominantly venous malformation in the caecum). However after 12 years of experience with this problem we have evolved a management strategy that is safe, effective and low cost – i.e. ideally suited to tropical countries.

Table 14.2   Causes of lower gastrointestinal haemorrhage in India and in Western countries.

India	Western countries
Enteric fever	Angiodysplasia
Non-specific ulcer	Diverticulosis
Tuberculosis	Neoplasms
Neoplasms	Meckel's diverticulum
Amoebic ulcer	Others
Angiodysplasia	
Others	

Management

After resuscitation by restoring intravascular volume (as previously described for patients with UGIH) an attempt is made to identify the bleeding source.

The history and examination may suggest that a patient has enteric fever, tuberculosis of the ileocaecal region, ulcerative colitis or colonic carcinoma but these are usually not of much help.

I have then found that the single most useful test is to look at the stool and note the darkest shade of the blood it contains. If the blood is red, the bleeding is from the rectum and left colon, if it is maroon (the frequent colour) the bleeding source is in the right colon or distal small bowel, and if it is brownish-black the bleeding is from the upper jejunum.

We then pass a nasogastric tube. A bile-stained aspirate that is free of blood excludes a bleeding source in the upper gastrointestinal tract.

Careful proctoscopy and sigmoidoscopy are used to examine for and exclude a lesion in the rectum and distal sigmoid colon. We have not found other investigations, such as colonoscopy, selective mesenteric angiography, radioisotope scanning and barium contrast studies to be very useful in acute massive bleeding. They necessitate the transfer of a patient from the ward to a diagnostic department where facilities for resuscitation are not readily available and the bleeding has often stopped by the time the patient reaches the facility. More importantly, it has been my experience that the results, if positive, may also be misleading, i.e. demonstrate a bleeding site that is not present at laparotomy. If the patient needs more than 6 units to replace the lost blood volume we transfer him to the theatre for operation. This is required in about 40 per cent of patients with lower gastrointestinal haemorrhage.

Operation

Through a long midline abdominal incision the small and large bowel are carefully inspected and palpated for a bleeding source. If the serosa is firmly rubbed with a dry swab punctate haemorrhages may reveal the presence of an underlying mucosal ulcer. Sometimes the lesion (such as a Meckel's diverticulum, tuberculous ulcer, leiomyoma or a large haemangioma) is obvious on gross inspection. If not the bowel can be examined from within by passing a sigmoidoscope inserted near the duodenojejunal flexure and gradually packing segments of the distal bowel onto the sigmoidscope in a concertina-like fashion till the ileum is reached. Usually two or three enterotomies are needed to examine the whole length of the small bowel.

If still no bleeding source is apparent we perform a 'blind' right hemicolectomy because we have found that most lesions, which cause lower gastrointestinal haemorrhage in India and are not obvious at laparotomy, are situated in the distal ileum and right colon.

Author's experience

We managed 145 patients with lower gastrointestinal haemorrhage at the All India Institute of Medical Sciences between January, 1981 and December, 1992. There were 112 males and 33 females (M:F=3.4:1) whose mean age was 38 years. The causes of bleeding are shown in Table 14.3 – the most common being enteric fever followed by non-specific ulcers in the ileum and caecum. The procedures carried out in 66 patients are listed in Table 14.4. The most

Table 14.3 Causes of lower gastrointestinal bleeding at the All India Institute of Medical Sciences (1981–1992).

Diagnosis	Number (per cent)	
Enteric fever	33	(23)
Non-specific ulcer	17	(12)
Vasculitis	11	(7.5)
Carcinoma	10	(6.8)
Tuberculosis	5	(3.4)
Angiomas	4	(2.8)
Ulcerative colitis	3	
Diverticulosis	3	
Angiodysplasia	3	
Miscellaneous	16	(11)
No cause found	40	(34)
Total	145	

Table 14.4 Operations performed for lower gastrointestinal bleeding at the All India Institute of Medical Sciences (1981–1992).

Procedure	Number
Right hemicolectomy	37
Ileal resection	8
Jejunal resection	7
Subtotal colectomy	6
Meckel's excision	2
Others	6
Total	66

frequently performed operation was a right hemicolectomy in 37 patients. In 16 of these we performed the operation 'blind' i.e. the lesion was not identified before resection. In these the opened specimen showed ulcers in nine, of which seven were non-specific, and two due to amoebic infection. In the other seven no cause was obvious yet bleeding did not recur.

Eight (12 per cent) of our patients died – three with continued bleeding, two from enteric septicaemia, one each from disseminated malignancy, pulmonary embolism and complications of mesenteric angiography (when we used to perform the investigation routinely in these patients).

In Western countries the operative mortality approaches 30 per cent mainly because the mean age of the patients is 60 years and also, I believe, because too many preoperative investigations are done to localise the bleeding site and this delays an effective procedure.

Summary

Patients with gastrointestinal haemorrhage are commonly seen in tropical countries where management options are somewhat restricted by the absence of sophisticated diagnostic and therapeutic facilities and the shortage of blood for transfusion. However our patients have the advantage of being approximately 20 years younger than those seen in Western countries. Upper gastrointestinal haemorrhage is most commonly due to portal hypertension rather than peptic ulcer and lower gastrointestinal haemorrhage due to typhoid and non-specific ulcers rather than angiodysplasia. Our experience has taught us that using a rational and stepwise approach consisting of resuscitation, diagnosis and bleeding control more than eight out of ten patients will leave hospital alive – a figure similar to those reported from the best Western centres.

Further reading

Chung SCS *et al*. Endoscopic injection of adrenaline for actively bleeding ulcers: a randomised trial. Br M J (Clin Res Ed) 1988; 296(6637):1631–1.

Kiire CF. Upper gastrointestinal bleeding in an African setting. JR Coll Physicians Lond 1987;21:107.

Shields R. Portal hypertension. Baillières Clin Gastroenterol 1992;6(3):425–634.

15

Upper Abdominal Pain

Upper abdominal pain is a common symptom occurring in up to a third of the normal population in the tropics. However, the symptom is non-specific and may be due to many different pathologies and originate in any organ of the upper abdomen or lower chest and mediastinum. The first priority in diagnosis and management is to exclude serious and life threatening disease. For example early gastric cancer presents with upper abdominal pain and can only be excluded by further investigation. Appropriate management is also important since many patients do not have serious pathology, and these require safe, simple and cheap management. Otherwise over-prescription of expensive treatments may cause more harm than the disease.

Practice points
- *Exclude serious and life-threatening disease.*
- *Do not burden the patient with expensive and unnecessary treatment.*

Clinical assessment

History

A full history must be taken to document the onset of the pain, its duration, frequency, character, exacerbating, and/or relieving features, radiation, associated phenomena, relation to food and importantly the effect on the patient's lifestyle. Always ask yourself the question 'Why has **this** patient consulted **me** today?' When there is vomiting the volume, content, frequency and timing in relation to eating are the main features to be elicited. Volume should be assessed in measures that the patient understands. Always take a careful drug history since some patients with dyspepsia mistakenly take aspirin or other non-steroidal anti-inflammatory drugs (NSAID) which may exacerbate or cause gastritis, duodenitis or ulceration.

Dyspepsia

Dyspepsia can be defined as upper abdominal pain related to eating. This can be further divided into several different categories according to the nature and associated features of the pain (Table 15.1). Studies in Europe and Africa suggest that almost one-third of the population have suffered dyspepsia within the preceeding 3 months. The cause will vary in different populations so it is important to know the common local causes of upper abdominal pain. A large proportion (up to 60 per cent) will have no detectable pathology on investigation, so called non-ulcer dyspepsia.

Table 15.1 Types of dyspepsia.

Ulcer-like dyspepsia
Gastro-oesophageal reflux dyspepsia
Dysmotility like dyspepsia
Idiopathic dyspepsia

In the absence of diagnostic physical signs dyspepsia may be classified as follows:

- **Ulcer-like dyspepsia:** characterised by epigastric pain, night waking and relief from eating, drinking milk or taking antacid.
- **Gastro-oesophageal reflux-like dyspepsia:** characterised by retrosternal discomfort, heartburn and regurgitation of acid. It is worse on lying down or after eating large meals.
- **Dysmotility-like dyspepsia:** characterised by early satiety, feeling bloated and nausea.
- **Idiopathic dyspepsia:** upper abdominal pain related to meals but without specific features on history or examination.

Examination

Often there will be no signs. Examine the eyes for the pale conjunctiva of anaemia, or the yellow sclera of jaundice. The mouth and pharynx should be inspected with the help of a bright light and tongue depressor, assessing hydration and looking for signs of oral candidiasis, leukoplakia or pigmented maculopapular lesions of Kaposi's sarcoma. Examination of the left supraclavicular fossa may reveal enlarged lymph nodes due to the metastatic spread of intra-adominal malignancy (Virchow's node or Troisier's sign). Abdominal examination may reveal an epigastric mass, enlarged liver or succussion splash.

Investigations

Not all patients need detailed investigation. Every patient presenting with dyspepsia should have a stool specimen examined microscopically for parasites which are treated if present. Upper abdominal pain in young people who are otherwise fit and whose lifestyle is unaffected may not need further investigation following a careful history and examination. In these it is reasonable to give a trial of antacids, which are cheap, readily available and often successful. The recent onset of upper abdominal pain over the age of 40 is more sinister and should be investigated by gastroscopy or barium meal to exclude gastric cancer. Persistent pain at any age warrants investigation, particularly if it is not relieved by H$_2$-receptor blockers or antacids. If facilities for investigation are not available be selective in choosing who to refer for special investigations.

Investigations include stool examination for parasites, liver function tests and gastroscopy. Barium meal examination (double contrast) may be used where upper endoscopy is not available or where the endoscopist is uncertain about the appearance (e.g. where a mass may be indenting the stomach or there has been previous gastric surgery). Ultrasound scanning allows the gallbladder, liver, spleen and kidneys to be assessed. The diagnostic approach to a patient with dyspepsia is summarised in Figure 15.1 and the differential diagnosis in Table 15.2.

Practice points

- *Upper abdominal pain in young people may not be associated with any serious pathology.*
- *The onset of dyspepsia over the age of 40 should be investigated to exclude gastric cancer.*
- *Many patients with dyspepsia are referred for endoscopy without stopping aspirin or other NSAID self-medication for pain.*

Table 15.2 Differential diagnosis of upper abdominal pain.

Condition	Diagnostic investigations
Parasites	Stool examination
Non-ulcer dyspepsia	Endoscopy, barium meal
Peptic ulceration	Endoscopy, barium meal
Gastric cancer	Endoscopy, barium meal
Gallstone disease	Ultrasound scan
Pancreatitis	Amylase, ultrasound scan
Pancreatic carcinoma	Ultrasound, CT, laparotomy
Hepatitis	Liver enzymes, serology
Cirrhosis	Ultrasound, liver biopsy
Epigastric hernia	Clinical examination
Splenic infarction, abscess	Ultrasound
Irritable bowel syndrome	Exclusion of other causes

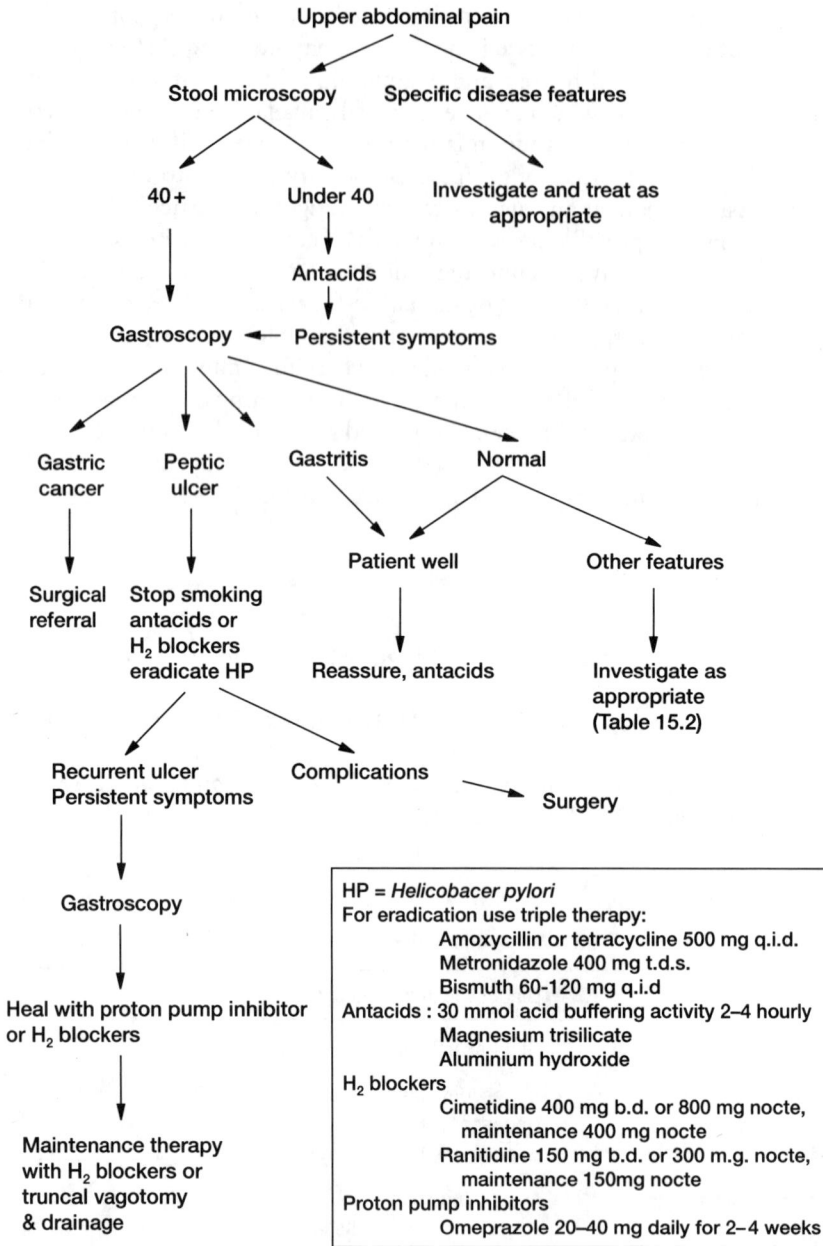

Figure 15.1 A practical approach to the diagnosis and management of upper abdominal pain.

Management of specific diseases

Parasites

Parasitic infection is common in the tropics and a common cause of dyspepsia. Hookworm is most commonly implicated as a cause of epigastric pain, but may be endemic and co-existent with other pathologies such as peptic ulceration. *Taenia* spp., *Ascaris lumbricoides, Giardia duodenalis* and *Entamoeba histolytica* may all cause abdominal pain, but the majority of people infected are asymptomatic.

Both dyspepsia and parasitic infection are common in the tropics. It is easy to assume that they are causally related, which is probably not true for many. Those with upper abdominal pain should have a fresh stool sample examined for intestinal parasites; if present, it is reasonable to treat these. If the pain resolves no further investigation may be required, but parasites may not be the cause of the pain.

Practice point
• *A finding of intestinal parasites dose not mean they are the cause of upper abdominal pain.*

Gastritis

The term gastritis is used loosely by doctors and patients to describe dyspeptic symptoms in the absence of an ulcer, and a clinical diagnosis of gastritis is one of the commonest reasons for admission in many parts of the tropics. However as a clinical diagnosis the term is meaningless and should be abandoned. Gastritis is a diagnosis that must be made on endoscopy. There is even a poor correlation between macroscopic appearances at endoscopy and a histological diagnosis of gastritis. Histological gastritis of the antrum will be found in most of the population in many countries in the tropics and is caused by *Helicobacter pylori* infection (pp 274–9). There is no guarantee to suggest that it is a cause of symptoms and other causes of upper abdominal pain should always be looked for. However if no other cause for pain is found treatment for *H. pylori* could be considered.

Practice point
• *A clinical diagnosis of gastritis without endoscopy is meaningless.*

Non-ulcer dyspepsia

Non-ulcer dyspepsia is by definition dyspepsia occurring in those without an ulcer visible on gastroscopy and in whom no other cause can be found for the symptoms.

Epidemiology

The prevalence of non-ulcer dyspepsia in the tropics is poorly documented, however where random surveys have been done 25 per cent of the 'normal' population report admit to experiencing dyspepsia within the preceeding 6 months. On investigation only a small proportion of these individuals will have demonstrable pathology.

Diagnosis

The symptoms cannot be distinguished from those of peptic ulceration and the definitive diagnosis is one of exclusion since there will be no signs present and the patient will be otherwise well.

Treatment

Antacids are safe and cheap but should only be prescribed if they relieve symptoms. Surgery is inappropriate and should be avoided. Many patients will be satisfied by being told they do not have a serious condition. Some will discover dietary factors that provoke their dyspepsia.

Gastric Helicobacter pylori *infection*

H. pylori is a spiral bacteria which lives in the stomach under the mucous layer. Having been first noticed in the last century it was forgotten until re-discovered and first cultured by Warren and Marshall in 1982 in Australia. It is a Gram-negative organism that needs a microaerophilic environment for its culture, and forms typical small grey colonies which are urease, oxidase and catalase positive.

Epidemiology

In the West approximately 20 per cent of 20 year olds and 60 per cent of 60 year olds are infected by *H. pylori,* but in the tropics over 80 per cent of the population are infected (Table 15.3, Figure 15.2). Infection is acquired at an early age – often before 5 years of age in the tropics. In the West infection is not acquired during adult life, and the differences in the prevalence of infection in adults are the result of cohort effect and reflect childhood levels of infection. In the tropics infection is associated with crowded living conditions and poor hygiene and continues to be acquired in adulthood. Infection is transmitted by the faecal–oral route and the organism has been isolated from the faeces in the Gambia.

Table 15.3 The world-wide prevalence of antibodies to *H. pylori*.

N. Australian Aborigines	2/274	1%
Manchester, UK	126/607	21%
Vietnam	225/365	62%
Ivory Coast	265/374	71%
Algeria	218/277	79%
Nigeria	228/268	85%

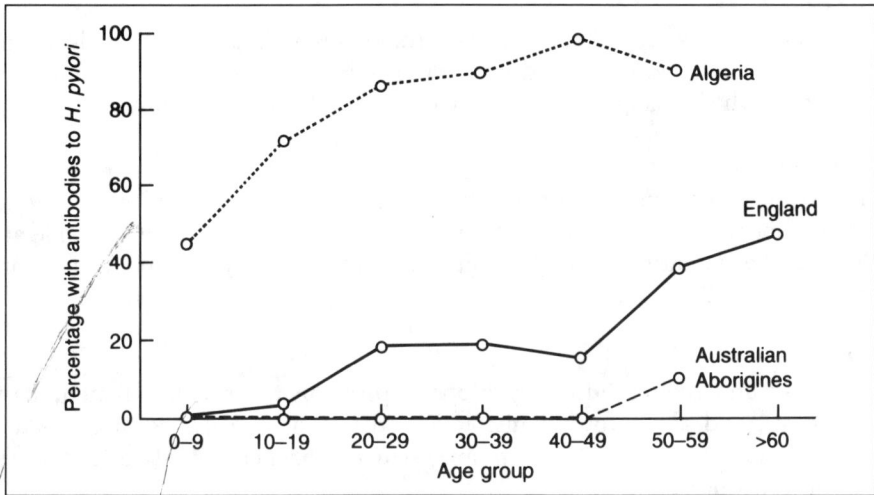

Figure 15.2 Exposure to *Helicobacter pylori* infection in different populations.

Diagnosis

Serology

Antibodies to *H. pylori* can be measured using an enzyme-linked immunosorbant assay (ELISA) which is now available commercially. This method of diagnosis is simple and reliable with a sensitivity of 95 per cent and specificity of 90 per cent. It is particularly applicable to large-scale epidemiological surveys and can be adapted for use in the tropics. Serum can be dried on filter paper, posted and eluted at the laboratory for measurement of antibodies.

Carbon urea breath test

This is a non-invasive test which detects the presence of ^{13}C or ^{14}C carbon dioxide formed by the action of *H. pylori* producing gastric urease after a labelled test meal. The test is more expensive and more difficult than others, but is the best method for assessing the effectiveness of *H. pylori* eradication and is the only method of diagnosis that is quantitative.

Table 15.4 Diagnostic tests for *Helicobacter pylori*.

Non-invasive: Serology
Carbon urea breath test
Invasive (endoscopic): CLO test
Histology
Culture

CLO test

This test is also is dependent on urease production by *H. pylori* . An endoscopic biopsy is taken and embedded in a commercially available gel containing an indicator which changes from yellow to red in response to urease.

Culture

H. pylori is not an easy organism to culture, requiring a microaerophilic environment and incubation for 5 days. Biopsies are streaked onto blood agar. This is the definitive method of diagnosis and the only method which can determine antibiotic sensitivities.

Histology

For those undergoing endoscopy, biopsy is probably the most useful method of diagnosis, and also allows a histological diagnosis of gastritis to be made. Various special stains have been suggested but haematoxylin and eosin are usually adequate.

Clinical significance of *H. pylori* infection

In their initial studies Warren and Marshall showed a strong association between *H. pylori* and antral gastritis. They also demonstrated that over 90 per cent of patients with duodenal ulcer have *H. pylori* infection.

Gastritis

Histologically diagnosed gastritis is very common in the tropics (Table 15.5) and shows a strong association with *H. pylori* infection. The association is particularly strong with active gastritis, in Nigeria 96 per cent of those with active gastritis had *H. pylori* infection as did 75 per cent of those with chronic gastritis. If the organism is eradicated gastritis resolves. Also volunteer studies have shown that subjects who have a normal gastric mucosa and ingest a culture of *H. pylori* develop gastritis. *H. pylori* is the cause of what was known as type B antral gastritis, and the causal role of *H. pylori* has been recognised in a new classification of gastritis the 'Sydney system' (Figure 15.3).

Peptic ulceration

Over 90 per cent of patients with duodenal ulceration have *H. pylori* infection. There has been much debate about whether *H. pylori* is the cause of peptic

Table 15.5 Prevalence of gastritis in some parts of the tropics.

Pakistan	96%
Ethiopia	100%
Nigeria	93%
Rwanda	100%

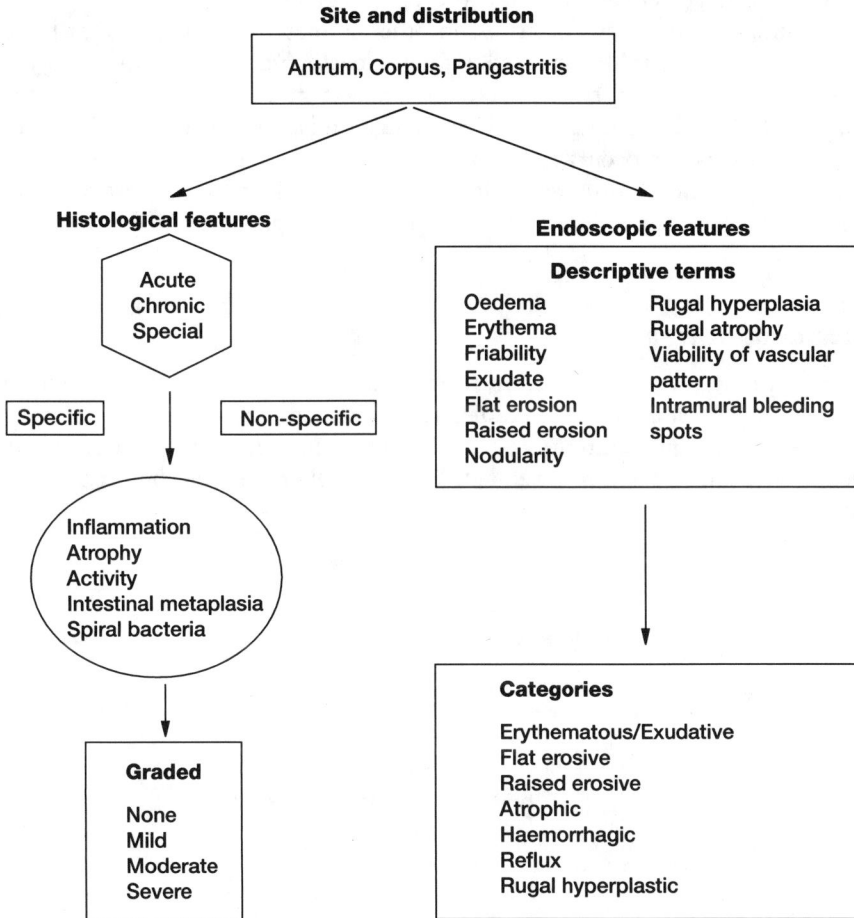

Site and distribution

Antrum, Corpus, Pangastritis

Histological features

Acute
Chronic
Special

Specific   Non-specific

Inflammation
Atrophy
Activity
Intestinal metaplasia
Spiral bacteria

Graded

None
Mild
Moderate
Severe

Endoscopic features

Descriptive terms

Oedema	Rugal hyperplasia
Erythema	Rugal atrophy
Friability	Viability of vascular
Exudate	pattern
Flat erosion	Intramural bleeding
Raised erosion	spots
Nodularity	

Categories

Erythematous/Exudative
Flat erosive
Raised erosive
Atrophic
Haemorrhagic
Reflux
Rugal hyperplastic

Figure 15.3 The Sydney classification of gastritis.

ulceration or just a commensal. However, eradication studies provide the strongest evidence for a causal role. Duodenal ulceration is a chronic relapsing condition and despite healing after treatment with standard H₂ antagonists, 70 per cent of ulcers recur within 1 year. In constrast if *H. pylori* is eradicated, duodenal ulceration is cured, with a recurrence rate of 0–8 per cent on long-term follow up.

However the majority of those infected by *H. pylori* do not develop duodenal ulceration and the mechanism by which *H. pylori* exerts its pathogenic effects is unknown.

Gastric cancer

Epidemiological studies have shown an association between *H. pylori* infection and gastric cancer. The first studies were done in China where varying rates of gastric cancer correlated with the prevalence of *H. pylori* infection. These initial findings have been confirmed in other studies which suggest that there is a two- to three-fold increased risk of developing gastric cancer in the presence of *H. pylori* infection, although a recent study has suggested that the risk may be as high as nine-fold. The association is with the intestinal type of gastric cancer which occurs most commonly in the gastric antrum. It is postulated that *H. pylori* causes superficial gastritis which initiates a process that leads, through atrophy, intestinal metaplasia and dysplasia to the development of gastric cancer (Figure 15.4).

Treatment of *H. pylori*

H. pylori is not an easy infection to treat and it is important to distinguish between suppression and true eradication. Initial studies suggested high rates of cure with a single antibiotic, but the organism was only suppressed and recurred as soon as treatment ended. With a single antibiotic the organism is

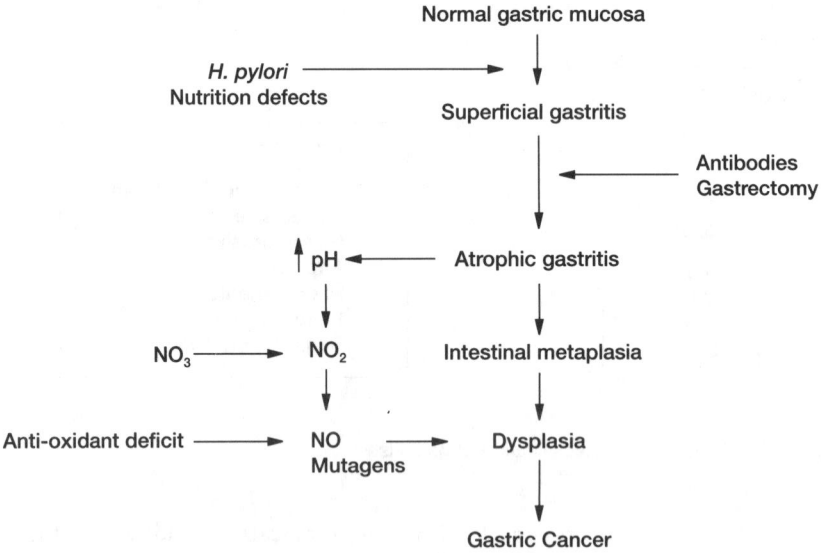

Figure 15.4 The role of *Helicobacter pylori* infection in the development of gastric cancer (adapted from Correa P. A human model of gastric carcinogenesis. Cancer Res 1988;48:354–60).

eradicated in 20 per cent or less. As a result treatment with three agents is now the gold standard, all the regimes contain bismuth e.g. De-Nol 1 tab q.d.s. for 1 month, with two antibiotics e.g. metronidazole 400 mg t.d.s. and amoxycillin 500 mg q.d.s. for the first 2 weeks. This regime gives good eradication rates of 80–90 per cent but at the cost of poor compliance and side effects in up to 30 per cent. It is also important to note that this regime has not been tested in the tropics where metronidazole resistance may be common. A new treatment is now emerging and is likely to become the most widely used, a combination of a proton-pump blocker and antibiotic. Omeprazole 20 mg b.d. and amoxycillin 500 mg q.d.s. give 70–80 per cent eradication rates, but it may well be that the newly released proton pump inhibitor lanzoprazole 30 mg b.d. for 4 weeks in combination with clarithromycin 500 mg t.d.s. for 2 weeks may be the regime of choice.

The question of who should be treated is even less clear as data from the tropics is scarce. The majority of patients in the tropics will have gastric *H. pylori* infection. At present eradication can only be recommended for the few with peptic ulceration, with the caveat that apart from a study in the New Territories of Hong Kong this is of uproven benefit in the tropical setting. In the future *H. pylori* eradication may become the norm for the treatment of all patients with peptic ulceration but clinical trials are urgently needed to determine the most effective treatment regime and to establish the re-infection rate, which is only 1 per cent per year in the West but may be much higher in the tropics. Certainly the mere finding of *H. pylori* infection is not an indication to treat, and would burden many with expensive and unnecessary treatment they could ill afford. There is no evidence that gastritis causes symptoms so that treatment of *H. pylori* gastritis may not be appropriate. There is also no convincing evidence that *H. pylori* is the cause of non-ulcer dyspepsia so that eradication cannot be recommended outside controlled trials.

Peptic ulceration

Peptic ulcers normally occur in the oesophagus, stomach, and duodenum, but may develop in the jejunum (Zollinger–Ellison syndrome or on the jejunal side of a gastrojejunostomy) or even rarely in the ileum if there is a Meckel's diverticulum with ectopic gastric muscosa. Ulceration in the stomach and duodenum are nearly always due to the action of acid and pepsin but other factors are also important. The dictum 'where there is no acid there is no ulcer' remains true unless there is gastric stasis, bile reflux, malignancy or ingestion of corrosives. Acid production is the key and is increased by vagal stimulation and gastrin secretion by the antrum. The role of *H. pylori* infection in the aetiology of duodenal ulceration is discussed on p 276. Diet, non-steroidal anti-inflammatory drugs (NSAIDs) and smoking are other important factors. Smoking and *H. pylori* infection also cause ulcer recurrence.

Epidemiology

The incidence of peptic ulceration varies enormously in different parts of the tropics and even within the same country. In South-East Asia duodenal ulcer is particularly common in major urban centres, particularly Hong Kong and Singapore. The incidence in Hong Kong appears to be highest in the cooler months. In Africa, Tovey and Tunstall identified areas of high prevalence along the West coast, in the Nile–Congo watershed, in Northern Tanzania and in Ethiopia, while the northern savannah of the West coast has a low prevalence (Figure 15.5). Gastric ulcer is generally rare throughout the tropics, an exception being the Eastern Highlands of Papua New Guinea. In India the duodenal to gastric ulcer ratio is 19:1 and in Africa it is 33:1. Dietary factors may be responsible for the differences, with white flour, polished rice and sugar being associated with an increased incidence while unrefined rice, millet and okra protect against ulcerations. There is no evidence that *H. pylori* infection accounts for these differences.

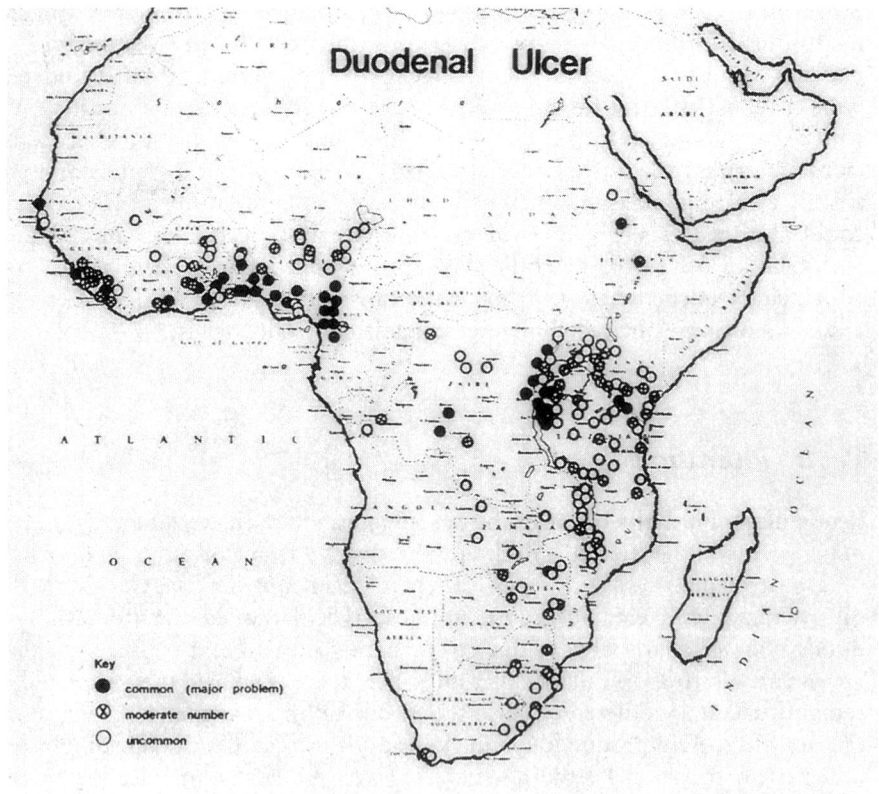

Figure 15.5   Duodenal ulcer in black populations in Africa south of the Sahara (from Tovey FI, Tunstall M, Gut 1975;16:564–76 with permission).

Presentation

The classic history of duodenal ulcer is upper abdominal pain related to meals, often occurring one to two hours after eating, and woken by pain at 2 a.m. in the morning. However, the presentation is variable and large ulcers may be painless and only attract attention once bleeding occurs when the patient may present with anaemia or haematemesis and melaena.

Diagnosis

Diagnosis requires upper gastrointestinal endoscopy or barium meal. It is normally appropriate to treat those under the age of 40 who respond to anti-ulcer therapy without definitive investigations. Those over 40 and those with recurrent or persistent symptoms need a definitive diagnosis. In the absence of endoscopy or barium meal a good knowledge of local disease patterns helps and may be used to select those who should be referred for endoscopy.

Duodenitis

Duodenitis does not have a distinct clinical presentation but can be recognised at gastroscopy as an inflamed and oedematous mucosa. At its most severe there is contact bleeding and multiple superficial ulcers. Practically it is an early form of peptic ulceration and should be treated in the same way as duodenal ulcer.

Management

A range of powerful anti-ulcer drugs is available. However following initial healing the ulcer will recur in 70 per cent within a year. There are two practical aspects to management, firstly which drug should be used to heal the ulcer and secondly, how can recurrence be prevented?

Ulcer healing

Antacids neutralise gastric acid and effectively heal peptic ulcers even in low doses. Four tablets of aluminium-magnesium antacid tablet per day give a healing rate of 74 per cent at one month, not significantly different from H_2 bockers, but at a fraction of the cost. H_2 blockers such as ranitidine and cimetidine act by blocking histamine mediated gastric acid secretion. More recently proton-pump blocking drugs (e.g. omeprazole) have been developed which suppress acid secretion even more effectively. This results in slightly faster healing rates and is particularly effective for severe oesophagitis. Pirenzepine is a selective antimuscarinic drug which inhibits gastric acid and pepsin secretion. Tripotassium dicitratobismuthate and sucralfate enhance the mucosal barrier, thereby protecting the mucosa from acid digestion. Tripotassium dicitratobismuthate also has an anti-*H. pylori* effect so that ulcers remain healed for longer. Misoprostol is a synthetic analogue of prosta-glandin E_1 which inhibits gastric acid secretion and protects against non-steroidal anti-inflammatory drug associated ulceration.

Table 15.6   Classes of ulcer-healing drugs.

Antacids
H$_2$-receptor antagonists
Proton-pump inhibitors
Selective antimuscarinics
Chelates and complexes
Prostaglandin inhibitors

Peptic ulcers may heal effectively with simple antacids; their cheapness, availability and efficacy must make them the first choice in poorer regions of the tropics. Wherever resources are limited the H$_2$ antagonists, cimetidine (400 mg b.d. or 800 mg nocte) and ranitidne (150 mg b.d. or 300 mg nocte), could be reserved for resistant ulcers.

Practice points
* *Antacids give effective ulcer healing.*
* *Patients with duodenal ulceration should be advised stop smoking to reduce the risk of recurrrence.*

Preventing recurrence
There is no agreed management strategy to prevent ulcer recurrence. Advice should be given to stop smoking, eat regular meals, minimise stress, and avoid aspirin or other NSAIDs. *H. pylori* infection should be eradicated. However since most of the population is infected in the tropics, eradication is sometimes difficult requiring multiple drug therapy and the reinfection rate is unknown. Given these uncertainties *H. pylori* eradication may not be indicated routinely. Long-term maintenance with ranitidine 150 mg or cimetidine 400 mg nocte is a possible but expensive alternative.

Persistent and recurrent ulceration
Twenty per cent of duodenal ulcers will fail to heal with 4–6 weeks of antacids or H$_2$ blockers. A further 4–6 week course will heal half of these, though it is wise to switch to a different drug such as a proton-pump inhibitor. Most ulcers will recur within 1–2 years unless eradication of *H. pylori* proves to be effective in preventing recurrence in the future. Even on maintenance therapy with H$_2$ antagonists 10–15 per cent of ulcers will recurr. Persistent or recurrent ulceration should be confirmed by endoscopy and a biopsy can be taken to test for *H. pylori* infection. Many in the tropics live in rural areas and do not have easy access to medical care, cannot afford maintenance treatment and are at greater risk of dying from perforation, bleeding or stenosis. Definitive surgery is often indicated for those with recurrent duodenal ulceration or complications. Persistent or recurrent gastric ulceration requires biopsy to exclude malignancy and definitive surgery. The choice of operation depends on the site and nature of the ulcer.

Complications

Pyloric stenosis

Persistent ulceration heals by fibrosis and can cause gastric outlet obstruction. There is usually a long history of dyspepsia, with more recent onset of vomiting occurring several hours after eating, of large volume and containing undigested food. Bile is absent from the vomit. On examination the patient is likely to be dehydrated and malnourished, and may have a succussion splash. The epigastrium may be distended.

The most important priority is to correct the fluid and electrolyte imbalance. These patients have been vomiting gastric contents rich in hydrochloric acid, sodium and potassium. They will be dehydrated, short of chloride and hydrogen ions – a hypochloraemic alkalosis. This should be corrected with normal saline with added potassium. In a very dehydrated patient fluid balance can be monitored by measuring urinary output hourly by means of a urinary catheter. The diagnosis can be confirmed by endoscopy or barium meal if available. It is wise to pass a large bore nasogastric tube to wash out the stomach, before surgery or endoscopy.

Definitive treament consists of truncal vagotomy and gastric drainage which should be performed within a few days of admission after rehydration. The patient may have a fluid deficit of several litres and should be passing at least 30 ml or more per hour before surgery. Operating before adequate rehydration is achieved is dangerous. These patients do not normally benefit from preoperative nutritional support which in any case may not be available.

Case history 1

A thin, malnourished 35-year-old smoker presented with a 5-year history of dyspepsia. Over the preceeding 6 weeks he had vomited twice each day 3 h after eating. The vomit, approximately of 1 litre, contained undigested food and no bile. On examination he was dehydrated, with a pulse of 110 and had a succussion splash. A clinical diagnosis of gastric outlet obstruction was made.

He was rehydrated with intravenous normal saline, 6 litres in the first 24 h (containing 160 mmol of potassium) and 4 litres in the following 24 h (containing 120 mmol of potassium). A wide-bore nasogastric tube was passed and the stomach washed out. At laparotomy 2 days after admission the gastric outlet obstruction was found to be due to a chronic ulcer in the first part of the duoenum. A truncal vagotomy and pyloroplasty was peformed. The patient was started on fluids at 24 h, made an uneventful recovery and was discharged well 7 days after his operation.

Table 15.7 Differential diagnosis of gastric outlet obstruction.

Pyloric stenosis
Antral carcinoma
Carcinoma of pancreas
Annular pancreas
Pancreatic psuedocyst
Bezoar

Perforation

Perforation presents with sudden onset of severe upper abdominal pain which rapidly spreads throughout the abdomen. The patient has signs of peritonitis with tenderness, guarding, rebound and rigidity (less marked in the old). The patient will have a tachycardia and unless treated rapidly will develop sepsis and hypotension. Erect chest X-ray is the most useful investigation and in about 70 per cent of cases shows a crescent of free gas under the diaphragm. The differential diagnosis includes acute pancreatitis which is discussed on pp 357–63.

Do not endoscope a patient with acute epigastric pain. This may blow off an omental plug sealing a perforation and result in generalised peritonitis. Defer endoscopy for 10–14 days. If there is doubt about the diagnosis a gastrograffin meal can be performed. Do not use barium as this is irritant to the peritoneal cavity.

The patient should be resuscitated with intravenous fluids and given antibiotics. A nasogastric tube should be passed to drain the stomach and a urinary catheter passed to monitor urine output. The patient should have a laparotomy or laparoscopy at which the perforated ulcer is patched with omentum. Gastric ulcers should be biopsied or excised. The aim should be for an efficient, fast operation but a truncal vagotomy and drainage should be done if the patient has chronic ulcer symptoms, and is fit for a more major procedure. Conservative management with nasogastric aspiration, intravenous fluids and antibiotics, is feasible in those who present early.

Posterior perforation of a gastric ulcer may present with less obvious signs without gas under the diaphragm. There is acute epigastric pain with guarding. The lesser sac must be opened and the stomach inspected from behind. Partial gastrectomy may be indicated.

Bleeding (see Chapter 14)

Posterior duodenal ulcers can erode into the gastroduodenal artery. This is a serious condition with a significant mortality. With definite haematemesis or melaena a large bore intravenous cannula should be inserted and 6 units of blood cross matched. If available, endoscopy should be performed to identify the source of bleeding. At endoscopy if the ulcer is spurting or oozing multiple injections with 1:10 000 adrenaline in 0.5 ml aliquots may stop the bleeding. If endoscopy is not available a careful clinical assessment as well as a local knowledge of the likely causes of upper gastrointestinal bleeding will help to determine the cause (p 261). Although bleeding from a peptic ulcer usually stops spontaneously a second bleed may be fatal, particularly in the elderly and those with other medical diseases or those who were severely shocked on admission. A total requirement for blood of over 4–6 units, recurrent bleeding or high risk of dying from a re-bleed are indications for surery. The ulcer and bleeding vessel should be underrun and a vagotomy and pyloroplasty performed. Where resuscitation facilities and blood are limited one should have a lower threshold to intervene, particulary if there is a visible vessel or large clot in the ulcer. When endoscopy became widely available in developed countries in the 1970s the mortality of upper gastrointestinal bleeding remained unchanged. Therefore a willingness to intervene surgically is likely to be the most important determinant of outcome in the tropics.

The management of upper gastrointestinal haemorrhage is discussed in detail on (pp 261–6).

Surgery for peptic ulceration

Surgery for duodenal and gastric ulceration is indicated for failed or unreliable medical treatment, life-threatening haemorrhage, gastric outlet obstruction or perforation.

Surgery limited to the treating the complication

Limited open or minimally invasive surgery may be performed for complications of ulcer and these may be performed at open operation, laparoscopically or endoscopically.

1. **Open operations**
   - Excision and primary suture of a perforated gastric ulcer.
   - Omental patch of a perforated duodenal ulcer.
   - Under-running of a bleeding ulcer with non-absorbable sutures (silk). (It is wise to combine this procedure with a definitive operation if technically feasible.)
2. **Minimally invasive procedures**
   - Laparoscopic omental patch for perforated ulcer.
   - Injection of a bleeding ulcer with alcohol and/or adrenaline or application of some other haemostatic agent such as a heater probe to the bleeding vessel.
   - Intrapyloric balloon dilatation for pyloric stenosis.

These operations limit their aims to dealing with the complication that has occurred and do nothing to prevent ulcer recurrence. However medical therapy may prevent ulcer recurrence and so may make definitive surgery with its attendant complications unnecessary.

Definitive surgery

None of the definitive procedures are ideal so surgeons and physicians need to carefully select who will benefit from definitive surgery which carries its own metabolic and mechanical complications. The definitive operations on the stomach for peptic ulceration include:

1. **Truncal vagotomy and drainage**

   This is a straightforward operation within the skills of the average general surgeon. Completeness of vagotomy can be assessed from histology of the vagus trunks though small nerve bundles may still be missed if the lower 5 cm of oesophagus is not completely cleared. The drainage procedure is necessary because truncal vagotomy interferes with gastric emptying in approximately 30 per cent of cases. Drainage is achieved by either pyloroplasty or gastrojejunostomy. The mortality rate for elective surgery should be below 1 per cent. Postvagotomy diarrhoea may occur in up to 20 per cent but reported series suggest it is rarely severe in the tropics. The ulcer recurrence rate is about 5–12 per cent but there are few long-term follow-up studies from the tropics.

2. **Highly selective vagotomy (HSV)**

   HSV is a safe operation which requires a specially trained surgeon. Unfortunately its recurrence rate is high, even in specialised units, and approaches 1 per cent per annum. This is unacceptable in the tropics where anti-ulcer drug therapy is not consistently available. Complications are rare often being related to technical error and complete vagotomy, dysphagia due to perioesophageal dissection or the very rare lesser curve necrosis (0.1 per cent). Mortality is in the region of 0.1 per cent. It may be the operation of choice in developed countries where elective ulcer surgery is rarely indicated. A variant of this operation, posterior truncal vagotomy combined with anterior lesser curve seromyotomy has also been developed.

3. **Truncal vagotomy and antrectomy**

   The vagotomy removes both the vagal stimulus to acid production and the antrectomy removes the ability to secrete gastrin. It is a 'belt and braces' operation with a recurrence rate of under 2 per cent but a slightly higher mortality rate of about 2 per cent. It is the operation of choice for recurrent ulceration after definitive surgery, antrectomy being added to a previous vagotomy.

4. **Partial gastrectomy**

   Partial gastrectomy can be performed with either a Bilroth I (gastroduodenal) or Pólya type (gastrojejunal) anastomosis and is indicated for duodenal ulcers which bleed persistently or for complicated gastric ulcers. Loss of stomach size produces early satiety but this is not usually a major problem. The patient should be advised to eat small meals more often. The mortality rate varies from 1–5 per cent in published series, being even higher when gastrectomy must be performed as an emergency for bleeding. Ulcer recurrence is rare after partial gastrectomy.

5. **Laparoscopic vagotomy**

   Some centres are now performing vagotomy laparoscopically. Congo red dye can be used to check for completeness of vagotomy. However, the majority of patients requiring definitive ulcer surgery in the tropics are still best treated by truncal vagotomy and a drainage procedure performed at laparotomy.

The role of truncal vagotomy in the tropics

A *British Medical Journal* editorial (9.3.91) questioned whether vagotomy has become an obsolete therapy for duodenal ulcer. Although vagotomy may be superseded in rich countries of the developed world this is not so in the developing world, particularly in sub-Saharan Africa. In poor countries the treatment of duodenal ulcer is restricted by lack of doctors, drugs and endoscopy. The cost of H_2-receptor antagonists or omeprazole makes long-term maintenance therapy unaffordable for most patients or their governments. Endoscopy for diagnosis or therapy is generally available only in major centres serving less than half their rapidly expanding populations.

In Sub-Saharan Africa complicated duodenal ulcer disease remains a common cause of emergency surgery and persistent or recurrent symptoms still require definitive surgery. Truncal vagotomy and either drainage or antrectomy remains the definitive operation of choice and the limited follow-up information available suggests this is a reasonable choice of therapy in tropical Africa. Thus some form of vagotomy will still be required for duodenal ulcer disease until Third World nations can afford a regular supply of anti-ulcer drugs including those for eradication of *Helicobacter pylori*. As the gap between rich and poor grows wider, it seems vagotomy will remain a necessary operation for many years to come.

Follow-up after definitive surgery

Patients being followed up after peptic ulcer surgery should be assessed by Visick grading (Table 15.8). It may not be possible to do sophisticated tests but every tropical doctor can inquire about dumping syndrome, diarrhoea, weight loss and anaemia and make an assessment as to whether the patient has benefitted from surgery or not. Diarrhoea and dumping syndrome are the most common complications of vagotomy and drainage. They are most likely to develop in the first few weeks. Where a major part of the stomach has been resected, or where there is a blind loop (Pólya gastrectomy) malabsorption, weight loss and anaemia may only develop some months or years after surgery. In the tropics long-term follow-up is difficult if not impossible so patients and their families must be advised about late complications.

Grading should ideally be done by someone other than the surgeon who did the original operation. The patient's diet, bowel frequency and consistency should be asked about and his weight recorded. Ask about early satiety/fullness, bloating, diarrhoea (number of stools, consistency and urgency), dumping (early and late in relation to meals), weight loss and lethargy. The patient should also be asked about recurrent pain and re-endoscoped if there is pain. Ulcer recurrence can only be easily diagnosed at endoscopy. True recurrence rates after surgery can only be properly assessed after 10–20 years. There is no such long-term follow-up published from tropical Africa or the South Pacific.

Patients complaining of recurrent pain, vomiting or bleeding require investigation which includes assessment by endoscopy and barium meal. An experienced endoscopist is needed particularly where details of the first operation are not available. Recurrent ulceration may be situated in the duodenum,

Table 15.8   Visick grading.

I	Asymptomatic
II	Much improved with minimal side-effects
III	Improved but has serious side-effects which interfere with lifestyle
IV	Worse than before surgery or has recurrent ulcer.

stomach or jejunum if there is a gastrojejunostomy. Recurrent duodenal or jejunal ulceration is probably due to an incomplete vagotomy. Gastric ulceration should be biopsied in case it is malignant, but is often the result of chronic inflammation due to bile refluxing into the stomach combined with stasis and poor motility. Bile refluxing into the oesophagus may also cause biliary oesophagitis.

Mild symptoms are treated as in Table 15.9. The management of patients suffering from severe complications requiring revisional gastric surgery is beyond the scope of this book. Despite the lack of long-term follow-up data it is my experience in the tropics that revisional gastric surgery is rarely required unless an ulcer recurs, in which case the cause may have been incomplete vagotomy. This can be assessed by acid studies using pentagastrin or insulin-induced hypoglycaemia in referral centres or crudely by testing gastric juice for acid using litmus paper. Antrectomy combined with a search for missed vagal trunks usually cures the patient.

Table 15.9 Some complications of surgery for peptic ulcer.

Complication	Comment	Management
Diarrhoea	20% mild, 1–2% severe	Dietary manipulation Codeine, Lomotil (co-phenotrope)
Dumping syndrome	Less than 5%	High roughage diet Timing meals to avoid it
Pernicious anaemia Iron deficiency	Total gastrectomy Total and partial Gx	Monthly cyanocobalamin Iron supplementation
Malabsorption		Treat diarrhoea or blind loop Exclude pancreatic, other causes
Blind loop syndrome	Pólya gastrectomy – bacterial overgrowth – afferent loop obstruct	Antibiotics Revisional surgery
Stomal ulceration	5–10%	Check completeness of vagotomy H_2-receptor blockers if incomplete May require revisional surgery
Biliary gastritis		Metoclopramide to promote emptying If severe, undo gastroenterostomy
Intestinal obstruction	As for other abdominal ops	Conservative or surgical treatment of adhesive obstruction.
Malignancy	20–30 years after surgery	Endoscopy, biopsy and surgery

Gastric cancer

Epidemiology

The incidence of gastric cancer varies throughout the tropics and is highest in Colombia, while of industrialised countries Japan has the highest incidence. Gastric cancer is relatively uncommon in Africa comprising 2–4 per cent of all tumours (p 182). The incidence in South African Asians (7 per 100 000) is similar to Madras (7.5 per 100 000).

Aetiology

Dietary factors are important including a high salt intake or lack of fresh fruit and vegetables (which are a good source of anti-oxidants). Chronic gastritis associated with ulceration, bile reflux from previous gastric surgery, ingestion of corrosives and are predisposing pathologies. Recently a higher incidence of gastric cancer has been reported in patients with gastric *H. pylori* infection (3–6 times the risk of those not infected). However most of the population of the tropics are infected by *H. pylori* for most of their lives and yet gastric cancer is not universally common.

Pathology of gastric carcinoma

Adenocarcinoma

The most common type is an adenocarcinoma which may be localised (intestinal type) or diffuse. The localised type tends to present with ulceration, a mass or gastric outlet obstruction. The diffuse type causes the thick walled (leather bottle) appearance of linitis plastica. Either type may present with widespread peritoneal metastases. Adenocarcinoma spreads to adjacent organs, by lymphatics, direct extension and transperitoneally.

Lymphoma

Lymphoma of the stomach may also present with a mass which sometimes ulcerates or with gastric outlet obstruction. In many series the stomach is the most common site of gastrointestinal lymphoma.

Leiomyoma

Leiomyoma is usually a benign tumour which may also present with a mass which may be ulcerated. The prognosis following resection is good, even if sarcomatous change has occurred.

Presentation

Patients can present with symptoms and signs from the primary tumour, secondary deposits or with the general features of malignant disease. Patients with gastric cancer often present will advanced, inoperable tumours, with emaciation, a large epigastric mass, ascites, or palpable lymph nodes in the left supraclavicular fossa (Virchow's node). Peritoneal metastases are sometimes palpable at the umbilicus (Sister Mary Joseph's nodule) or on pelvic examination. Spread of gastric carcinoma to the ovary is called a Kruckenberg tumour.

The patient may well have had dyspepsia for months or years before presentation. Indeed in one series from Africa 60 per cent of patients with gastric cancer had been wrongly treated for peptic ulcer. Every effort should be made to make a definitive diagnosis in those over 40 with dyspepsia of recent onset. Most patients with gastric cancer are over 60 years of age although 15 to 25 per cent occur in patients under 45.

Practice point
- *At operation large inflammatory masses may appear similar to gastric carcinoma particulary where perforation was localised and contained adhesions by the liver or pancreas. Always biopsy a gastric ulcer or mass.*

Management

It is important that the treatment of patients with advanced malignancy is appropriate. It is inappropriate to operate on patients who are moribund from advanced malignancy. A very clear understanding of what can realistically be achieved is needed. The prognosis is grim in patients with advanced disease. Few live beyond 6 months without at least palliative resection.

Symptomatic relief
In those with advanced disease, analgesia alone may be the most appropriate management. Those with gastric outlet obstruction may benefit from a gastrojejunostomy to relieve vomiting. This requires some uninvolved stomach.

Palliative surgery
Exclusion gastroenterostomy (Devine) provides better palliation than gastrotenterostomy alone. Palliative resection offers the best relief and a Bilroth I anastomosis can usually be carried out since anastomotic recurrence is rare as the patient normally dies of metastasis rather than local recurrence.

Practice point
- *Radial resection of gastric cancer can be curative.*

Radical gastrectomy
The Japanese have led the way in gastric cancer detection and surgery. They have described in detail the lymph drainage of the stomach and on the basis of this advised the 'R2' radical gastrectomy, which removes the tumour and the draining lymph nodes. In short this involves excision of the greater omentum, peritoneum over the pancreas with dissection of the nodes around the porta hepatis and the coeliac axis. Japanese results using this technique are excellent.

However these results have not been matched in the West, partly due to the increased morbidity of this major surgery in the obese elderly Western patient. However in appropriate patients R2 gastrectomy gives a better chance of achieving a curative resection and long-term survival, and was achieved in about 10 per cent of cases in Nigeria.

Lymphoma
The treatment is excision of the tumour, staging after investigating for other sites of involvement and chemotherapy.

Leiomyoma
The tumour should be excised. Further therapy is unnecessary. A leio-myosarcoma should be widely excised as for an adenocarcinoma removing the lymph node drainage of the stomach.

Case history 2
A 65-year-old man presented with a 4-month history of dyspepsia. He had lost 20 kg in weight in the preceding months, and had taken to his bed. In the preceding week he had vomited small amounts of blood and eaten little. On examination he was pale and dehydrated. He had a large palpable epigastric mass and a fixed mass in the left supraclavicular fossa. He was dehydrated and his haemoglobin was 6 mg/dl. A clinical diagnosis of gastric cancer was made. This was confirmed at gastroscopy which revealed a tumour involving most of the gastric antrum. The patient was kept comfortable and given water to drink. The diagnosis was explained to the relatives. No further treatment was offered so the relatives took the patient home with adequate oral analgesics. The patient died one week later.

Gastro-oesophageal reflux and hiatus hernia

Hiatus hernia is a herniation of the stomach through the oesophageal hiatus into the thorax. There are two types. A sliding hiatus hernia is the common type in which the gastro-oesophageal junction slides up through the hiatus and may be complicated by reflux oesophagitis, stricture and shortening of the oesophagus. A shortened oesophagus results in the gastro-oesophageal junction moving into the thorax which increases the likelihood of reflux, further inflammation and fibrosis. The finding of a sliding hiatus hernia means little without also demonstrating reflux oesophagitis.

A rolling or para-oesophageal hernia is one in which the gastro-oesophageal junction remains in position in the abdomen but the rest of the mobile stomach herniates alongside the oesophagus into the chest. It may be complicated by gastric volvulus and may present as acute chest or upper abdominal pain.

Hiatus hernia and gastro-oesophageal reflux are rare in the tropics, so careful thought should be given to other possible causes of the patient's symptoms, common oesophageal disorders are discussed in Chapter 12.

Clinical presentation

Gastro-oesophageal reflux is characterised by burning retrosternal pain, worse on lying down, bending over and after large meals. If severe and prolonged it can cause oesophageal ulceration and stricture formation which leads to dysphagia. Barrett's oesophagitis – an extension of the gastric mucosa at least 3 cm above the gastro-oesophageal junction also occurs with severe reflux. This is of importance in that it may become dysplastic or frankly malignant. There are no specific signs to be found on examination.

Diagnosis

Although a fluid level may occasionally be seen behind the heart on chest X-ray, hiatus hernia is best diagnosed by barium meal. Oesophagitis is recognised at endoscopy. It is graded mild (red longitudinal streaks at the lower oesophagus), moderate (tongues of shallow ulceration which bleed on contact), and severe (deep, often contiguous ulceration and oedema, possibly with early stricture formation).

Treatment

Treatment with antacids, mucosal protectants and alginates (e.g. the combination tablet Gastrocote) is usually effective particularly if combined with advice to loose weight, eat small meals and sleep propped up. Coffee, fats, alcohol and smoking all increase the likelihood of reflux and should be avoided if possible. Constipation, by increasing intra-abdominal pressure on defecation, may also encourage reflux of gastric acid into the oesophagus. In severe gastro-oesophageal reflux treatment with omeprazole represents a real therapeutic advance with very good symptom relief and stabilising of stricture formation. When a stricture is present it is treated by dilatation and medical or surgical measures to prevent reflux. Surgery is usually reserved for severe cases and usually involves a fundoplication which is performed either at open operation or laparoscopically. If the oesophagus is markedly shortened then a gastroplasty can be used to lengthen it and restore the gastro-oesophageal junction to the abdomen.

A paraoesophageal hernia is treated by urgently inserting a nasogastric tube to deflate the stomach if there is acute pain. Definitive treatment involves surgical repair of the hiatus to prevent further herniation into the chest.

Gallbladder disease (see Chapter 20)

Gallbladder disease can be difficult to distinguish from dyspepsia of other causes and should always be considered in the differential diagnosis. Gallstones are particularly common in South-East Asia but the prevalence varies enormously and can increase very rapidly as has recently occurred in Saudi Arabia, Zambia and Papua New Guinea.

Epigastric hernia

It is always important to thoroughly examine the patient. Herniation of preperitoneal fat can occur due to a small defect in the linea alba through which omentum protrudes causing intermittent pain. A small midline lump is usually palpable and this is exacerbated by asking the patient to sit up. Surgical treatment is by closure of the defect with a non-absorbable suture.

Pancreatitis

Acute and chronic pancreatitis are discussed on pp 357–65.

'Gas-bloat syndrome'

Many patients complain of 'too much gas', either passing what they consider to be excessive quantities of flatus or of belching, associated with feelings of being bloated and satiety after eating small quantities of food, sometimes with nausea and vomiting. This benign syndrome is called the gas-bloat syndrome. The absence of signs in a patient who is otherwise well means that firm reassurance is all that is necessary.

Irritable bowel syndrome

Although this syndrome is a common cause of abdominal pain in the West, its prevalence is poorly documented in the tropics. It is mentioned here as an occasional cause of upper abdominal pain due to distension or spasm of the bowel. It often affects the affluent, urban dwellers in the tropics and is aggravated by stress. It is a chronic condition which waxes and wains over many years, characterised by pain relieved by defecation, abdominal distension and looser, more frequent motions with the onset of the pain. The passage of mucus and a sensation of incomplete evacuation are also common. Pharmacological treatment is unrewarding. The patients requires firm reassurance and an explanation of the chronicity and benign nature of the disease. Parasitic infestation and colorectal neoplasia must be excluded.

Further reading

Epidemiology and dyspepsia

Holcombe C, Okolie H. Incidence of duodenal ulcer in the northern savannah of Nigeria. Trop Doct 1991;21:16–18.

Holcombe C, Omotara BA, Padonu MKO, Bassi AP. The prevalence of symptoms of dyspepsia in North Eastern Nigeria. Trop Geog Med 1991;43:209–14.

Holcombe C. The aetiology and management of dyspepsia in Africa. Trop Doct 1991; 21:107–12.

Jayaraj AP, Tovey FI, Clark CG. Possible dietary factors in relation to the distribution of duodenal ulcer in India and Bangaladesh. Gut 1980;21:1068–76.

Talley NJ, Phillips SF. Non-ulcer dyspepsia: potential causes and pathophysiology. Ann Intern Med 1988;108:865–79.

Tovey FI, Tunstall M. Duodenal ulcer in black populations in Africa south of the Sahara. Gut 1975;16:564–76.

Tsega E editor. Non-ulcer dyspepsia and gastritis in Ethiopia. Addis Ababa: Research Publications Office, Addis Ababa University.

Helicobacter pylori

Dixon M. Acid, ulcers and *H. pylori*. Lancet 1993;342:384–5.

Eurogast Study Group. An international association between *Helicobacter pylori* infection and gastric cancer. Lancet 1993;341:1359–62.

Glupczynski Y, Bourdeaux L *et al*. Prevalence of *Helicobacter pylori* in rural Kivu, eastern Zaire: a prospective endoscopic study. Eur J Gastroenterol Hepatol 1991;3:449–55.

Holcombe C, Omotara B A, Eldridge J, Jones DM. The commonest bacterial infection in Africa: *Helicobacter pylori*, a random serological survey. Am J Gastroenterol 1992; 87(1):28–30.

Holcombe C. *Helicobacter pylori*: the African enigma. Gut 1992;33:429–31.

Holcombe C, Tsimri S, Eldridge J, Jones DM. The prevalence of antibodies to *H. pylori* in children in northern Nigeria. Trans R Soc Trop Med Hyg 1993;87:19–21.

Marshall BJ, Warren JR. Unidentified curved bacilli in the stomach of patients with gastritis and peptic ulceration. Lancet 1984;i:1311–15.

Sullivan PB, Thomas JE *et al*. *Helicobacter pylori* in Gambian children with chronic diarrhoea and malnutrition. Arch Dis Child 1990;65:189–91.

Walker SJ, Murrary AE. Review of *Campylobacter pylori* in upper gastrointestinal disease. Br J Hosp Med 1988; July:27–36.

Working Party Report to the World Congress of Gastroenterology, Sydney 1990. *Helicobacter pylori*: causal agent in peptic ulcer disease? Journal of Gastroenterology and Hepatology 1991;6:103–40.

Surgery for duodenal ulcer

Dewulf E. Abdominal emergencies: a four year experience in Central Africa. Trop Doct 1986;16:129–31.

Huizinga WKJ, Robbs JV, Simjee AA. Surgery for duodenal ulcer: acid secretory profile and selection of procedure. S Afr Med J 1985;68:514.

Mabogunje OA. Perforated duodenal and gastric ulcers in the Nigerian Savannah. Int Surg 1985;70:327–30.

Makuria T. Ulcer surgery in 720 patients in Ethiopia. Ethiop Med J 1985;23:75.

Watters DAK. Surgery for duodenal ulcer in Zambia. Trop Doct 1992; 22:181–2.

Gastric cancer

Arigbabu AO. Gastric cancer in Nigeria. Trop Doct 1988;18:13–15.

Correa P. A human model of gastric carcinogenesis. Cancer Res 1988;48:354–60.

Desai Y, Seebaran AR, Mars M. Gastric carcinoma in Durban's Indian population. S Afr Med J 1991;79:68–9.

McCulloch P. Description of the Japanese method of radical gastrectomy. Ann R Coll Surg Engl 1994;76:110–14.

Hiatus hernia

Bassey OO, Eyo EE, Akinhanmi GA. Incidence of hiatus hernia and gastro-oesophageal reflux in 1030 prospective barium meal examinations in adult Nigerians. Thorax 1977;32:356–9.

List of Drugs

Diazepam: (non-proprietary) 5 mg/ml for intravenous use.

Lignocaine: Spray for pharyngeal anaesthesia, lignocaine 10%.

Antacids: Many different proprietary preparations, commonly containing aluminium and magnesium e.g. Maalox or Gelusil.

Ranitidine: H_2 blocker made by Glaxo (Zantac), 150 mg b.d. for 4–8 weeks in peptic ulceration.

Omeprazole: Proton pump inhibitor made by Astra (Losec). 20 mg daily for 4 weeks in peptic ulceration. 20 mg daily for 4 weeks in gastro-oesophageal reflux, continued if necessary. 40 mg daily for four weeks combined with amoxycillin to treat *H. pylori*.

Pirenzepine: Selective anti-muscarinic drug made by Boots (Gastrozepin). 50 mg b.d. for peptic ulceration.

Bismuth: Tripotassium dicitratobismuthate made by Brocades (De-Nol) 240 mg b.d. for peptic ulceration, also has an anti-*H. pylori* action.

Sucralfate: A mucosal protectant made by Wyeth (Antepsin). 2mg b.d. for peptic ulceration.

Misoprostol: A prostoglandin E_1 analogue made by Searle (Cytotec). 400 mg b.d. for peptic ulceration.

Ethanolamine oleate: A sclerotherapy agent, used in 1 ml aliquots for sclerosing bleeding vessels seen in peptic ulceration.

Amoxycillin: (Non-proprietary) antibiotic used in combination with omeprazole for *H. pylori* eradication, 500 mg q.d.s. for the first 2 weeks.

Metronidazole: (Non-proprietary) antibiotic used in combination for *H. pylori* eradication. 400 mg t.d.s.

16

Acute Abdominal Pain

This chapter discusses the recognition and management of acute abdominal conditions in which peritoneal inflammation or hollow-tube obstruction, or both, dominate the clinical presentation. Medical conditions which mimic acute abdominal pathology will be discussed under abdominal pain.

Patients with an 'acute abdomen' present with one or more of the following complaints:

- pain and tenderness,
- vomiting,
- distension,
- constipation.

These four are general symptoms, which are also features of diseases outside the gastrointestinal tract, so it is essential to make a thorough clinical assessment. In busy tropical hospitals some patients with fever are never examined lying down. Abdominal pain may be misinterpreted as body aches and treatment given for malaria. Sadly it is not uncommon for a surgeon to be asked to see a patient with generalised peritonitis only after 2–3 days in a medical ward.

Case history 1

A 40-year-old obese man complained of malaise and fever. He was treated for malaria by a health clinic but because he was not improving he was referred to the teaching hospital. He was admitted as a case of 'partially treated malaria'. The doctor performing abdominal examination stated that the liver and spleen were not enlarged but made no comment in the notes concerning palpation of the lower abdomen or right iliac fossa. The patient's malaria slide was negative so he was discharged home. A few days later he was readmitted with high fever, toxaemia and in respiratory distress. Surgical opinion was sought and he was found to have distension with little rigidity and generalised abdominal tenderness maximal in the right iliac fossa. He was resuscitated and antibiotics were commenced. At laparotomy he had a ruptured appendix with generalised peritonitis of a few days' duration. Postoperatively he developed adult respiratory distress syndrome and died despite ventilatory support.

His lower abdomen had never been properly examined during his first admission and his doctor had not reconsidered the referring diagnosis of malaria. The patient died of a curable condition and certainly came to hospital in good time to be treated.

Case 1 illustrates the importance of good clinical assessment. Specific points regarding the history of pain, vomiting, distension and constipation will be discussed in the section on clinical presentation. This chapter does not deal with abdominal trauma except where it forms part of the differential diagnosis of an acute abdomen since sometimes a patient will not remember his initial episode of trauma, as occurred in case 2.

Case history 2
A 24-year-old male, smelling strongly of alcohol, was admitted with abdominal distension following a drinking bout 24 hours earlier. He had been found lying in a ditch. He denied any history of trauma and had no external bruising. He complained of upper and generalised abdominal pain but was not shocked. Examination revealed generalised abdominal tenderness, most marked throughout the upper abdomen, and rigidity in the upper abdomen but a softish abdomen in the flanks and iliac fossae. Bowel sounds were present. A working diagnosis of acute pancreatitis was made and he was treated overnight by nasogastric tube and intravenous fluids. His haemoglobin was 10.1 g/dl and serum amylase was normal. Over the next 48 h he developed distension and his bowel sounds disappeared; tenderness persisted but was lessening and his pain improved. His vital signs remained stable but there was a low-grade fever of 37.5°C. He was thought to have paralytic ileus and observations were continued for the next 3 days during which he improved. At this time he looked mildly jaundiced and pale. Liver enzymes were normal and he resumed a normal diet. His repeat haemoglobin was found to be 4.7 g/dl. Abdominal ultrasound scanning demonstrated an enlarged, ruptured spleen. Since he was stable he was treated non-operatively by transfusion and a further 10 days of bed-rest. He made an uneventful recovery but could never remember his initial bout of trauma which must have occurred when he was drunk and fell into the ditch.

Clinical presentation

Abdominal pain and tenderness

The character of the pain should enable you to determine whether the patient has peritonitis or obstruction. The site of pain and its radiation will suggest the organ or structure involved. Other aspects to note in the history of abdominal pain are listed in Table 16.1.

Character

Intestinal and ureteric are true colics in that pain comes in waves and disappears between bouts. Biliary colic and renal pain are constant pains lasting

Table 16.1 Points to note in the history of abdominal pain.

Site	Character	Radiation, referred pain
Onset	Severity	Aggravating and relieving factors
Duration	Progress	Associated symptoms

some hours or days; the severity of pain reaches a plateau and then subsides gradually. Peritonitis causes severe, constant pain which gets progressively worse as the acute inflammation increases.

Site

Ask the patient to point to the site of maximum pain and tenderness. Pain from the foregut is experienced in the central upper abdomen; pain from the midgut around the umbilicus; and pain from the hindgut in the hypogastrium. Pain is normally experienced centrally when only the visceral peritoneum is inflamed. Once inflammation affects the parietal peritoneum, pain is experienced at the site of inflammation. For example, acute cholecystitis may be experienced as an epigastric pain until inflammation of the parietal peritoneum causes localised right upper quadrant pain and tenderness. Acute appendicitis is experienced as a central pain that shifts to the right iliac fossa. Someone with an obstructed inguinal hernia containing small bowel may only complain of colicky periumbilical pain.

Radiation and referred pain (Table 16.2)

Radiating pain spreads from its site of origin in continuity to another place, whereas referred pain may be experienced only at a distant site. In each case the point of radiation or referral is supplied by the same nerve root as the site of origin. In ureteric colic, loin pain radiates to the iliac fossa and groin. Shoulder-tip pain due to diaphragmatic irritation is an example of referred pain and is caused by blood, pus or some other inflammatory process in adjacent organs such as the liver, spleen or lung.

Patients at the extremes of life, those with severe medical disease and those who have had an acute abdomen for some days may not complain of much abdominal pain and it may be the systemic effects of their illness (fever, sweating, confusion, tachypnoea, tachycardia) that dominate the presentation. In these cases there is usually abdominal distension but guarding and rigidity may not be marked.

Medical conditions mimicking acute abdominal pathology

Herpes zoster

Herpes zoster (shingles) causes pain in the affected dermatomes 2–3 days before the development of vesicles. There will be no abdominal signs accompanying the severe pain.

Table 16.2 Diagnositic features of abdominal pain.

Referred and radiating pain	Probable diagnosis
Shoulder tip (referred) irritation	Diaphragmatic
Epigastric radiating to the back:	Pancreatitis Posterior DU
Central or epigastric radiating to back (May also be predominantly back pain)	Aortic aneurysm
Loin radiating to iliac fossa, groin and genitals	Ureteric colic
Loin pain, fluctuating, usually no radiation	Renal pain
RUQ to back or right infrascapular area	Acute cholecystitis
Scrotum to groin and iliac fossa	Testicular torsion
Back, loin, iliac fossa and groin (?flexed hip)	Psoas abscess

DU = duodenal ulcer; RUQ = right upper quadrant

Diabetic ketoacidosis

In diabetic ketoacidosis hypovolaemia and poor splanchnic flow may cause acute abdominal pain and tenderness which quickly subsides as the diabetes is treated. All patients with acute abdominal pain should have a urinalysis for glycosuria to screen for possible diabetics. Unnecessary laparotomy will be disastrous in a severely ill diabetic.

Sickle crisis

Sickle crisis may also cause acute abdominal pain. The diagnosis may be suspected from the medical history and can be confirmed with a blood film.

Acute intermittent porphyria

This condition is sometimes termed the little imitator and is an autosomal dominant failure of haem synthesis with world-wide distribution. It may present with colicky abdominal pain, nausea, and vomiting without fever or leukocytosis. Women are more often affected than men and attacks may be related to the menstrual cycle. An attack may also be triggered by drugs such as barbiturates, sulphonamides, oestrogens, steroids and griseofulvin, or starvation and infection. The diagnosis should be suspected from the history. Fresh urine left standing in the light turns dark. Porphobilinogen and aminolevulinic acid are increased in the urine. The treatment includes intravenous haem, good nutrition, control of intercurrent infections and avoidance of porphyrogenic drugs.

Chest diseases

Acute chest diseases such as myocardial infarction or pulmonary embolism may present as acute upper abdominal and retrosternal pain. Right heart failure often causes a tender congested liver. Pneumonia may cause upper abdominal pain in children. The younger the child the poorer is the localisation of the pain.

Other conditions to consider

Opiate addicts undergoing withdrawal may complain of acute abdominal pain. Tetanus may cause rigidity and spasm of the abdominal wall musculature. Patients with Munchausen's syndrome seek unnecessary medical attention and this may be expressed by claiming to have severe abdominal pain and exhibiting voluntary guarding in the hope of inducing a surgeon to operate. There may be scars of previous surgery. Examination of the abdomen when the patient is asleep will be normal.

Vomiting

The doctor should inquire about the colour, content and amount of the vomit and, if possible, inspect it. Always determine if the vomit contains blood which may be fresh or altered by gastric digestion ('coffee grounds'). The amount of blood and vomit is often exaggerated and may only be estimated from the patient's general condition. Epistaxis may be confused with haematemesis and with epistaxis swallowed blood may later be vomited. Haematemesis is discussed in detail on pp 259–65. Exclude dysphagia and food regurgitation due to carcinoma of the oesophagus or pharyngeal pouch. Vomit should contain gastric juice including acid. Food is normally partially digested.

Persistent vomiting that is not bile-stained suggests gastric outlet obstruction or duodenal obstruction above the ampulla of Vater. Bile-stained vomit without abdominal distension suggests any obstruction is between the ampulla of Vater and proximal or upper jejunum. Bile-stained vomit with abdominal distension suggests small or proximal large bowel obstruction. Faeculent vomiting suggests a gastrocolic fistula or vomiting of distal small bowel contents in well-established obstruction.

If a nasogastric tube has been inserted always examine the aspirate. High nasogastric aspirates are a sign of obstruction or ileus.

In acute cholangitis or bile-duct obstruction nasogastric aspirate frequently does not contain bile until the bile duct starts to drain and the patient begins to improve.

Vomiting is also a symptom of many illnesses outside the gastrointestinal tract such as viral infection, myocardial infarction, raised intracranial pressure and side-effects of drugs.

Distension (Table 16.3)

The abdomen may be distended by gas, fluid, and intestinal contents in the stomach, intestine or colon or by fluid in the peritoneal cavity which may be

Table 16.3   Causes of abdominal distension

Common causes of paralytic ileus
Peritonitis from any cause, viz:
  Haemoperitoneum
  Perforated viscus
  Intra-abdominal abscess
  Leaking anastomosis
  Strangulated or ischaemic bowel
Postoperative abdominal surgery
Retroperitoneal haematoma
Fractured lumbar spine
Spinal cord injury
Electrolyte imbalance, esp. hypokalaemia, uraemia
Head injury

Causes of painless distension of the abdomen
Large cysts
  Ovarian
  Dermoid
  Pancreatic psuedocyst
  Renal
Megacolon
  Hirschprung's
  Anorectal atresia with fistula
  Idiopathic
  Chagas' disease
Solid tumours
  Ovarian tumour
  Fibroids
  Gross splenomegaly
  Gross hepatomegaly
  Teratoma
Fluid distension
  Gross ascites
  Hydronephrosis

Painful distension
Peritonitis or intra-abdominal abscess
Intestinal obstruction
Paralytic ileus (discomfort and tightness rather than pain)
Haemoperitoneum
  Ruptured ectopic pregnancy
  Bleeding hepatoma
  Ruptured aneurysm
  Abdominal trauma

ascites, blood or pus. The distension may be associated with an abdominal masses or occasionally a huge abdominal mass or cyst may appear like generalised abdominal distension.

Gastric distension

Gastric distension may be so gross that it fills most of the abdomen, or it may only distend the upper abdomen. Sometimes the stomach has a long mesentery and can lie in the central and lower abdomen (the so-called J-shaped stomach). The stomach may contain food residue which gives a characteristic X-ray picture (Figure 16.1). There may also be visible peristalsis travelling from left to right in the upper abdomen. Gastric distension may be acute and cause respiratory embarassment and mimic myocardial infarction. Often the cause is not appreciated until the distended stomach is noticed on X-ray but this is often because the upper abdomen has not been inspected, palpated or percussed.

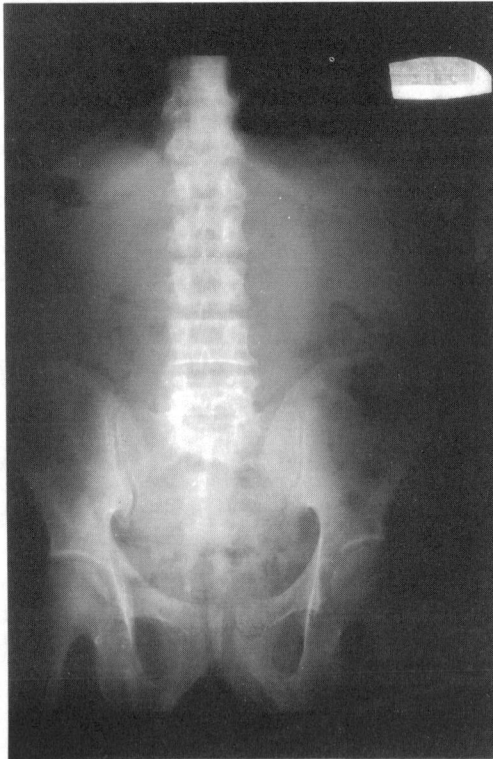

Figure 16.1 Distended stomach in 55-year-old male with gastric outlet obstruction. The stomach is full of food residue which has a mottled appearance. The rest of the abdomen has little intestinal gas.

Bezoar

In patients with a bezoar the stomach contains food, hair or vegetable matter and this may lead to persistent vomiting often with gastric distension.

Gastric volvulus

Gastric volvulus, which may complicate a paraoesophageal (rolling) hernia, may cause acute retrosternal or upper abdominal pain and distress, and the stomach may also become gangrenous.

Intestinal distension

Small bowel obstruction and paralytic ileus

Distension of the central part of the abdomen more than the flanks is characteristic of intestinal distension. The abdomen is often highly tympanitic. There may be visible small bowel loops in a thin patient and also visible peristalsis. The bowel sounds are hyperactive, high-pitched and tinkling if the bowel is still viable. In paralytic ileus there are visible bowel loops but inactive or absent bowel sounds. Distension is associated with gas fluid levels in both small bowel obstruction and paralytic ileus. In small bowel obstruction the gas fluid levels occur in step-ladder pattern from upper left descending to lower

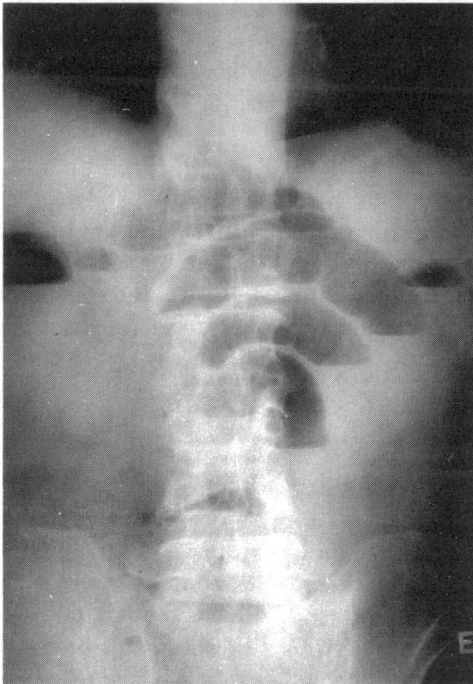

Figure 16.2 Small bowel fluid levels showing a step-ladder pattern in a patient with intestinal obstruction.

right (Figure 16.2) whereas in paralytic ileus they occur at the same level across the abdominal film.

In the early postoperative period (2–10 days) it may be difficult to differentiate between paralytic ileus or obstruction. To determine the cause the first step is to correct potential causes of paralytic ileus such as hypokalaemia. Paralytic ileus should resolve within a few days. Persistence of paralytic ileus may suggest an intra-abdominal abscess, leaking anastomosis, peritonitis or retained foreign body. Colicky pains are common in the resolution phase of paralytic ileus. These are caused by some segments of bowel contracting against others which are still 'paralytic'. These pains resolve within 24 h with passage of flatus. Persistent colicky pains or a high aspirate suggests postoperative intestinal obstruction due to a twist, kink or adhesions.

Large bowel obstruction

Gross colonic distension (e.g. sigmoid volvulus) results in a highly tympanitic abdomen on percussion and a characteristic X-ray appearance (Figure 16.3). In large bowel obstruction the caecum will be grossly distended if the ileocaecal valve is competent. A distended caecum greater than 10 cm should be considered at risk of rupture (Figure 16.4).

Differentiating small and large bowel obstruction on X-ray

On the supine abdominal film when valvae conniventes are visible crossing the entire bowel lumen (Figure 16.5) the distension is due to small bowel. In large bowel obstruction haustrations do not cross the whole lumen but only partially encroach on each side (Figure 16.3). When the ileocaecal valve is incompetent the appearance of small bowel obstruction will be superimposed on that of large bowel obstruction.

Ascites

Another problem is to distinguish between small bowel distension and ascites. In ascites the flanks are more prominently distended than the central abdominal and there is usually a fluid thrill. Shifting dullness is normally present. The X-ray picture shows a ground glass appearance and absence of gaseous distension.

Constipation

Determine whether the patient has absolute constipation (no faeces or flatus). Absolute constipation suggests complete intestinal obstruction or paralytic ileus. In patients with small bowel obstruction the onset of pain may be followed by a single bowel action as the rectum empties its contents. However constipation will normally develop within a few hours.

Always determine the nature of bowel action in the preceding days or weeks. A recent change in bowel habit, or passage of mucus or blood might suggest a colonic neoplasm. Blood in the stool in young children may suggest intussusception.

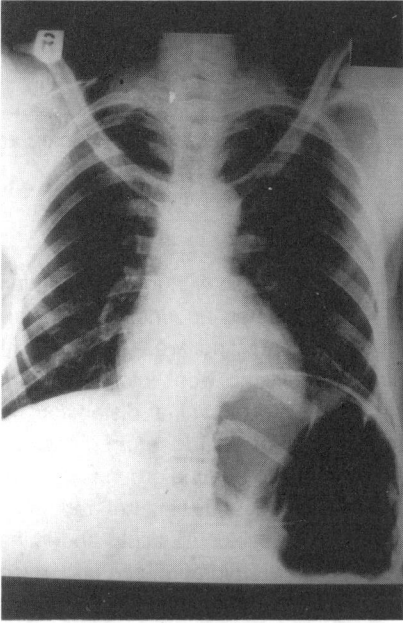

Figure 16.3 Sigmoid volvulus. The distended large bowel is evident beneath the left hemidiaphragm.

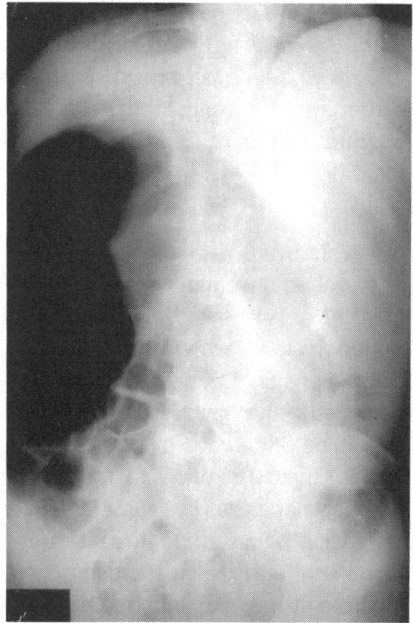

Figure 16.4 Distension of the caecum due to carcinoma of the proximal transverse colon. The distended caecum is at risk of rupture, particularly if it is greater than 10 cm in diameter.

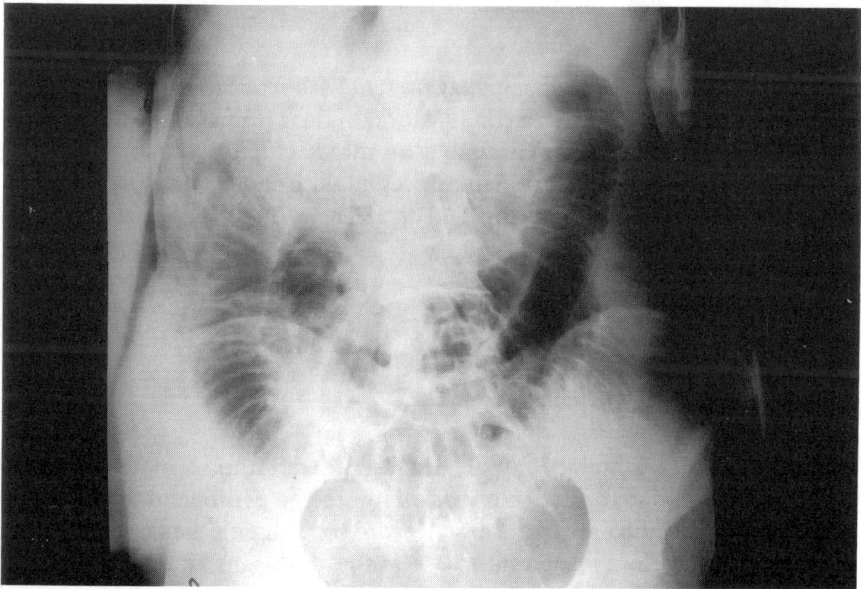

Figure 16.5 Small bowel distension due to intestinal obstruction. Valvae conniventes are seen traversing the whole lumen.

Diarrhoea may complicate intra-abdominal sepsis or a retroileal appendicitis. Patients with typhoid or salmonella enteritis may complain of either diarrhoea or constipation. If the patient has diarrhoea it may sometimes be difficult to distinguish between generalised peritonitis or gastroenteritis. Rectal examination may reveal a pelvic abscess or ultrasound scanning may locate an intraloop abscess.

Case history 3
A 34-year-old woman was 36 weeks pregnant. She presented with lower abdominal pain, fever and some diarrhoea. The obstetrician suspected appendicitis. Her abdominal signs were equivocal so she was observed and was treated with chloramphenicol and metronidazole. The following day she went into labour and delivered a live child. Her recovery was complicated by abdominal distension but abdominal and rectal examination did not suggest peritonitis. Her serum potassium was 2.7 mmol/l so she was treated with a potassium infusion on the grounds that she probably had paralytic ileus. Her fever subsided and she felt better but her abdominal distension persisted. Four days later she deteriorated, developing acute abdominal pain in her right iliac fossa and generalised rigidity. After rehydration she underwent laparotomy and was found to have two perforations in her terminal ileum. The Widal test was negative, probably excluding typhoid. Her abdominal symptoms must have been due to some other enteritis which was difficult to diagnose until perforation and generalised peritonitis ocurred. She made an uneventful recovery and was discharged home on the tenth postoperative day.

Shock

Patients with acute abdominal pain may present with septicaemia, hypovolaemic shock or respiratory failure as a complication of their primary pathology in the abdomen. Occasionally a patient with a ruptured ectopic pregnancy, bleeding hepatoma or abdominal aneurysm may present with sudden collapse or confusion; shock, abdominal distension and tenderness only being discovered on examination.

Early management

Initial assessment

Acute abdominal pathology rapidly leads to deterioration in the patient's general condition due to fluid extravasation into the peritoneum or intestinal lumen, electrolyte imbalance or sepsis. Before focusing on the acutely painful abdomen it is therefore important to assess the vital signs and general condition of the patient. Look particularly for respiratory distress (alar flaring, rapid and shallow breathing with use of accessory muscles) and hypovolaemia (rapid pulse with low volume and cold, clammy hands). Fever, hypotension, respiratory distress, confusion, restlessness or coma are signs that indicate the severity of the patient's condition, and how urgently resuscitation is required.

Often the cause of an acute abdomen cannot be accurately determined by history and examination alone. It is more important to decide whether emergency surgery is required by recognising the signs and symptoms of peritonitis or intestinal obstruction. Most surgeons will be able to decide on clinical grounds whether a laparotomy is needed. The actual cause can then be diagnosed during laparotomy. Investigation may be helpful but should not be ordered if it means delaying an urgent laparotomy for conditions such as appendicitis, peritonitis or intestinal obstruction where gangrenous bowel is suspected. Zachary Cope aptly made this point in rhyme:

> We all have to confess, though with a sigh
> On complicated tests we much rely
> And use too little hand and ear and eye.

Investigations

Specific investigations

The most important diagnostic investigation is an erect chest radiograph which will demonstrate gas or fluid levels under the diaphragm or concomitant pulmonary disease. Pneumonia may cause acute abdominal pain, particularly in children. Abdominal radiographs in the erect and supine positions are the best diagnostic tools in intestinal obstruction (Figures 16.2–16.5). Wherever biliary tract disease is common look carefully for aerobilia on the abdominal films (Figure 16.6). Aerobilia suggests cholecystoduodenal fistula or severe biliary tract sepsis. A serum amylase greater than 3–4 times upper limit of normal is diagnostic of acute pancreatitis. Liver enzymes may help differentiate between acute hepatitis and acute cholecystitis, and between hepatitic and obstructive jaundice. Since most causes of acute abdominal pain have an inflammatory component the white count should be measured, but a raised white count is never diagnostic in its own right. Ultrasound scanning may demonstrate free fluid, an abdominal mass or abscess. It is particularly useful for pancreaticobiliary disorders and for excluding genital tract pathology in the female pelvis. The role of other investigations including paracentesis is discussed in the section on specific diseases.

General investigations

Patients with acute abdominal pathology are prone to fluid and electrolyte imbalance because of gastrointestinal losses and fluid sequestration in the bowel and peritoneal cavity. The urea, electrolytes and creatinine should be checked to ensure the patient is made fit for theatre. Hypokalaemia is particularly important to recognise. Urinalysis should be routinely performed, to-

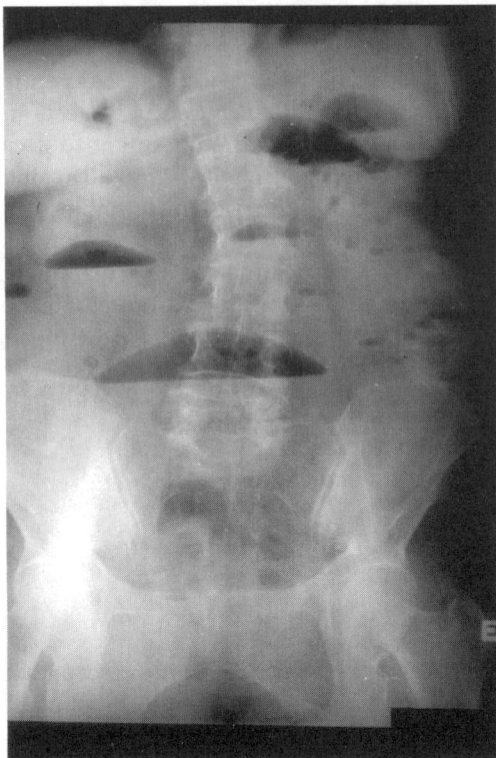

Figure 16.6 Small bowel obstruction and aerobilia in a Chinese patient with cholecystoduodenal fistula and gallstone ileus.

gether with urine microscopy where urinary tract pathology forms part of the differential diagnosis. The haemoglobin or haematocrit levels should be checked or at least estimated clinically. Blood should be cross-matched in preparation for theatre.

Immediate management

The priority is resuscitation to make the patient fit for surgery. This involves intravenous fluid therapy with Hartmann's solution, normal saline, colloid or blood as appropriate. The response to resuscitation should be monitored by repeated assessment of the pulse, blood pressure, peripheries and urine output. In patients with generalised peritonitis, gastric distension or intestinal obstruction, the stomach and upper gastrointestinal tract should be decompressed by nasogastric tube to minimise pressure on the diaphragm (which interferes with ventilation) and to reduce the risk of aspiration of gastric contents on induction of anaesthesia. Where infection is present, broad-spectrum antibiotic therapy should be commenced.

Blood gases or oxygen saturation should be measured in patients with respiratory distress if possible. If they are not available decisions about airway management, oxygen therapy and ventilatory support must be made clinically. In the critically ill patient urethral catheterisation allows measurement of urine output and specific gravity to provide an estimate of circulating volume and renal function. If there is doubt about fluid management after initial resuscitation the central venous pressure can be monitored. If there is a bleeding tendency or severe septicaemia, measure the clotting time and order a coagulation profile.

Analgesia

Give generous analgesia early unless the cause of pain is a distended bladder. A number of studies have shown that analgesia does not interfere with clinical assessment of the acute abdomen. Do not delay the administration of analgesia awaiting referral or a senior opinion. Give pethidine 1 mg/kg or morphine 0.1 mg/kg by intravenous bolus. The actual dose should be titrated against its effect on the patient.

17

Intestinal Obstruction

Intestinal obstruction implies a blockage to the distal flow of intestinal contents. The onset may be acute, subacute or chronic. Psuedo-obstruction is a condition in which the bowel is distended and inactive but there is no blockage. Megacolon implies gross distension of the colon and may be due to chronic obstruction or impaired bowel motility.

Pathophysiology

Considerable collection of fluid in the intestinal lumen may occur proximal to the site of the obstruction. Abdominal distension impairs ventilation by upward pressure on the chest and there is also the risk of aspiration. Once strangulation of the bowel occurs micro-organisms cross the intestinal wall and enter the portal circulation and the peritoneal cavity. Endotoxaemia or peritonitis may complicate the picture. Once the bowel is ischaemic and becomes gangrenous signs of peritonitis are superimposed on those of intestinal obstruction so that the obstructed, high-pitched, hyperactive bowel sounds diminish in frequency and the abdomen eventually becomes quiet. By this stage the patient normally has severe toxaemia.

Clinical presentation (see also pp 297–304)

The presentation of acute intestinal obstruction varies according to the site of blockage and whether or not there is gangrene of the bowel.
The following presentations will be seen:

1. **Vomiting without generalised distension.** There may still be epigastric fullness or distension. Pain is variable. The site of obstruction is in the duodenum or proximal jejunum.
2. **Colicky pain, vomiting, generalised distension and constipation.** Bowel sounds are high pitched, tinkling and hyperactive. The site of obstruction is in small bowel or ileocaecal region.

3. **Cramping colicky central or lower abdominal pain, constipation and distension.** Vomiting is variable. The site of obstruction is in the large bowel. If the ileocaecal valve is incompetent, small bowel obstruction may be superimposed on the large bowel obstruction.
4. **Pictures 2 or 3 above with signs of peritonitis and absent bowel sounds.** Bowel strangulation has occurred. The patient may have toxaemia and hypotension and be in respiratory distress.

The clinical features of vomiting, distension and constipation have already been fully discussed in the context of acute abdominal pain (pp 300–306).

Duodenal and proximal jejunal obstruction

The causes are pancreatic neoplasm, anular pancreas causing duodenal obstruction, pancreatic pseudocyst or abscess, obstruction of the third part of the duodenum by the superior mesenteric artery (Wilkie's syndrome), neoplasm of the transverse colon, fibrosis associated with a gastroenterostomy, masses pressing on the proximal jejunum, adhesions, malrotation and jejunal volvulus.

The patient has persistent bile-stained vomiting (unless due to pancreatic neoplasm with obstructive jaundice), and gastric rather than abdominal distension (full epigastrium with a succussion splash). Endoscopy is normal but barium meal and follow through will show the site of the lesion or at least failure of contrast to progress through the small bowel. Surgical resection or bypass of the obstructing lesion will be required.

Small bowel obstruction

The commonest causes of small bowel obstruction are hernia and adhesions in the adult and intussusception (ileoileal and ileocaecal) (Figure 17.1a & b) and worm bolus (ascaris) in children (p 383). Table 17.1 shows other causes for bowel obstruction which may be classified as luminal, mural and extramural. The incidence of different causes varies from region to region. For example, in adults in West Africa inguinal hernia is the commonest cause of small bowel obstruction.

Large bowel obstruction

Sigmoid volvulus is common throughout sub-Saharan Africa but is rare in the South Pacific and South-East Asia. In Hong Kong and Singapore, where a high proportion of the population is elderly, colorectal carcinoma is the commonest cause of large bowel obstruction. Colocolic intussusception in both adults and children is much more common in the tropics than developed nations and is often due to infection rather than a tumour.

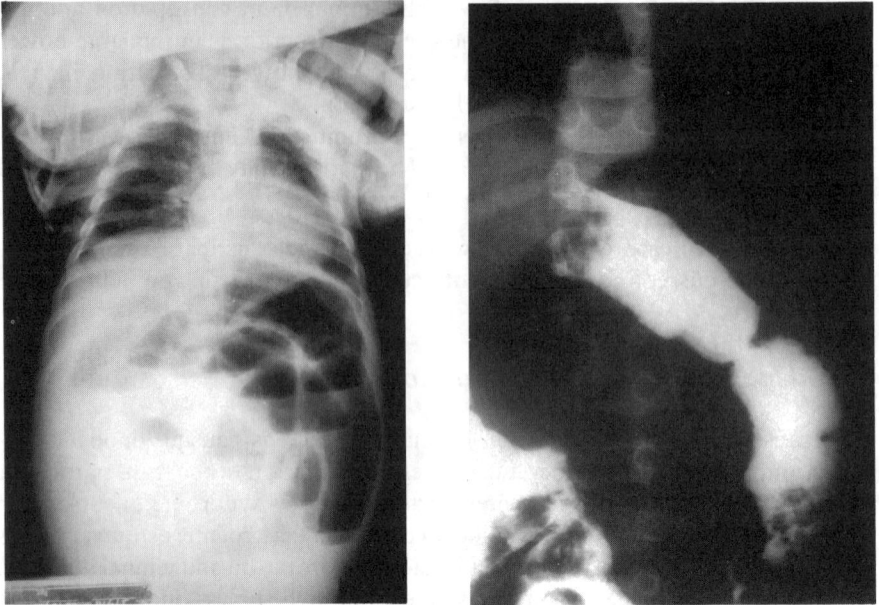

Figure 17.1 *Left* Gas-fluid levels of small bowel obstruction in a Melanesian child with intussusception. Note the absence of gas in the right iliac fossa.
Right Barium enema showing the point of the intussusception in transverse colon. In this case operative reduction of the intussusception was required because the intussusception had been present for 72 hours and barium enema reduction was not successful.

Table 17.1 Causes of intestinal obstruction.

Luminal
  Worm bolus
  Food bolus
  Gallstone
  Foreign body (Figure 17.2 abc)
  Imperforate anus

Mural
  Intussusception
  Tumour, e.g. lymphoma, adenocarcinoma
  Stricture – ischaemic, amoebic, schistosomal, radiation, tuberculous, malignant
  Diverticular disease (rare)
  Hirschprung's disease
  Congenital atresias

Extramural
  Adhesions
  Hernia, internal (e.g. paraduodenal, obturator, sciatic), external (inguinal, femoral, paraumbilical)
  Volvulus
  Abdominal masses, abscesses and tumours
  Duplications

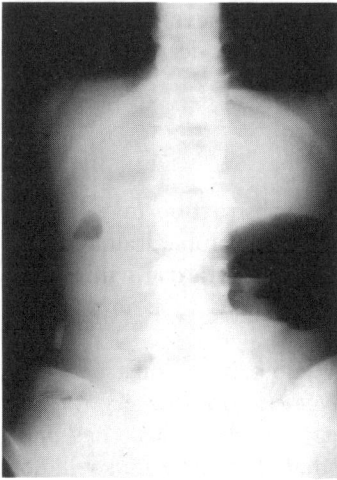

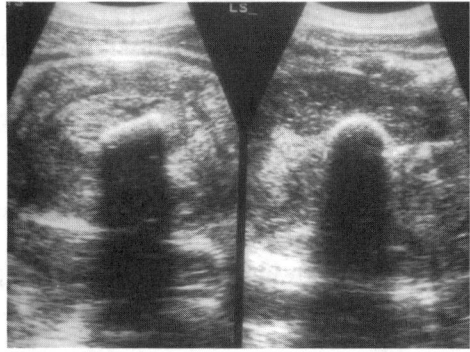

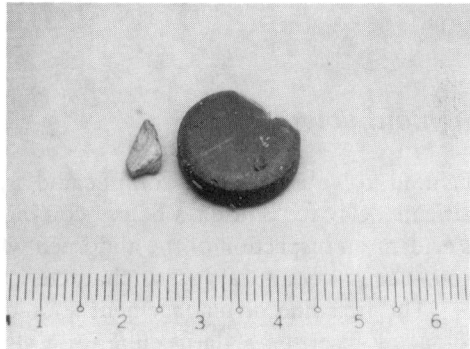

Figure 17.2 Small bowel obstruction. A foreign body is visible in the right iliac fossa on plain X-ray (*above*) which was also demonstrated on ultrasound (*above right*) and proved to be a tablet blocking the ileo-caecal junction at laparotomy (*right*). (*above right* courtesy of Dr R. Evans).

Management

The cause of intestinal obstruction may often not be known before operation. It is therefore important to recognise obstruction so that surgery is not delayed, particularly when strangulation of the bowel is likely. Gangrene of the bowel is associated with a higher mortality.

The first priorities in management are resuscitation with rehydration and correction of electrolyte abnormalities. The aim is to make the patient fit for theatre and then operate early (within 12 h) if there is a complete obstruction and adhesions are not the most likely cause. Operate even earlier if there are signs of strangulation.

Hernia

Inguinal hernia is by far the commonest reason for small bowel obstruction in most parts of the tropics. An obstructed hernia requires emergency surgery, hopefully before strangulation occurs. An irreducible hernia without complications requires elective surgery. In the tropics many patients have long-standing hernias which are never repaired due to lack of surgical services.

Previous abdominal surgery

If the patient has an abdominal scar, the cause of obstruction may be adhesions. Adhesive obstruction may settle with nasogastric tube drainage and rehydration with intravenous fluids. The patient should improve within 24–48 h. If he or she does not, or there are signs of strangulation, the obstruction must be relieved surgically.

The reason for a more conservative approach with adhesive obstruction is that there is more chance of spontaneous improvement, and surgery for adhesions becomes more hazardous the more operations the patient has had. Dividing one set of adhesions offers no guarantee that more adhesions will not form.

Sigmoid volvulus

Sigmoid volvulus is often complicated by strangulation, particularly where patients delay for 3–4 days before coming to hospital. The colonic distension is evident on inspection of the abdomen which is grossly tympanitic to percussion. The X-ray appearance is characteristic (Figure 16.3).

The first line of management should be to try and deflate the sigmoid colon, by inserting a flatus tube up a sigmoidoscope. This strategy is often successful in early cases but once the volvulus has been present for some days or strangulation has occurred it will not succeed, and persistence may perforated the colon. Once the colon has been deflated, the obstruction is relieved, the volvulus untwists and the urgency of surgical resection is gone. However, the author believes it is best to perform sigmoid resection and primary anastomosis during the same hospital admission. Many patients, if discharged with a date for elective surgery, may not reattend, and then suffer a recurrence and die. Studies suggest that sigmoid volvulus recurs in 75–90 per cent of cases. Elective resection with primary anastomosis can be performed a few days later after bowel preparation.

When deflation is unsuccessful or contraindicated by strangulation emergency laparotomy is undertaken. The operative management depends on whether the bowel is viable or not.

Gangrenous bowel

If the bowel is gangrenous it is wise not to untwist it during resection since untwisting would infuse a large amount of toxic products into the circulation. Primary anastomosis is difficult in the presence of gangrenous bowel and most surgeons advocate Hartmann's procedure, which involves a temporary colostomy. This operation is safe for all surgeons in the emergency situation. Leaving a long rectal stump tagged to the anterior abdominal wall by a non-absorbable suture makes subsequent identification and closure much easier. Later, closure of the colostomy demands a formal large bowel anastomosis and should be performed by an experienced surgeon. Colostomies are particularly difficult to manage in the tropics because of erratic supplies of colostomy bags but these difficulties should not endanger the life of the patient by making the surgeon feel he must 'anastomose at all costs'. If the patient will not go home with a colostomy the Hartmann's can be closed after 3 weeks.

Viable bowel

When the bowel is viable resection should still be performed. There is no place for sigmoidopexy operations or just undoing the twist because recurrence is almost certain. Only if the doctor performing the surgery is not able to resect the bowel safely should the volvulus be undone and the abdomen closed. Resection and primary anastomosis is safe for viable bowel providing the operator can confidently perform an anastomosis. Primary anastomosis will save patients the problems of a temporary colostomy in the tropics.

Abdominal cocoon and peritoneal encapsulation

Abdominal cocoon is a rare cause of acute or subacute obstruction affecting girls in which small bowel becomes coiled up inside a thick membrane. The membrane should be incised and resected to relieve the obstruction.

Peritoneal encapsulation is a similar but distinct condition affecting both sexes. The entire small bowel lies within an accessory but otherwise normal peritoneal membrane. It is probably a derivative of the peritoneum of the yolk sac.

Acute psuedo-obstruction

Acute colonic psuedo-obstruction (Ogilvie's syndrome) describes a clinical condition in which the symptoms, signs and radiological appearances of large bowel obstruction are present but without any mechanical cause. There is transient impairment of bowel motility, probably due to failure of the sacral autonomic parasympathetic nerves. The diagnosis should be considered in a hospitalised patient with colicky abdominal pain, progressive distension and constipation, who is recovering from childbirth, pelvic surgery, spinal trauma or some systemic illness. A large number of pathologies and drugs including opiates and antidepressants have been implicated. The abdomen is often grossly distended but tenderness and signs of peritonism are less than expected. The rectum is normally empty. The abdominal radiograph will show a grossly dilated colon, mainly distended by gas rather than fluid. Perforation may occur and result in pneumoperitoneum.

If the diagnosis is suspected and the patient does not show signs of perforation or peritonitis, a contrast enema and sigmoidoscopy or colonoscopy should be performed to exclude other pathologies and perhaps decompress the colon. Saline enemas should precede these procedures. Fluid and electrolyte imbalances should be corrected and potentiating drugs such as opiates stopped. Conservative management with nasogastric drainage and intravenous fluids is advised. Failure to resolve, increasing dilatation of the caecum beyond 12 cm or signs of perforation or peritonitis are indications for surgery. Caecostomy may be the simplest form of decompression in a sick patient with a viable caecum. Ischaemia of the caecum requires right hemicolectomy.

Megacolon

Megacolon presents with constipation and abdominal distension. There will be faecal loading and often faecal impaction.

In a child, megacolon is normally the result of short-segment Hirschprung's disease or missed incomplete anorectal malformation. The diagnosis is made by appropriate perineal examination, proctosigmoidoscopy and rectal biopsies at the anorectal ring and lower rectum.

In adults, megacolon following childbirth or uterine prolpase may be due to stretching of the pelvic parasympathetic nerves. In developed countries chronic constipation and straining may also predispose to pelvic floor descent and parasympathetic impairment. Chronic laxative abuse or application of enemas may compromise bowel motility.

Chagas' disease

In South and Central America Chagas' disease due to *Trypanosoma cruzi* is endemic. In the chronic phase of the disease denervation of the colon may develop due to destruction of the myenteric plexus. This phase normally develops in the fourth and fifth decades of life. There are considerable regional variations in the incidence of megacolon in Chagas' disease. Clinically, megacolon manifests as constipation, difficulty in discharging even soft faeces and distension, often with palpable faecal masses. The rectoanal reflex may be absent on anorectal manomery. Diagnosis is by serology and xenodiagnosis or haemoculture, the latter two being successful in no more than 45–50 per cent of cases.

There is no evidence that chronic disease can be reversed by chemotherapy with Nifurtimox and Benzonidazole, although they may suppress parasitaemia. The management is similar to other causes of megacolon and begins with diet, laxatives and judicious use of enemas to prevent faecal impaction and gross abdominal distension. Where failure of the internal sphincter to relax is a major factor myectomy or sphinctertomy may be indicated.

Other large bowel emergencies

Colorectal carcinoma commonly presents with obstruction in the tropics and is discussed on pp 403–5. Western large bowel diseases are beginning to emerge in the urbanised population of some developing countries (pp 177–9).

Diverticular disease

Diverticular disease is characterised by thickening of the muscle coat of the colon and the presence of diverticula, which are mucosal pouches prolapsing through the colon wall between the mesenteric and antimesenteric taenia. Diverticula are created by a combination of high intraluminal pressures and weakness of the wall. They usually develop in elderly caucasians in sixth or seventh decades. There are sporadic reports of diverticular disease from sub-Saharan Africa including Ghana, Zimbabwe, Uganda and Nigeria.

Clinical presentation

Diverticula may become inflamed (diverticulitis) and present with lower abdominal pain and peritonitis. Inflammed diverticula may perforate and cause generalised peritonitis. Alternatively the perforation may be contained by omentum and surrounding structures and so form a diverticular abscess which may present as a tender mass in the left iliac fossa. Adherence of an inflammed diverticulum to an adjacent structure such as bladder or small bowel may result in an internal fistula developing. Diverticulitis may also present with haemorrhage due to erosion of the adjacent blood vessel in the wall of the colon.

Management

If generalised peritonitis or intestinal obstruction develops the patient will require emergency laparotomy and a Hartmann's procedure. A tender diverticular mass or abscess usually settles on bed rest, nil by mouth and antibiotics. Bleeding usually settles with conservative treatment. The diagnosis can then be confirmed by barium enema after the acute episode has settled. The openings of the diverticula can often be seen on sigmoidoscopy or colonoscopy which should be performed to exclude malignancy. The patient should be treated by high roughage diet to lower intracolonic pressures. A small proportion of cases who suffer recurrent attacks require elective resection of the affected colonic segment. Recurrent attacks of diverticulitis may shorten and narrow the bowel so that a stricture develops and results in subacute or acute intestinal obstruction.

Inflammatory bowel disease

Both Crohn's disease and ulcerative colitis are rare in the tropics. Cases have been reported from Southern Africa, and the Indian sub-continent. Patients with inflammatory bowel disease may present with weight loss and bloody diarrhoea, associated joint, skin or eye inflammation, intestinal obstruction, anorectal problems (fissure or fistula), or toxic dilatation of the colon. The diagnosis is made by colonoscopy or sigmoidoscopy, biopsy and barium enema. Treatment is largely medical using topical or systemic steroids (10–30 mg prednisolone per day) to induce remission and Salazopyrin (sulphasalazine) (1–3 g per day) to maintain remission. Complications such as intestinal obstruction or toxic dilatation of the colon may require emergency surgery. A detailed description of inflammatory bowel disease and its treatment is beyond the scope of this book.

Further reading

Archampong EQ. Diverticular disease in an indigenous African community. Ann R Coll Surg Engl 1978;60:464–70.

Dorudi S, Berry AR, Kettlewell MGW. Acute colonic psuedo-obstruction. Br J Surg 1992;79:99–103.

Ihekwaba FN. Diverticular disease of the colon in black Africa. J R Coll Surg Edinb 1992;37:107–9.

Iwatt AR, Inyang UE, Udoeyop UW, Essiet A. Emergency large bowel surgery in a tropical environment: approach and outcome. Int Surg 1990;75:191–4.

Sengupta SK, Sinha SN. Clinicopathological features of primary gastrointestinal lymphomas: a study of 42 cases. Aust N Z J Surg 1991;61:133–6.

Sigmoid volvulus

Faranisi CT. Primary resection and anastomosis for sigmoid volvulus. Proc Assoc Surg E Afr 1989;12–15.

Ofiaeli RO. Volvulus of the sigmoid colon – a reappraisal. Trop Doct 1993;23:23–4.

Shepherd JJ. Treatment of volvulus of the sigmoid colon: a review of 425 cases. Br M J 1968;2:280–3.

18

Peritonitis and Pigbel

Peritonitis

In the tropics the commonest non-traumatic causes of peritonitis are appendicitis, perforated duodenal ulcer, tubo-ovarian infection, typhoid perforation and amoebic colitis. A ruptured amoebic liver abscess and ruptured abdominal tubercular lesion are common causes of peritonitis at the All India Institute. Perforation or inflammation of any intra-abdominal viscus may give rise to peritonitis which may then be complicated by septicaemia. Death may result without urgent treatment. Where the patient survives the acute phase of peritonitis without treatment he may present with a subphrenic or intra-abdominal abscess. Despite surgery, peritonitis has a high mortality, often in excess of 10 per cent in many tropical hospitals. Long duration of peritonitis is correlated with a high mortality as is a distal gastrointestinal source of inflammation – faecal peritonitis from a perforated colon is worse than chemical peritonitis from a perforated duodenal ulcer. Postoperative peritonitis is associated with a mortality rate of around 30 per cent and when peritonitis complicates the ascites of chronic liver or renal disease the rate is even higher.

Blood also irritates the peritoneal cavity. Common causes of intraperitoneal bleeding include ruptured ectopic pregnancy, bleeding hepatoma and delayed rupture of a traumatised spleen. Ruptured aortic (retroperitoneal) or an intra-abdominal aneurysm may also occur.

Clinical recognition

History

The patient complains of generalised abdominal pain. The speed and site of onset may suggest a possible cause. The clinical features of each cause are described elsewhere in the book. Table 18.1 provides a summary. If the pain was initially due to distension of a tubular structure (e.g. the appendix or fallopian tube), rupture may be characterised by a lessening in the intensity of

319

Table 18.1 Symptoms associated with different causes of peritonitis.

Symptoms	Probable cause
Acute epigastric, severe, rapid onset	Perforated duodenal or gastric ulcer
Acute epigastric, severe, radiating to back history of alcohol intake	Acute pancreatitis
Jaundice, upper abdominal pain, fever (Charcot's triad)	Acute cholangitis
Central abdominal pain for 7–10 days, headache	Typhoid
Central abdominal pain shifting to right iliac fossa	Appendicitis
Vaginal discharge, lower abdominal pain	Tubo-ovarian sepsis
Bloody diarrhoea for a few days	Amoebic colitis
Recent criminal abortion	Perforated uterus
Lower abdominal pain, missed period, faint	Ruptured ectopic pregnancy
Faint, collapse, shock	Intra-abdominal haemorrhage

pain, which gradually becomes more generalised as the whole peritoneal cavity becomes involved.

Examination

The patient with peritonitis looks toxic, anxious, restless and in obvious pain. Movement aggravates the pain so he lies immobile and uncomfortable. Sweating, tachycardia, tachypnoea with flaring of the nares, use of the accessory muscles of respiration and fever are evident on general examination. Fluid extravasation into the peritoneal cavity and intestinal lumen due to paralytic ileus cause hypovolaemia. Septicaemia may result in initially hyperdynamic, peripheral circulation (warm hands, feet and nasal tip), though later vasoconstriction (cold and clammy hands, feet and nasal tip) supervenes due to hypovolaemia. If there is a delay in presenting to hospital the anxious, restless look is replaced by a haunted, disinterested one in which the eyes are sunken. After a few days there may be a tinge of jaundice due to cholestasis.

> The sunken cheeks, the dark rings round the eyes,
> The beads of sweat which on the forehead rise,
> The haunted look, all tell at any age
> Peritonitis in the latest stage
> (Zachary Cope)

The abdominal signs of peritonitis are listed in Table 18.2.

In chemical peritonitis (bile, gastric acid or pancreatic enzymes), pain is often intense and the abdomen is board-like in its rigidity. There is so much rigidity that there may be little obvious distension. In infective or faecal peritonitis there is generalised tenderness and guarding combined with increasing distension due to peritoneal exudate and ileus. The peritoneal reaction to

Table 18.2 The abdominal signs of peritonitis.

Abdomen moves poorly or not all with respiration
Distension
Guarding and rigidity
Tenderness and rebound tenderness
Absent bowel sounds

blood is more variable and sometimes abdominal rigidity is less marked with only generalised tenderness, a little guarding and distension (Case history 2, p 297). Patients with hepatomegaly, distension and shock may be bleeding from a hepatoma. Abdominal rigidity and guarding arise as a result of acute inflammation of the peritoneal cavity. Once the intensity of acute inflammation starts to subside and reflex muscle contraction becomes exhausted the abdominal wall softens. The abdomen remains distended but feels a little thick. If the patient survives and presents later during the resolution phase, 2–3 weeks after the onset of bacterial peritonitis, the abdomen feels thick, firm and doughy. Bowel sounds return and as the temperature swings, the patient seems to step out of the grave. There may be signs of a localised subphrenic, pelvic or other intra-abdominal abscess which requires aspiration or drainage.

Practice point
- *Do not forget to perform a rectal or vaginal examination in patients with suspected peritonitis. A pelvic abscess or female genital tract source of sepsis may be detected.*

Critically ill patients and those who have had recent surgery may be particularly difficult to assess. In critically ill patients the abdominal signs of peritonitis may be vague. Peritonitis may present as unexplained renal or respiratory failure or hypotension. In spontaneous bacterial peritonitis secondary to hepatic cirrhosis with acites, abdominal signs are absent in at least a third of patients. Nausea, vomiting and diarrhoea associated with a deterioration in renal or hepatic function may be the only indicator of the development of peritonitis. Postoperative peritonitis may be suspected when distension and tenderness persist after abdominal surgery, often with a swinging fever and raised white count. Rigidity and guarding are often absent so that differentiating postoperative peritonitis from paralytic ileus may be difficult. Always consider the possibility of peritonitis or intra-abdominal abscess if the original reason for laparotomy was sepsis or where an anastomosis may be leaking. Relaparotomy is best performed early not after days of indecision. Where the peritoneal cavity was originally very septic with multiple pockets of thick pus, a planned relaparotomy 48–72 h later is sometimes better than waiting for deterioration to occur. In selected cases of severe established peritonitis the abdomen may not be closed normally but rather the wound edges approximated with tension sutures or a Marlex mesh with a zipper to facilitate multiple relaparotomies and peritoneal toilet.

Investigations

Investigations are not normally necessary to diagnose the presence of peritonitis but may suggest a cause.

Radiographs

A chest X-ray in the erect position may show gas or a fluid level under the diaphragm. There may be basal atelectasis or a small pleural effusion accompanying a subphrenic abscess. A supine abdominal X-ray may show fluid between thickened bowel loops if peritonitis is established (Figure 18.1). Gaseous distension and fluid levels all at the same level across the abdomen are characteristic of paralytic ileus on an erect abdominal X-ray. A plain film may show calcification in an aortic aneurysm.

Paracentesis

Paracentesis should not be performed routinely, but only in doubtful cases

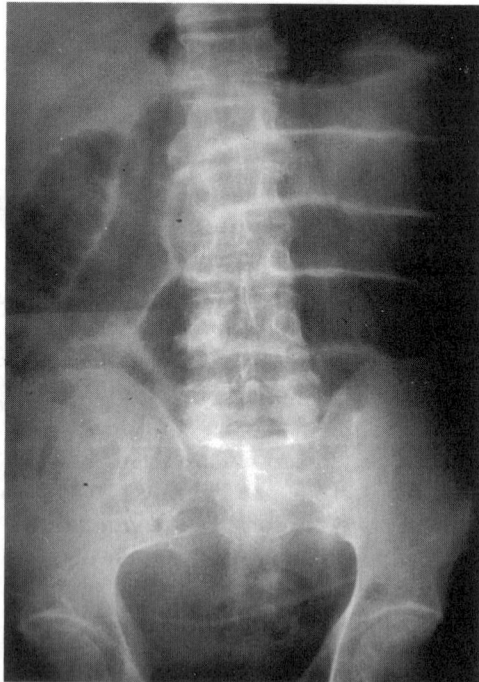

Figure 18.1 Distended small bowel loops are thickened and there is free fluid between the loops of bowel. Patients with this X-ray appearance normally require surgery.

with abdominal distension and suspected free fluid. A four-quadrant tap with a 21-gauge needle is unlikely to cause iatrogenic damage to the intestines. It may be impossible to aspirate thick pus through such a thin needle so a negative tap does not exclude peritonitis.

Ultrasound scanning

Ultrasound scanning may show intraperitoneal fluid or an abscess collection but resuscitation and laparotomy should never be delayed awaiting an ultrasound in cases where the diagnosis of peritonitis is obvious.

Blood tests

The blood count will show leucocytosis. Blood should be cross-matched in preparation for surgery and urea and electrolytes checked.

Serum amylase should be measured if acute pancreatitis is a possible cause and if the reagents are available. It is often difficult to distinguish between acute pancreatitis and a perforated duodenal ulcer without an amylase, since 30 per cent of cases of perforated ulcer do not have gas under the diaphragm. The serum amylase level must be 3–4 times the upper limit of normal before it can be considered diagnostic of acute pancreatitis as other causes of the acute abdomen including perforated peptic ulcer, acute cholecystitis, intestinal obstruction and ruptured aortic aneurysm can also raise the level of serum amylase.

Management

Generalised peritonitis

Before surgery the patient must be resuscitated so that hypovolaemia, electrolyte imbalance and respiratory failure are treated. The urine output should be monitored by indwelling catheter in critically ill patients. Oliguria may not improve until after the peritoneal cavity has been cleared of sepsis. Broad-spectrum systemic antibiotics should be commenced.

The aim of laparotomy is to eradicate the source of contamination. Peritoneal lavage with saline or tetracycline in saline (1 g/l) is effective in cleaning the peritoneal cavity. Localised abscess cavities should be drained, but normally drains are not inserted because drainage of the peritoneal cavity as a whole cannot be achieved. Sometimes a tube drain to the pelvis or subphrenic space is advisable if there is thick pus in a partially walled-off cavity.

After surgery some patients are critically ill, needing oxygen therapy and mechanical ventilation. Renal failure may develop so it is important to monitor the urine output. In the tropics a bleeding tendency due to disseminated intravascular coagulation (DIC) is best managed by transfusion of fresh whole blood.

Female genital tract sepsis

In tubo-ovarian sepsis where peritonitis is localised to the pelvis a trial of 24–48 h antibiotic therapy may be indicated in stable patients. However if the patient is deteriorating or a tender mass is enlarging, earlier laparotomy is mandatory. Rupture of a tubo-ovarian abscess carries a high risk of mortality. In the absence of generalised peritonitis a pelvic abscess can sometimes be drained through the vaginal fornix (culpotomy) or rectum. If it is suspected that the uterus is perforated or gangrenous, then laparotomy with a view to hysterectomy should be performed as soon as the patient is resuscitated. Failure to remove the source of sepsis often results in inadequate control of peritonitis and, ultimately, death of the patient.

Intra-abdominal and subphrenic abscess

Recognition

The key to diagnosis is to suspect it. There is usually a known potential cause even though the surgeon may be reluctant to admit it in a patient after surgery. Abdominal tenderness, distension and paralytic ileus are common signs. The patient may be febrile and confused. A mass may be palpable abdominally or rectally. Sometimes the abscess will cause diarrhoea due to its proximity to the bowel or vomiting if it presses on the stomach or duodenum. Ultrasound examination may demonstrate the abscess and allow aspiration. Leucocytosis with markedly increased neutrophils will be present. Subphrenic abscess may also be accompanied by intercostal tenderness with signs of atelectasis in the lower chest. A chest X-ray may show a gas-fluid level under a raised hemi-diaphragm, basal atelectasis and sometimes a small pleural effusion. Diaphragmatic movement may be absent on the affected side when viewed on X-ray screening. Ultrasound or computed tomography (CT) scanning may demonstrate the abscess cavity and allow aspiration. In around 10 per cent of cases a subphrenic abscess may be complicated by empyema which is treated by intercostal drainage.

Management

Solitary intra-abdominal abscesses without signs of generalised peritonitis should be managed by aspiration if this can be accurately performed under ultrasound or CT control. Aspiration can be repeated if the cavity persists on follow-up scanning. In the absence of ultrasound or CT scanning it is often worthwhile to perform blind aspiration at the site of maximum intercostal tenderness (for subphrenic or liver abscess) or into a tender, fluctuant mass. A 21-gauge needle rarely does any harm in this situation. If the condition of the patient deteriorates, the pus is too thick to aspirate or aspiration is not possible, then localised drainage of the abscess cavity by open operation should be performed. It is often possible to obtain extraperitoneal drainage which spares contamination of the rest of the peritoneal cavity. Drainage is normally accompanied by a marked improvement in the patient's condition. Where an abscess is associated with generalised peritonitis urgent laparotomy is required.

Intestinal fistula

Free drainage of faeces or intestinal contents through the drain site denotes an intestinal fistula. In the absence of generalised peritonitis the fistula should be treated conservatively in the first instance. The patient should be given nil by mouth (for a small bowel fistula) and receive parenteral nutrition. A distal small bowel or large bowel fistula can often be managed without central feeding.

Intestinal fistulae heal spontaneously in about three-quarters of cases provided there is no distal obstruction, no persistent intra-abdominal sepsis and the patient receives nutritional support. The absence of obstruction in the distal bowel can be established by contrast studies performed through the fistula. Supportive care includes protection of the skin by good stoma care, maintaining fluid and electrolyte balance and giving nutritional support.

Surgery is indicated to drain intra-abdominal infection, if the bowel mucosa is visible at the fistula site on the skin, if there is distal obstruction or if the fistula fails to close within 6 weeks. If parenteral nutrition is not available then early surgery with closure of the fistula is advised for high output fistulae discharging more than 500 ml per day. Surgery for intestinal fistula is difficult and tedious and should be undertaken by someone with experience.

Typhoid peritonitis (see also page 38)

The rate of perforation varies throughout the tropics, from approximately 5 per cent in Cairo and South Africa to 8–18 per cent in West Africa. Perforation most commonly affects children and young adults and has traditionally conferred a high mortality. In Ghana, where perforation is a common problem the mortality has been reduced to 5 per cent by an aggressive surgical approach to management.

The diagnosis depends on awareness of the possibility in endemic areas. Typical symptoms include prodromal fever, headache, joint pains, vomiting and distension with abdominal tenderness and variable guarding. The diagnosis may be difficult when perforation occurs while the patient is already on medical treatment which may mask or delay the signs of peritonitis in an already sick patient. Also, when perforation occurs days before admission the dominant clinical presentation is distension rather than tenderness and guarding. Leukocytosis is the norm and usually gross, though about 5 per cent will have leukopaenia. Abdominal and chest radiographs only show pneumoperitoneum in 10–20 per cent of cases.

The treatment of typhoid perforation is resuscitation, laparotomy and support of failing systems. At surgery the perforated ulcer (or ulcers) can be biopsied and closed by suture. Resection is not normally required despite the gross appearance of multiple ulcers. The patients are usually critically ill and respond best to swift and simple surgery after being well resuscitated. Postoperative complications occur frequently, the commonest being wound infection, bronchopneumonia and enterocutaneous fistula. Reperforation occurs in about 3 per cent.

Fulminating and complicated amoebic colitis

The clinical presentation is variable and mimicks many other conditions in endemic areas. Distal bowel disease presents with diarrhoea, blood and mucus in the stool but lesions of the right colon may present with normal bowel actions or even constipation. Abdominal pain and distension are present, tenderness is often mild, even when there is perforation. When amoebic colitis is suspected multiple tissue biopsies should be taken at proctosigmoidoscopy and fresh stools should be examined for haematophagous amoebae (p 45).

Mucosal amoebiasis usually responds to metronidazole. Transmural disease involves the entire thickness of the colonic wall and results in ischaemic necrosis which can be complicated later by perforation. Metronidazole will not cure ischaemic necrosis. Transmural disease that fails to respond to antibiotics or is complicated by perforation, colonic dilatation or bleeding requires surgery. Failure to respond within 48 h to metronidazole given in a dose of 800 mg 8-hourly orally or 500 mg 8-hourly intravenously indicates that transmural disease is present and surgery is required. A satisfactory response is indicated by disappearance of distension, reduction in abdominal tenderness, improved well-being and decrease in diarrhoea.

Where surgery is indicated the colon will be covered with omentum. These omental wraps should be left intact. The peritoneal cavity should be lavaged, the colon washed out and a loop ileostomy performed to decompress the colon. After 6 weeks a gentle barium enema should be performed to assess the patency of the colon. If there is a stricture, it should be resected before the ileostomy is closed.

Pigbel: enteritis necroticans

Pigbel is the colourful name given to the condition of enteritis necroticans as it occurs in Papua New Guinea. The first description of a case of pigbel was recorded in 1959, and thereafter it rapidly became apparent that 'necrotising jejunitis', 'necrotic enteritis' or 'necrotising enteritis' was a highly important cause of mortality and morbidity in the Highlands provinces of Papua New

Guinea. In Goroka hospital it was second only to pneumonia as a cause of death in children over the age of 12 months. It was apparent at an early stage that there was a close relationship between the condition and the occurrence of feasting in the highlands communities, at which large amounts of pig meat were consumed, hence the name pigbel ('bel' means stomach). Pathologically, and clinically, the condition appeared to be the same as 'Darmbrand' or Hamburg Disease, an epidemic of necrotising enterocolitis described in Germany in the late 1940s.

Necrotising enterocolitis was apparently well known to and described by ancient and medieval medical writers. The circumstances resulting in gut necrosis by toxins produced by an overgrowth of anaerobic organisms are certainly not unique to Papua New Guinea, and necrotising enteritis has been described in other countries including Uganda, Solomon Islands, Bangladesh, and People's Republic of China. It is therefore important that all doctors – and particularly those working in the poorer and less 'developed' areas of the world are aware of the possibility of necrotising enterocolitis as a possible cause of abdominal pain and unexplained peritonitis.

Pathophysiology

The unravelling of the aetiology of pigbel – involving surgeons, physicians, paediatricians, epidemiologists, microbiologists and veterinarians makes fascinating reading. The factors involved appear to be:

1. A high environmental prevalence of *Clostridium perfringens* type C resulting in food contamination and possibly the presence of this organism in the human gut.
2. A changed intestinal environment caused by a sudden and unaccustomed high animal protein load in a person whose normal diet consists of sweet potato and other vegetables.
3. Rapid proliferation of the *Clostridium perfringens* type C in this changed environment and its production of B toxin.
4. Low levels of upper intestinal proteolytic activity resulting from proteolytic inhibitors in the dietary staple – the sweet potato – and produced by intestinal parasites, principally *Ascaris*, which fail to destroy the increased levels of clostridial B toxin.
5. B-toxin-mediated damage to the gut surface, impairing gut motility, and resulting in adherence of the clostridia with further toxin production, damage and the characteristic necrosis.

The final aspect of the fascinating story of pigbel was the introduction of a toxoid vaccine, given to infants at the same time as the triple antigen vaccine, which has been highly successful in preventing what was once a common, feared, and often fatal disease. Cases of pigbel are still seen, but the incidence has been greatly reduced.

Presentation

There is a spectrum of presentation from mild, with spontaneous recovery, to fulminating and death within a matter of hours. Pain is a constant feature. It is usually severe. It is often continuous, but may have colicky exacerbations. Vomiting is common and the presence of flecks of altered blood indicates a severe form of the disease. Abdominal distension is also common. In general, the more distended the abdomen, the more severe the disease. Diarrhoea is an early feature. Blood staining is a marker of severity and frank bleeding may be a serious complication. Constipation follows diarrhoea in all but mild cases.

Loops of thickened, tender bowel may be palpated in some severe cases presenting early. At a later stage the abdomen is diffusely tender with rebound tenderness and other signs of peritonitis. Bowel sounds may be normal or increased in the early stages, but with the development of peritonitis disappear. Poor peripheral circulation, apathy, and other signs of toxaemia are usually associated with extensive and severe disease and a poor outcome.

A 'chronic' form of pigbel is described in which patients present months or years after mild disease – or with no obvious previous history – with signs of subacute obstruction or malnutrition secondary to malabsorption. Acute obstruction from adhesions secondary to pigbel may also occur.

Diagnosis

In the Papua New Guinean context, a recent history of a pig feast in the area would make the diagnosis of pigbel in a child or adult presenting with abdominal symptoms and signs highly likely. Without such a history, the diagnosis would be less secure. The differential diagnosis necessarily includes typhoid, dysentery, gastroenteritis, intussusception, appendicitis, other causes of acute bowel obstruction, ectopic pregnancy, pelvic inflammatory disease and severe malaria.

Treatment

In general, mild cases can be successfully managed conservatively while severe cases, including those with recurrent severe bleeding or signs of peritonitis, require surgery after adequate resuscitation. In cases of moderate severity, the general principle is to treat conservatively initially, with surgery if there are signs of deterioration, or if there is no resolution of signs and symptoms within 48 h.

Mild cases

Give intravenous fluids. Half strength Darrow's solution is used for children in

Papua New Guinea, but other glucose and electolyte solutions for correction of bowel losses and maintenance of daily fluid and electrolyte requirements are satisfactory. Pass a nasogastric tube. Aspirate, then leave on free drainage. Give a single dose of an antihelminthic effective against *Ascaris*. If the child is malnourished, a dose of tinidazole, if available, can be given. Otherwise give nothing by mouth for the first 24 h. Give a course of benzyl penicillin – intravenously at first – until the patient has fully recovered. After 24–48 h of improvement the intravenous line and nasogastric tube can be reviewed and oral rehydration solution, given if available, or other clear fluids if it is not.

After a further 24 h milk and other oral fluids can be given, progressing to soft foods and finally the normal solid diet.

Severe cases

Resuscitate and prepare for surgery. Correct fluid and electrolye depletion. Use half strength Darrow's, half normal saline with potassium or other suitable fluid. Cross-match the patient and transfuse if necessary. Insert a nasogastric tube, aspirate and leave on free drainage. Give nothing by mouth. Commence intravenous benzyl penicillin and chloramphenicol or other broad-spectrum parenteral antibiotics. The indications for surgery are the likelihood of the presence of gangrene or perforation of the bowel, persistent obstruction or severe or recurrent haemorrhage.

At operation, perforated or gangrenous areas of the bowel are resected and reanastomosed by end-to-end anastomosis. The lesions are usually in the small bowel, particularly the jejunum; the colon is rarely affected.

Case history 1
A 10-year-old girl presented with acute abdominal pain, vomiting and passage of dark red blood per rectum following ingestion of pig meat. On examination she was febrile and had toxaemia, abdominal distension, tenderness with rebound but minimal guarding. Abdominal X-rays showed multiple fluid levels.

She was resuscitated, the upper gastrointestinal tract decompressed by nasogastric tube and antibiotics given. Her toxaemia subsided and abdominal distension lessened gradually over 5 days. Her Widal test was negative. Had there been evidence of deterioration in abdominal signs, further gastrointestinal bleeding or signs of perforation on X-ray, laparotomy would have been performed with a view to resecting necrosed bowel.

Further reading

Peritonitis

Archampong EQ Surgical complications of enteric fever. Baillière's Clin Trop Med Comm Dis 1988;3:301–10.

Luvuno FM. Surgery for complicated amoebiasis. Baillière's Clin Trop Med Comm Dis 1988;3:349–66.

Richens J. Management of bowel perforation in typhoid fever. Trop Doct 1991;21: 149–52.

Sharma L *et al.* Generalised peritonitis in India – the tropical spectrum. Jpn J Surg 1991;21:272–7.

Watters DAK. Severe peritoneal sepsis. Baillière's Clin Trop Med Comm Dis 1988;3: 275–300.

Pigbel

Davies MW, editor. Pigbel. Monograph Series No 6. Papua New Guinea Institute of Medical Research. November 1984.

Enteritis necroticans – Papua New Guinea Medical Journal 1979;22(1) – various articles.

19

Right Iliac Fossa Pain and Acute Appendicitis

Epidemiology

The incidence of appendicitis is increasing in the tropics, particularly in urban areas where a low-residue, highly refined diet is consumed. In Port Moresby, Papua New Guinea, over 200 appendicectomies were performed in 1993, an incidence of about one per thousand, and appendicectomy has become the commonest emergency abdominal operation. Many African countries also report over 100 cases per annum in their urban teaching hospitals and the number of appendicectomies is rising in African district hospitals which in the 1970s reported only 1 to 5 cases per year.

The male to female ratio is usually around 2:1. The rate of perforated appendices in most studies is around 20 per cent but perforation is more likely to occur at the extremes of life when the symptoms and signs are harder to recognise. The mortality rate is also higher at the extremes of life and in the tropics young adults still die because the diagnosis is missed (Case 1, p 296).

Aetiology and pathology

The majority of cases are probably due to a faecolith or lymphoid hyperplasia obstructing the appendiceal lumen, resulting in mucosal and then transmural inflammation. Although some cases of appendicitis settle spontaneously, progression to gangrene and perforation with peritonitis occur in at least a fifth of cases. Without surgical removal of the acutely inflamed appendix the perforation rate would undoubtedly be higher. The peritoneum, omentum, small bowel and mesentery may encase an inflamed appendix resulting in an inflammatory mass which is often palpable. When pus resulting from a perforated appendix is localised by the surrounding tissues an appendix abscess forms. A rare cause of appendiceal pain is an appendiceal mucocoele, which is an obstructed, enlarged appendix, full of mucus. Occasionally worms, schistosomal or other granulomas, carcinoma of the caecum or foreign bodies

331

may obstruct the appendix and result in acute inflammation. Appendiceal tumours such as carcinoid or adenocarcinoma may present as acute appendicitis.

When appendicitis settles spontaneously, regardless of whether there was a palpable mass, recurrent attacks are likely. Occasionally chronic inflammation will develop, resulting in repeated bouts of low-grade pain in the right iliac fossa. Chronic appendicitis is a fairly uncommon cause of recurrent pain but is difficult to diagnose without removing the appendix for histology.

Clinical presentation

History

Pain is the dominant symptom though it is often not severe. Classically the patient suffers from colicky, periumbilical pain which shifts after a few hours to the right iliac fossa. Occasionally the patient may suffer from epigastric pain which shifts to the right iliac fossa. Often the preceeding central abdominal pain is not remembered, and the patient's only complaint is pain in the right iliac fossa. Absence of central pain is rare unless the patient is a fit muscular individual who has ignored it. The pain usually gets progressively worse until perforation occurs. Then the intensity may subside as pain becomes generalised. Vomiting seldom occurs more than once or twice though the patient may be anorexic and nauseous. Constipation is variable. Diarrhoea may occur in 5 per cent of cases in which the appendix lies retroileal or hangs in the pelvis. Headache suggests another diagnosis such as mesenteric adenitis or typhoid.

Examination

The patient is not usually distressed. Fever is low-grade (37.2–37.4°C) until gangrene and perforation ensue. Oral fetor and tachycardia are typical findings. The abdomen is maximally tender in the right iliac fossa, usually at McBurney's point, accompanied by guarding, rigidity and rebound tenderness. In the interests of the patient's comfort it may not be necessary to test for rebound tenderness if one is convinced about the diagnosis on the basis of the history, local tenderness and guarding. Other signs such as Rovsing's (pain experienced in the right iliac fossa when the left iliac fossa is deeply palpated) are sometimes present. Rectal examination may reveal pelvic appendicitis that is not evoking inflammation or signs in the right iliac fossa. Bowel sounds may or may not be present. Absent bowel sounds should make one look for other signs of generalised peritonitis. During pregnancy the caecum and appendix are pushed higher in the abdomen, which means the maximum point of tenderness is higher. Rigidity and guarding are less obvious in pregnancy.

Practice point
• *Never exclude appendicitis without performing a rectal examination.*

Investigations

Investigations, including a white blood count, are not necessary to diagnose the majority of cases of appendicitis. Once the decision is made to perform appendicectomy there is little to be gained by performing further tests. Leukocytosis occurs in a wide range of pathologies to be considered in the differential diagnosis of acute appendicitis. Early on, the white count may be normal but it does rise as acute inflammation intensifies. In doubtful cases it is wise to perform urinalysis and urine microscopy, particularly in women to exclude urinary tract pathology. A urine culture dipstick will take 18–24 h before it can be read so it is of little help on the day of admission. Abdominal radiographs are indicated only to exclude other pathologies. A faecolith is rarely present on a plain abdominal X-ray but when present, it is diagnostic of appendicitis. Its appearance may be confused with a calcified mesenteric node or phlebolith. Ultrasound scanning is only indicated to exclude other pathologies, especially in the female genital tract. You should not delay operating on a case of obvious appendicitis to merely to perform an ultrasound. Laparoscopy increases the accuracy of diagnosis in some centres, especially where it has been performed for suspected tubo-ovarian pathology in young women. Although laparoscopy may save some unnecessary appendicectomies it is not possible to recognise inflammation limited to the mucosa by viewing the appendix from the serosal surface.

Differential diagnosis (Table 19.1)

The differential diagnosis of right iliac fossa (RIF) pain depends on the age of the patient.

Mesenteric adenitis

Mesenteric adenitis affects children and is a viral inflammation of the mesenteric nodes. Vomiting, high fever, a history of upper respiratory tract infection, and cervical lymphadenopathy are characteristic features. The abdominal signs are often minimal and usually subside with overnight observation. To avoid missing a pelvic appendicitis perform a rectal examination. Ensure the child does not have meningitis.

Urinary tract infection and ureteric colic

Ureteric pain radiates up or down the line of the ureter and is not preceded by central pain. Since the ureter lies retroperitoneally, abdominal signs are usually limited to tenderness without guarding or rebound. Suprapubic tenderness suggests cystitis. Ask about a history of dysuria, frequency and haematuria.

Table 19.1   The differential diagnosis of right iliac fossa pain and tenderness.

Pathological process	Clinical features
Inflammation and infection	
Mesenteric adenitis (children)	High fever, vomiting, cervical nodes abdominal signs unremarkable and improve with observation
Meckel's diverticulitis	Usually discovered at appendicectomy, present in 2% individuals, may bleed, cause obstruction, or become inflammed
Caecal diverticulum (adults)	May be inflammed, perforate or bleed. Usually discovered at surgery unless unexplained bleed
Inflammatory masses	Barium enema if inflammation settles, may be diagnosed only at laparotomy. Cause of mass may be need histology, weight loss, abdominal mass, long history
• Tuberculosis, Yersinia	Signs of tuberculosis elsewhere.
• Crohn's disease	Caucasian patients with systemic, eye, joint or anorectal manifestations.
• Gastroenteritis	Abdominal tenderness without peritonitis, history food poisoning or diarrhoea, vomit
• Infestation	Worms or ova in stool, may be chronic history, rarely acute
• Amoebic colitis	Blood and slough with pus in stool, *Entamoeba histolytica* cysts or organisms in stool, patient may be critically ill and deteriorating
Malignancy	
Lymphoma	Lymphoma elsewhere, weight loss
Caecal carcinoma	Anaemia, weight loss, intermittent pain. Ba enema required
Large bowel tumour	Obstruction causing caecal distension
Genital tract pathology	
Salpingitis	Vaginal discharge, sexual contact with STD, consider HIV infection
Pelvic abscess	Previous salpingitis, history of criminal abortion? perforated uterus. ?HIV infection
Ectopic pregnancy	Missed menses, vaginal bleeding, distended abdomen may be pale or shocked, ultrasound may diagnose
Torsion or bleed into ovarian cyst or fibroid	Severe pain, minimal signs, ultrasound may diagnose
Testis (normal)	Torsion with referred pain, testis tender and swollen
Testis intra-abdominal	Torsion or malignancy (teratoma/seminoma)

Always perform urinalysis and examine the urine microscopically for cells and casts. This investigation will avoid unnecessary appendicectomy for urinary tract pathology. A pelvic appendicitis lying against the bladder may cause dysuria and frequency and may be suspected on rectal examination.

Tubo-ovarian pathology

The maximum point of tenderness is typically lower in the pelvis. It takes longer for the anterior parietal peritoneum to become inflamed so that guarding and rigidity develop later. A twisted ovarian cyst often causes severe pain out of all proportion to the abdominal signs. Salpingitis is often accompanied by vaginal discharge and venereal disease. An ectopic pregnancy may present with right iliac fossa pain and shock. Consider such a diagnosis in every adult female with right iliac fossa pain, take a menstrual and sexual history, and perform a pregnancy test. Abdominal distension or shock may suggest haemoperitoneum, and, when the abdomen is distended, paracentesis of the right iliac fossa may yield blood. Do not merely observe a female in whom ectopic pregnancy is a strong possibility. Confirm the diagnosis by ultrasound scanning, laparoscopy or laparotomy. Shock is an indication for urgent surgery.

Practice point
- *Always consider the diagnosis of ectopic pregnancy in a female with right iliac fossa pain. If you suspect a ruptured ectopic pregnancy cross-match blood and organise urgent laparotomy.*

Occasionally RIF pain may be due to perforated duodenal ulcer or ruptured liver abscess tracking down the right paracolic gutter, acute cholecystitis in a low lying, pendulous gallbladder or sigmoid diverticulitis when the inflamed sigmoid is lying across the right iliac fossa.

Retroperitoneal infection may also cause RIF pain. Pyomyositis of the iliacus muscle may present as a tender mass and high fever. Formerly this was a more common cause of RIF pain than appendicitis in tropical hospitals. A psoas abscess may track down the retroperitoneum and present anywhere from the iliac fossa to the groin. The hip is usually flexed and there will sometimes be vertebral disease visible on X-ray.

Management

The management of acute appendicitis is appendicectomy which is best performed before gangrene or perforation occur. Undoubtedly some patients with acute appendicitis settle with conservative management, but this should not be considered correct except when attempted appendicectomy may be difficult and injure the caecum, particularly where appendicitis has been present for a few days and there is a mass.

Suspected acute appendicitis without a mass

Give metronidazole suppositories (500–1000 mg) with the premedication to reduce the wound infection rate. Appendicectomy should be performed through a skin-crease, muscle-splitting, incision in the right iliac fossa. It is sometimes difficult to locate the appendix and the surgeon may have to extend the incision, follow the taenia coli to the base of the appendix, and in difficult, retrocaecal cases, mobilise the caecum. Meticulous haemostasis and avoidance of contact between the inflamed appendix or appendix stump and the wound also minimises the wound infection rate. If the appendix appears normal at operation, remove it, but search the right iliac fossa for other possible causes of right iliac fossa pain: the most likely diagnoses you will recognise on exploration include Meckel's diverticulum, ileitis, torsion of the omentum or tubo-ovarian pathology. Deal appropriately with any pathology you discover. Aim for a 80–90 per cent success rate in diagnosing appendicitis. In centres where laparoscopic facilities are available appendicectomy can be performed laparoscopically.

Appendiceal mass

It is difficult and dangerous to perform an appendicectomy in the presence of a mass. The patient should be treated with antibiotics (metronidazole suppositories 1 g 8-hourly and intravenous gentamicin 80 mg 8-hourly or chloramphenicol 500 mg 6-hourly) and observed. If a mass is palpated under anaesthesia and the patient's condition is otherwise stable, it is sensible to defer appendicectomy and observe. Surgery is only indicated if the patient's condition is deteriorating (as determined by rising pulse rate, temperature, deteriorating general condition, increasing right iliac fossa tenderness, and size of mass). It may not be possible to differentiate clinically between an appendix mass and appendix abscess. Although ultrasound may show an abscess cavity it rarely influences decision making. Both an appendix mass and an abscess are initially managed conservatively. However deterioration suggests an abscess is leaking or expanding. Drainage of the cavity without appendicectomy is indicated and can often be achieved without spreading pus throughout the peritoneal cavity since the abscess is walled off. Interval appendicectomy should be performed after 3 months once the inflammatory adhesions have subsided.

Suspected perforation and generalised peritonitis

Antibiotics should be prescribed as described in the preceding section on appendiceal abscess. The patient should be resuscitated and made fit for theatre. Surgeons vary as to whether they will operate through a right iliac fossa or midline incision. If peritonitis is generalised and has been present for some time adequate peritoneal lavage cannot be performed through a right iliac fossa incision. When there is some doubt about the cause of peritonitis it is wise to perform a midline incision. If the perforation is recent then an incision in the right iliac fossa is usually adequate, particularly in children.

The management of peritonitis is further discussed on p 323.

Further reading

Adebamowo CA, Akang EE, Ladipo JK, Ajao OG. Schistosomiasis of the appendix. Br J Surg 1991;78:1219–21.

Gelfand M. Acute appendicitis, an urban disease in Africans. Trop Doct 1981;11: 22–33.

Ogbonna BC, Obekpa PO, Momoh JT, Obafunwa JO, Nwana EJ. Laparoscopy in developing countries in the management of patients with an acute abdomen. Br J Surg 1992;79:964–6.

Ojo OS, Udeh SC, Odesanmi WO. Review of histopathological findings in appendices removed for acute appendicitis in Nigerians. J R Coll Surg Edinb 1991;36:245–8.

Otu AA. Tropical surgical abdominal emergencies: acute appendicitis. Trop Geogr Med 1989;41:118–122.

20

Right Upper Quadrant Pain

Right upper quadrant pain may be due to cholecystitis or liver pathology. Occasionally it may be due to cardiac failure causing liver congestion or right lower lobe pneumonia.

Cholecystitis

Cholecystitis is due to gallstones in about 95 per cent of cases. In about 5 per cent of cases acalculous cholecystitis occurs, particularly in severely ill patients. Cholecystitis may also complicate typhoid fever.

Gallbladder stones

Aetiology

Stones form in the gallbladder when components in the bile exceed the capacity of the bile to keep them in solution. Stasis in the gallbladder (e.g. in pregnancy) and a nidus for seeding (e.g. parasites) contributes to their formation. Cholesterol is normally kept in solution in the bile mixed with bile salts and phospholipids. Cholesterol stones form in the gallbladder when the bile becomes supersaturated with cholesterol. Cholesterol stones may be pure or mixed. Pure cholesterol stones are pearly white in colour and often solitary (the so called cholesterol solitaire). Mixed stones, composed of variable quantities of cholesterol, calcium bilirubinate and calcium carbonate, are typically multiple and have faceted surfaces. Cholesterol stones are more common in Europeans than Asians and Africans.

Pigment stones may be divided into two groups. Black pigment stones, often occurring as a complication of haemolytic anaemia due to increased production of bilirubin, are hard, small and brittle. Brown pigment stones, associated with biliary infection, are composed of calcium bilirubinate trapped in glycoprotein matrix. They are soft and pliable. Infecting organisms of the biliary tract such as *Escherichia coli* produce β-glucuronidase. This enzyme hydrolyses conjugated bilirubin to the unconjugated form that combines with calcium to precipitate as the water insoluble calcium bilirubinate. Stasis, infestation of the biliary tract and cirrhosis are also thought to be important factors in the aetiology of pigment stones. In Asia and the Orient pigment stones are more common than cholesterol stones although the latter are becoming more frequently encountered. This is particularly so in younger patients, reflecting changes in diet, environmental conditions and a reduced incidence of parasitic infestation.

Clinical features

Silent gallstones

Approximately 10 per cent of the population carry stones in their gallbladder, the incidence increases with age. The number of people with asymptomatic gallstones greatly exceeds those with symptomatic stones and the vast majority of stones will not cause symptoms during life.

Acute biliary pain

When a gallstone obstructs the outlet of the gallbladder 'biliary colic' occurs. The term biliary colic is a misnomer because the pain is not intermittent (Figure 20.1). Typically it is brought on by a meal rich in fat. It is a constant aching pain located in the epigastrium or right upper quadrant, sometimes radiating through to the interscapular area. It lasts for a few hours and if severe may be associated with nausea or vomiting. The pain is relieved when the stone disimpacts itself.

Acute cholecystitis

If the obstructing stone fails to disimpact the gallbladder may become infected with bacteria, usually Gram-negative organisms. Pain fails to subside, fever develops and there is tenderness in the right upper quadrant. Murphy's sign (the patient catches his breath because of pain during deep inspiration when the right upper quadrant is palpated) may be present. In severe cases the distended, inflamed gallbladder may be palpable as a tender mass. In neglected cases the gallbladder may rupture, leading to generalised peritonitis. In other cases a localised abscess may form. These complications are more likely to occur if the patient is diabetic.

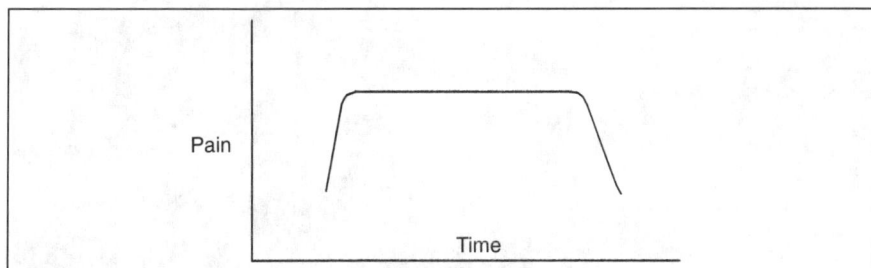

Figure 20.1 Biliary pain is constant in severity and lasts for several hours.

Cholangitis and pancreatitis

Gallbladder stones may migrate into the bile duct and cause biliary obstruction. Superimposed infection in the bile duct leads to cholangitis (see next section). Stones may also impact at the ampulla of Vater, causing acute pancreatitis.

Investigations

Ten per cent of the gallstones are radio-opaque and may be seen on a plain abdominal radiographs. The diagnosis is best confirmed by ultrasonography. The stones are seen as echogenic foci casting acoustic shadows (Figure 20.2). In acute cholecystitis, in addition to the stone(s), the gallbladder is distended and thick walled. There may be fluid collections around the gallbladder and tenderness may be elicited by pressure with the ultrasound probe. Other investigations such as oral cholecystography and intravenous cholangiography are less sensitive and rarely used nowadays.

Often ultrasonography is the only imaging investigation necessary. Coexisting common bile duct stones should be suspected if there is a history of jaundice or cholangitis, the serum bilirubin or alkaline phosphatase levels are elevated, or if dilated bile ducts are found on ultrasonography. Further investigations such as endoscopic retrograde cholangiopancreatography (ERCP) may be indicated, especially if laparoscopic cholecystectomy is to be performed.

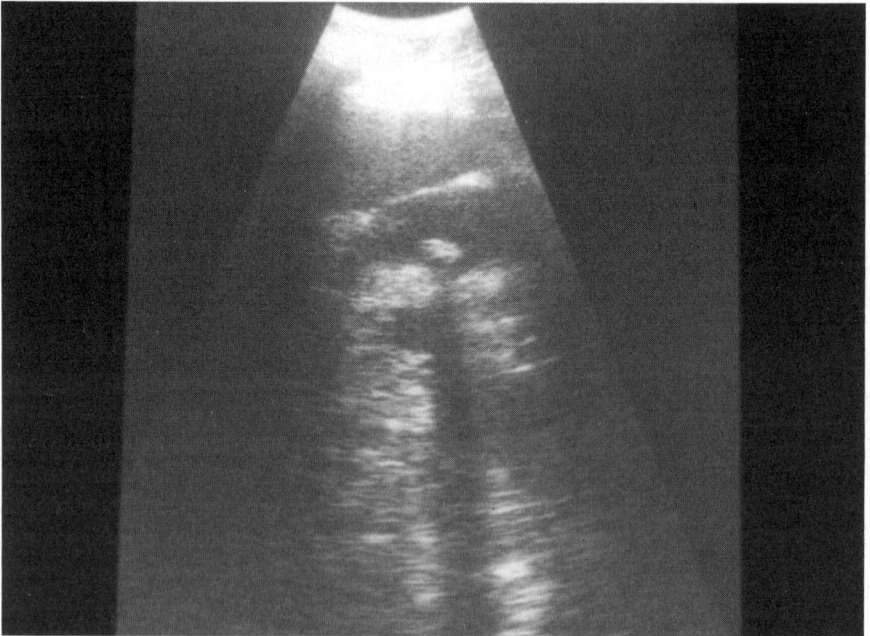

Figure 20.2 Ultrasound scan showing a gallstone casting a typical acoustic shadow.

Management

Asymptomatic gallstones

Asymptomatic gallbladder stones do not require any treatment. Although gallstones have been associated with gallbladder cancer this is a rare occurrence. The risks associated with cholecystectomy are greater than expectant management. There is no sound surgical argument for performing cholecystectomy for asymptomatic gallbladder stones. An uncommon exception is the patient with calcification in the gallbladder wall (porcelain gallbladder) who is at greater risk from gallbladder cancer. For ill-understood reasons acute cholecystitis frequently occurs after laparotomy, even in patients who have had no previous trouble from their gallstones. For this reason the gallbladder should be removed when gallstones are found during laparotomy if the patient's condition permits.

Acute biliary pain

Biliary 'colic' is usually self-limiting. Relief may be hastened by analgesics and intramuscular anti-spasmodics (hyoscine butylbromide (Buscopan) 40 mg IMI). In the long-term patients should be advised to have the gallbladder removed as recurrent attacks are likely. The results of non-operative treatments such as dissolution therapy or extra-corporeal shock wave lithotripsy (ESWL) are disappointing. Bile salt dissolution therapy is slow, and works only if the gallbladder functions, the stones are small and lucent and the compliance is good. Lithotripsy also requires a functioning gallbladder and adjuvant dissolution therapy. With both techniques reformation of stones occurs if bile salt therapy is discontinued.

Acute cholecystitis

Patients presenting with acute cholecystitis should be admitted to hospital, kept nil by mouth, and treated by IV fluids and IV antibiotics. A broad-spectrum antibiotic covering Gram-negative organisms (e.g. cephalosporin or aminoglycoside) is appropriate. There is no overall consensus when it comes to the surgical management of acute cholecystitis. About 80 per cent of patients will respond to conservative treatment, as evidenced by rapid resolution of pain and fever. The traditional approach is to perform delayed cholecystectomy some 2 to 3 months later, once the inflammation has subsided. There is an increasing trend, however, to perform early cholecystectomy during the same hospital admission rather than adopting an expectant policy. The patient undergoes surgery within 48 h of presentation, preferably on an elective operating list. Although the surgery can be more difficult during the acute phase this early approach causes no greater morbidity or mortality than elective cholecystectomy providing it is performed by an experienced surgeon. There are advantages in that the disease process is aborted right away and the risk of the patient being readmitted in the interim with a further attack is removed. The overall time spent in hospital is reduced because the patient does not require another admission for elective cholecystectomy.

If fever and pain do not subside, there are signs of spreading peritonitis or evidence of septicemia, urgent surgery is indicated. Cholecystectomy in such circumstances may be technically very difficult. If structures in Calot's triangle cannot be identified it may be wise to perform a cholecystostomy rather than running the risk of damaging the common bile duct. If expertise is available, another alternative in elderly unfit patients is percutaneous cholecystostomy under ultrasound guidance.

Case history 1
A 79-year-old male presented with a 2-day history of progressive right hypochondrial pain. The examining surgeon noted a fever of 38.5°C but no jaundice. There was a tender mass beneath the right costal margin. An urgent ultrasound scan showed a grossly distended gallbladder containing debris. The gallbladder wall was thickened and there was surrounding pericholecystic fluid. Tenderness was elicited directly over the gallbladder with the ultrasound probe. The common bile duct was normal. Empyema of the gallbladder was diagnosed. In view of coexistent medical problems a percutaneous cholecystostomy was performed under ultrasound guidance. The drain yielded pus. The patient's general condition rapidly improved over the next 24 h with resolution of pain and fever. Intravenous antibiotics (a cephalosporin and metronidazole) were continued for 5 days. As the patient remained without symptoms no further treatment was planned. Note: Urgent laparotomy and cholecystectomy is an option in younger patients, but if cholecystostomy is chosen then delayed cholecystectomy should be advised.

Cholecystectomy
The traditional approach to gallstone disease is open cholecystectomy. This procedure is the gold standard to which all other procedures should be compared. It is a safe operation with the added flexibility of being able to deal with common bile duct stones without any undue difficulty. The disadvantages are the postoperative wound pain and protracted recovery period required before the patient can return to useful activity. The operating time is probably no quicker than laparoscopic cholecystectomy.

Laparoscopic cholecystectomy
The operative approach to gallstones has radically changed over the last 4 years with the advent of laparoscopic techniques. In many hospitals throughout the world laparoscopy is now the standard approach for cholecystectomy. This procedure requires specialised equipment and operating theatre layout (Figure 20.3). A CO_2 pneumoperitoneum is established and a laparoscope is introduced through an umbilical cannula. Three additional access ports are required for operating instruments; one in the midline epigastrium, one subcostally in the mid-clavicular line and a third subcostally in the anterior axillary line. The procedure is viewed from a television monitor linked to a compact video camera attached to the laparoscope. The operative principles are the same as with open cholecystectomy. After defining the biliary anatomy

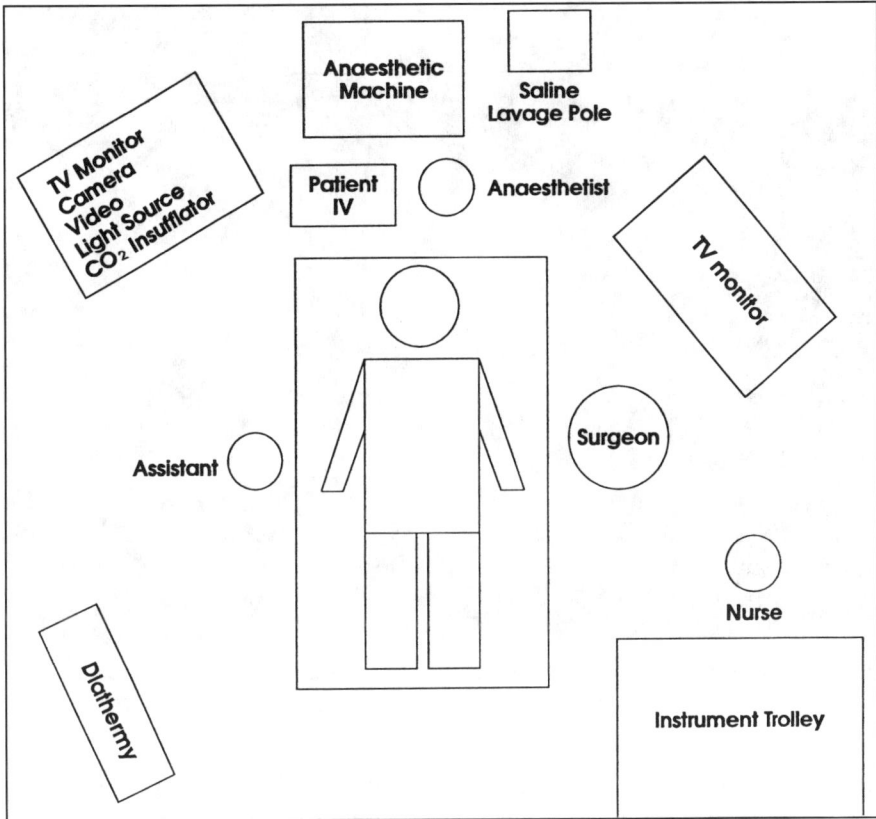

Figure 20.3 Operating theatre layout for laparoscopic cholecystectomy.

the cystic duct and cystic artery are ligated with endoscopically placed clips (Figure 20.4). Operative cholangiography can be performed if indicated. The gallbladder is dissected from the liver by diathermy and usually extracted through the umbilical wound.

The advantages of laparoscopic cholecystectomy are a quicker postoperative recovery, very little postoperative pain and early return to normal activity. A reduction in hospital stay results in more efficient use of limited resources. Most patients are discharged from hospital within 24 h of surgery and return to work within a week. The initial capital outlay and recurrent cost of disposable equipment is high. In experienced hands the procedure takes no longer than open cholecystectomy. The conversion rate to open surgery is low (around 5 per cent). Complications are few although the chance of bile duct damage during the learning phase may be higher than at open cholecystectomy. This is due to inexperience on the part of the operator and can be overcome by proper training. This technique can be applied to all patients with symptomatic gallstones who are fit for surgery. Acute cholecystitis was initially considered

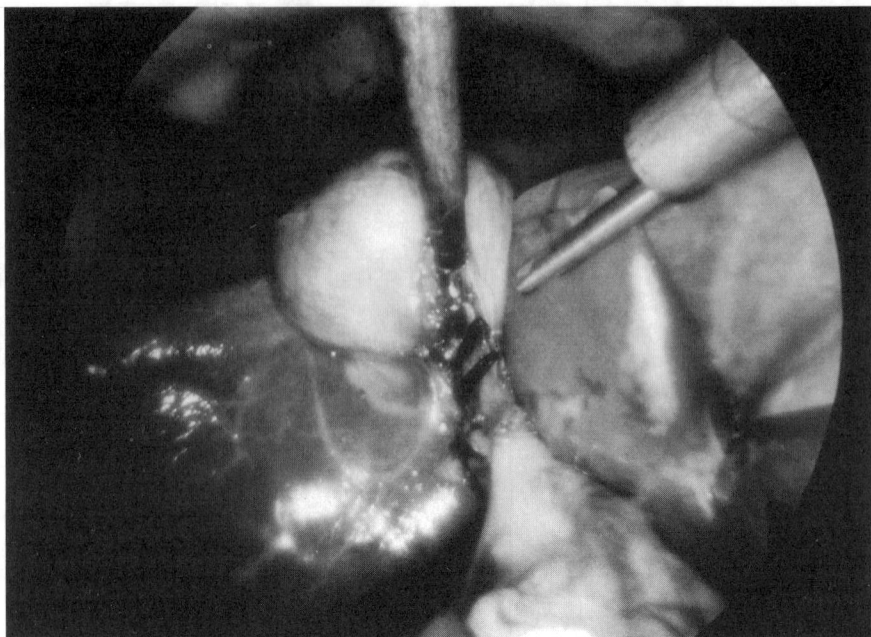

Figure 20.4   Surgeons view during laparoscopic cholecystectomy. Clips on cystic duct.

to be a contraindication to laparoscopic surgery although experienced surgeons are now dealing with acute cases with no extra morbidity.

Common bile duct stones

The management of patients with both gallstones and common bile duct (CBD) stones has changed considerably since the advent of laparoscopic techniques. The traditional approach is open cholecystectomy and exploration of the common bile duct. However, the introduction of laparoscopic surgery has forced surgeons to reconsider their management of CBD stones. Laparoscopic techniques for common duct exploration are not well established although laparoscopic transcystic duct CBD exploration is being evaluated in specialised centres. Preoperative biliary endoscopy has, therefore, been employed more extensively to detect and remove CBD stones. ERCP is indicated in the presence of CBD dilatation on ultrasound, elevated alkaline phosphatase and/or bilirubin, a history of cholangitis and possibly pancreatitis. If ERCP is unavailable such patients should undergo operative cholangiography. If common duct stones are found conversion to open cholecystectomy and common duct exploration will be necessary unless the patient can be referred elsewhere for postoperative ERCP.

Elderly patients with gallbladder stones may become asymptomatic after endoscopic common duct clearance. Cholecystectomy can, therefore, be avoided. This is a perfectly acceptable option in the elderly as only 5 per cent of patients will develop further symptoms requiring surgery.

Sickle cell disease and cholelithiasis

Haemolysis results in the secretion of bile that has a high bilirubin content and results in the formation of pigment stones. However the incidence rises with age but is lower in West African patients (around 5–10 per cent) with sickle cell disease than in North American blacks where 50 per cent of those affected over the age of 10 years may have gallstones. This difference may be due to differences in the cholesterol content of the diet and consequently in the bile. Thus with urbanisation the incidence of cholelithiasis in Africans with sickle cell disease may rise.

Management

Pigment stones should be managed similarly to other gallstones. Symptomatic stones require appropriate surgical treatment though care should be taken to avoid a sickle crisis during surgery and anaesthesia by avoiding hypoxia, hypothermia and infection. The preoperative haemoglobin should be at least 8 g/dl. Asymptomatic stones can be observed.

Typhoid cholecystitis

This occurs more frequently than is generally recognised during an attack of typhoid fever. It presents with acute epigastric or right upper quadrant pain with signs of acute cholecystitis in the second week of the illness. The patient is more ill than is normal for acute cholecystitis due to gallstones. The treatment is conservative, with appropriate antibiotics for *Salmonella typhi* unless empyema supervenes.

Chronic carriers with typhoid may have *S. typhi* lodging in the gallbladder. All patients convalescent from typhoid should be screened and cholecystectomy advised if there is persistent isolation of *S. typhi* in the stools.

Acalculous cholecystitis

This may occur in elderly, malnourished or critically ill patients where infection complicates stasis and sludge formation. Signs of right upper quadrant peritonitism are often, but not invariably, present. Ultrasound scanning will show a distended gallbladder with a thickened, oedematous wall, sometimes with gas. The management is similar to cholecystitis due to gallstone cholecystitis

– nasogastric tube, intravenous fluids and broad-spectrum antibiotics. Urgent cholecystectomy is indicated if the patient fails to improve or it is suspected that the gallbladder is gangrenous.

Biliary sludge

The sludge consists of supersaturated bile containing cholesterol monohydrate crystals, calcium bilirubinate crystals and mucin glycoprotein. Those at risk include patients receiving total parenteral nutrition, those with AIDS, the critically ill in intensive care units and those suffering prolonged fasting following abdominal surgery. Supersaturation of the bile and poor gallbladder contractility due to fasting are important in the pathogenesis. The presence of biliary sludge during a critical illness may predispose to the later development of gallstones so that these patients should be carefully followed up by ultrasound scanning though the decision to perform cholecystectomy will be made according to clinical symptoms.

Recurrent pyogenic cholangitis

Aetiology

Recurrent pyogenic cholangitis is a common cause of acute hospital admission in Asia. This disease is characterised by the *de novo* development of pigment stones in the intrahepatic and extrahepatic biliary tree and the development of strictures in the intrahepatic bile ducts (Figure 20.5). The calculi consist predominantly of calcium bilirubinate, glycoprotein matrix and bacteria. They are muddy, brown and soft, often growing to several centimetres in diameter.

These stones are endemic in Asia but are now being reported with increasing frequency in Asian immigrants to Western countries. The condition has been named Oriental cholangiohepatitis, primary cholangitis, hepatolithiais and recurrent pyogenic cholangitis. The exact aetiology is uncertain but bacterial infection, worm infestation of the biliary tree and a protein deficient diet have all been implicated. The disease predominantly affects the lower income groups and the incidence appears to be declining over recent years. It used to be a disease of young adults but in more affluent countries it has become a disease of the elderly. The mean age of people admitted to hospital with this condition in Hong Kong is now around 70 years of age.

Clinical features

Patients with stones in the bile duct present with recurrent attacks of cholangitis. The three most important clinical features are abdominal pain, fever and

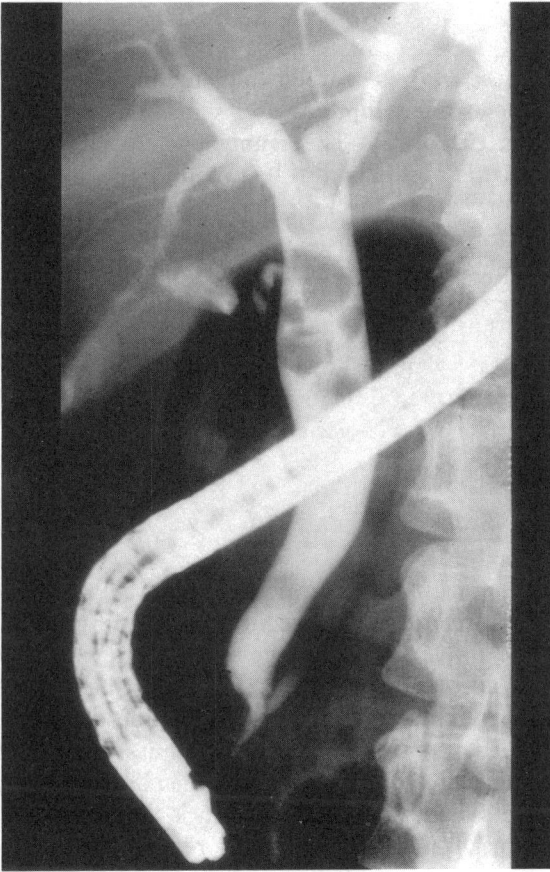

Figure 20.5 Multiple common bile duct calculi found at ERCP.

jaundice, i.e. Charcot's triad. The urine is dark brown or 'tea coloured' during an acute attack. The abdomen may bear scars of previous biliary surgery. Guarding in the epigastrium and upper quadrant may be present. In the elderly the presentation may be atypical and not immediately recognisable as abdominal pain and/or fever may be absent.

Although at the time of presentation the general condition may be good, sudden deterioration into septicaemia shock with associated mental confusion occurs frequently. The addition of confusion and hypotension to Charcot's triad has been termed 'Reynold's pentad' and denotes acute obstructive supportive cholangitis. This is due to coexistent infection, usually with Gram-negative organisms, in an obstructed high pressure biliary system. In these circumstances cholangiovenous reflux can occur resulting in septicaemia. Without urgent decompression of the biliary system the outcome is fatal.

Investigation

In most patients the diagnosis can be made on clinical grounds alone on the basis of the characteristic symptoms and signs. Blood count may show a polymorphonuclear leucocytosis. The serum bilirubin and alkaline phosphatase are elevated. Transaminases may also be raised in an acute attack, reflecting the inflammatory process in the liver parenchyma. A raised serum amylase indicates concomitant pancreatitis.

Plain radiography of the abdomen is generally unhelpful except occasionally when air is seen in the biliary tree. This indicates either a spontaneous fistula between the bile duct and the duodenum or a previous biliary enteric bypass. Ultrasonography may show a dilated biliary tree. Brown pigment stones are soft and are often difficult to image as they do not always cast as dense an acoustic shadow as cholesterol stones.

Management

Initial management consist of giving nothing by mouth, nasogastric suction, intravenous fluid replacement, blood cultures and intravenous antibiotics. In view of the possible development of acute renal shutdown as a result of septic shock, aminoglycosides should be avoided if possible. Cephalosporins or quinalones are the antibiotics of choice. Coagulation disturbances should be screened for and corrected accordingly with vitamin K or fresh frozen plasma depending upon the degree of urgency and impending endoscopic or surgical intervention. Those patients with a severe attack should have a urethral catheter inserted and their urinary output monitored.

More than three-quarters of the patients respond to conservative treatment. For those patients not responding as judged by the presence of deepening jaundice, persistent pain, high fever, signs of peritonitis or impending shock, urgent biliary decompression is necessary. Endoscopic drainage by ERCP, if available, is now the procedure of choice in these circumstances. As the procedure is less invasive than surgery and no additional morbidity accrues from its use in the acute situation, ERCP should be performed early to abort the attack rather than adopting an expectant attitude. In most cases the biliary system is readily decompressed via a nasobiliary catheter (Figure 20.6). In critically ill patients and those with a coagulopathy, nasobiliary drainage can be achieved without a prior sphincterotomy. Bile should be aspirated from the drain to decompress the biliary tree and sent for bacteriological culture. The response to endoscopic drainage is usually dramatic. Stone extraction is only attempted when the patient is clinically stable.

After the acute episode is over the aim of treatment is to clear the bile ducts of any calculi and improve biliary drainage. An endoscopic sphincterotomy is performed by bowing a wire over the sphincter of Oddi and applying diathermy current to incise the sphincter. With an adequate sphincterotomy most stones less than 1 cm in diameter will pass spontaneously but most

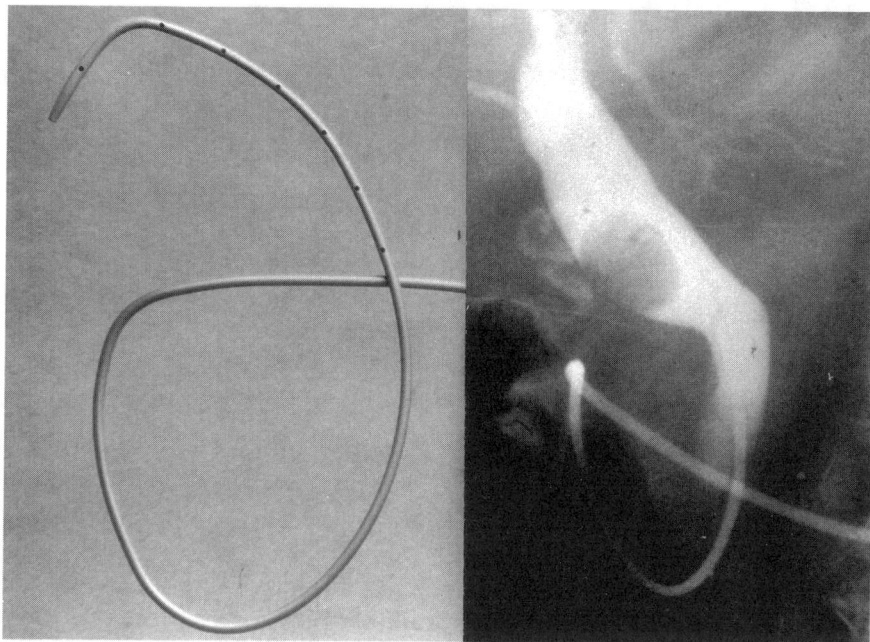

Figure 20.6 Naso biliary drain.

endoscopists will usually pursue a more active extraction policy due to the risk of further cholangitis from stone impaction at the sphincterotomy. Stones can be extracted by balloon catheter or Dormier basket, however, the calculi of recurrent pyogenic cholangitis are often too large to be extracted intact and frequently have to be broken up before removal (Figure 20.7). Fortunately they are usually soft and fragmentation is easily achieved by the use of a mechanical lithotriptor which can pass down the channel of the larger endoscopes (Figure 20.8). Following lithotripsy the fragments can be removed with a standard basket. In patients who are more stable, drainage, sphincterotomy and stone removal may be achieved during one session. Once the offending stone is disimpacted and the biliary tree decompressed the pain disappears and sepsis rapidly subsides.

Case history 2

A 65-year-old oriental female presented with a 12-h history of upper abdominal pain, chills and tea coloured urine. On examination she was mildly jaundiced, febrile and the upper abdomen was tender to palpation. The urine was dark and bile was present on analysis. Pyogenic cholangitis was diagnosed. Blood cultures were taken and intravenous antibiotics given. Her clinical condition quickly deteriorated with hypotension and confusion. ERCP was performed immediately. The common bile duct was dilated and contained multiple calculi. A nasobiliary drain was inserted. She responded quickly to decompression of the biliary tree and antibiotics. Three days later

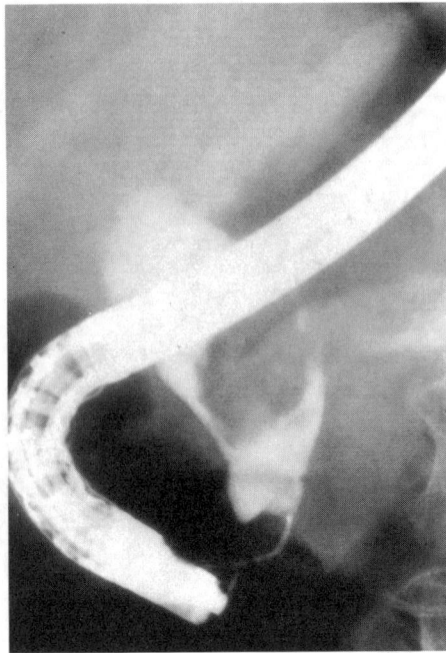

Figure 20.7   Large common bile duct stone requiring lithotripsy prior to extraction.

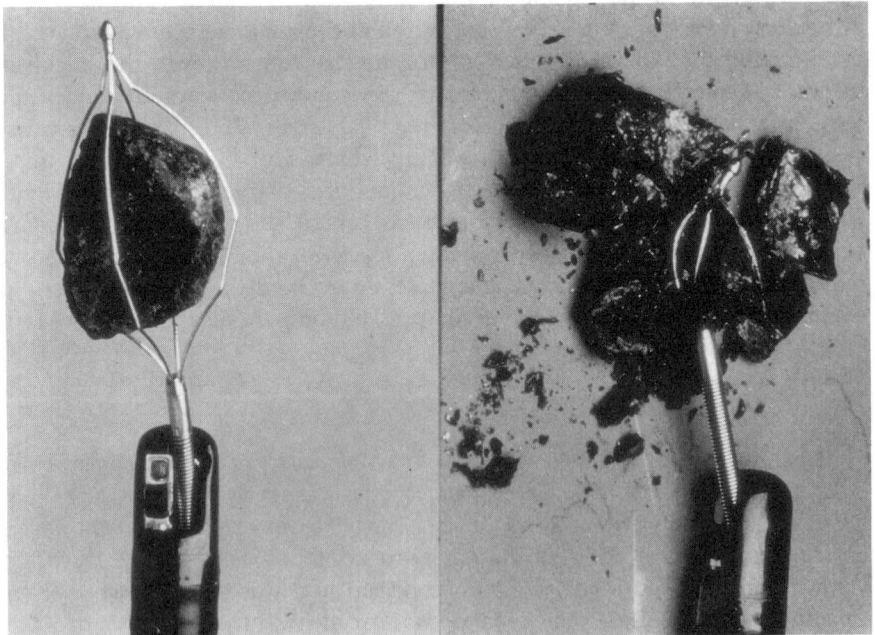

Figure 20.8   Lithotripsy basket.

she underwent another ERCP. An endoscopic sphincterotomy was performed and all the common duct calculi were extracted. Note: In urgent cases such as this, where the clinical diagnosis is almost certain, establishing biliary drainage is essential and takes priority over further diagnostic investigations.

In patients who are too ill to undergo repeated endoscopic procedures the insertion of a 10 Fr biliary stent will ensure biliary drainage and prevent stone impaction. Such stents can be left *in situ* indefinitely or removed at a later date when the patient's condition improves, at which time stone extraction may be possible.

If ERCP is unavailable and surgery is the only available option then the procedure performed will depend upon the operative findings and the condition of the patient. If the patient has responded to conservative management then elective surgery can be performed. The aim is to remove stones and improve biliary drainage so that the chance of recurrence is decreased. The presence of gallstones is an indication for cholecystectomy. Operative cholangiography will reveal the number and site of intraductal stones which can then be removed through a choledochotomy. Completion cholangiography, or preferably choledochoscopy, should be preformed to ensure that there are no residual stones in the common bile duct and that there is free drainage into the duodenum. If simple common duct exploration is performed a T tube should be inserted and the completeness of clearance checked by T tube cholangiography in the postoperative period. Unfortunately the stones will inevitably reform after simple common duct exploration. If the patient is fit enough a biliary enteric bypass (choledochoduodenostomy, choledocho-jejunostomy or transduodenal sphincteroplasty) should be performed to improve biliary drainage so that any small stones that reform can be passed without symptoms. Impacted stones at the lower end of the common bile duct are an absolute indication for transduodenal sphincteroplasty or choledochoduodenostomy.

In the emergency situation the objective of surgery is to achieve adequate drainage of the proximal biliary tract and to avoid protracted operative procedures and operative cholangiography. For this purpose choledochotomy and insertion of a T tube is usually adequate, the bile often looks like pus and gushes out once the bile duct is incised. Any impacted stones at the lower end of the bile duct may be left to be extracted later, however, one must be sure that the proximal ductal system is adequately drained. In the past, surgical drainage with T-tube decompression was, for many patients, the only option, and in this group of sick patients, the morbidity and mortality was high, in the region of 16 per cent to 40 per cent. This contrasts with a mortality of 5 per cent associated with urgent endoscopic drainage so explaining the preference for the latter when available. Another alternative is urgent percutaneous transhepatic drainage. Good results have been reported with this procedure but there is a greater risk of haemorrhage, bile leakage and peritonitis in this sick group of patients.

Intrahepatic stones and strictures

Recurrent pyogenic cholangitis is often complicated by the presence of intrahepatic stones and intrahepatic strictures (Figure 20.9). The management of such cases still presents a challenge for both the therapeutic endoscopist and the surgeon. Intrahepatic stones occurring within the right or left main ducts along the axis of the common bile duct are more accessible to extraction but difficulties arise when the stones are in the more peripheral segments of the liver. Stones that develop proximal to intrahepatic strictures may be tightly packed within the intrahepatic duct leaving little room for manipulation with therapeutic devices. Balloon dilatation of the stricture can be performed to improve access for instruments.

When endoscopic expertise is unavailable percutaneous transhepatic cholangiography, tract dilatation and percutaneous choledochoscopy may allow successful stone extraction. The technique is easier as the working distance is shorter and selective puncture of the diseased segment allows better access.

Unfortunately, despite successful endoscopic treatment, stricture and stone recurrence is common. For those cases with recurrent strictures and stones in a localised segment, liver resection is the most effective and often only treatment.

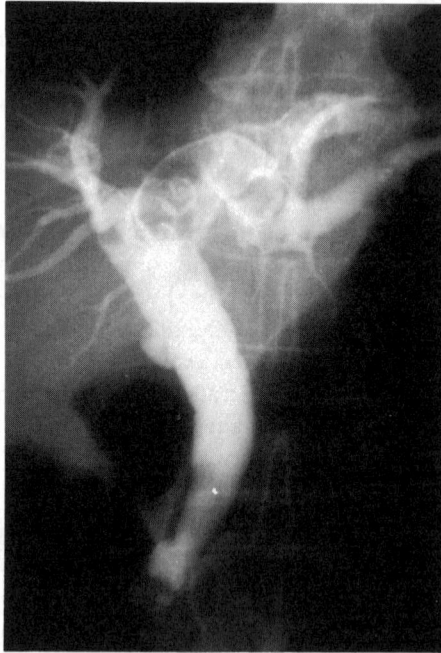

Figure 20.9 Multiple intrahepatic stones.

Case history 3

A 49-year-old female, with a history of recurrent pyogenic cholangitis, was admitted with a 2 day history of upper abdominal pain and chills. On examination she febrile but not jaundiced. There was mild tenderness in the epigastrium. Another attack of cholangitis was suspected and she was treated accordingly. Biochemistry showed mildly elevated serum alkaline phosphatase and bilirubin levels. On ultrasound scanning the left lobe of the liver was shrunken and contained multiple calculi within dilated intrahepatic ducts. ERCP was performed. The common bile duct was dilated but contained no stones. There were multiples stones in the left intrahepatic ducts proximal to a tight stricture. A nasobiliary drain was inserted through the stricture into the left ducts. The attack resolved following nasobiliary drainage. Her previous records showed that she had undergone endoscopic dilatation of the intrahepatic stricture twice in the last 3 years. 99mTc-EHIDA isotope scintigraphy showed little function in the left lobe, therefore, she underwent left hepatic lobectomy.

Sclerosing cholangitis

This is a rare condition with an incidence in Western countries of 2–3 per 100 000. The aetiology is obscure but 70 per cent have ulcerative colitis. The diagnosis is established by biopsy. Patients tend to survive 5–10 years with repeated dilatations and maintaining drainage of the biliary system. Cholangiocarcinoma may develop. The only hope of cure is liver transplantation.

Cholangiocarcinoma

Cholangiocarcinoma and its association with opisthorchiasis is discussed on pp 187–9.

Hepatic disease as a cause of right upper quadrant pain

Acute hepatitis

This condition may present with epigastric or right upper quadrant pain a few days before jaundice develops. Liver enzymes will be diagnostic and ultrasound of the gallbladder will be normal.

Liver abscess

Liver abscesses are usually due to amoebiasis or bacterial infection. Clinical manifestations include a palpable mass or intercostal tenderness. On radiograph of the erect chest the right diaphragm may be elevated (Figure 20.10)

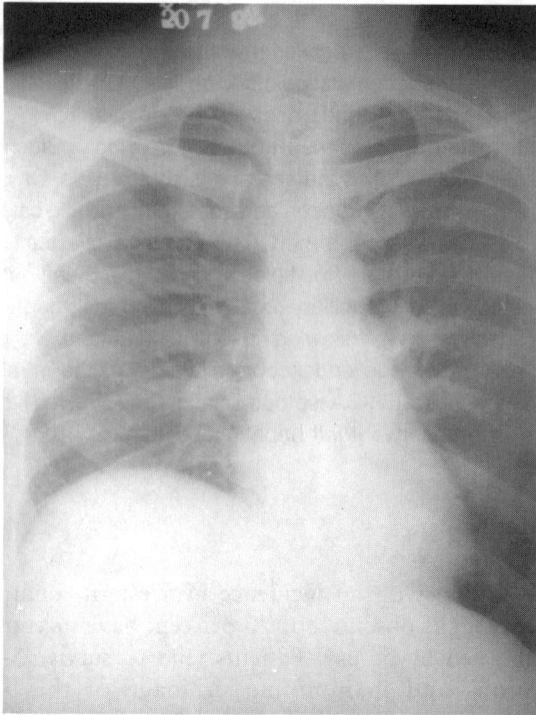

Figure 20.10   Raised right hemidiaphragm due to amoebic liver abscess.

and occasionally there is an obvious fluid level. Ultrasound examination is diagnostic and may allow ultrasound-guided aspiration. If ultrasound examination is unavailable a diagnostic aspiration (21-gauge needle) can be performed at the site of maximum tenderness or into a tender mass. Treatment is appropriate antibiotics, which means metronidazole or tinidazole 800 mg t.d.s. in areas where amoebiasis is endemic, and gentamicin or a cephalosporin for a pyogenic infection. Failure to improve or signs of impending rupture are an indication for urgent drainage by open surgery or percutaneously with guidance by ultrasound or computed tomography scanning. Check the clotting profile before intervention (see pp 43–5 and Figures 3.1–3.4 pp 46–50).

Hydatid cyst (pp 109–12 and Figure 3.7 p 52)

Hepatoma (hepatocellular carcinoma – see pp 184–7)

This common tumour may sometimes present with a tender right upper quadrant mass due to necrosis and bleeding within the tumour. A hepatoma may also bleed into the peritoneal cavity causing localised peritonitis if it is oozing around the tumour or distension and shock if bleeding is massive. Bleeding hepatomas are normally advanced, often with associated cirrhosis, so that the management is aimed at resuscitation and stopping the bleeding. If the bleeding does not stop spontaneously, intervention by tumour embolisation, application of suture and surgicel or injection with absolute alcohol is indicated. Only very rarely is the bleeding from a hepatic adenoma or localised carcinoma which may be suitable for resection. The hospital mortality in ruptured hepatocellular carcinoma is around 50 per cent.

Practice points

- *Asymptomatic gallbladder stones do not merit any treatment.*
- *Gallstones are common and their presence does not necessarily mean that they are the cause of current symptoms. Peptic ulceration and stomach cancer should be considered.*
- *Patients with acute cholangitis may deteriorate very rapidly.*
- *In elderly patients cholangitis may present without abdominal pain. A high index of suspicion for the diagnosis is necessary.*
- *Urgent biliary decompression is life saving in patients with suppurative cholangitis.*
- *In elderly patients the gallbladder can be left* in situ *after endoscopic common duct clearance.*

Further reading

Gallbladder stones

Adeji A, Rotimi VO, Akande B, Olumide F. The bacteria flora of gallbladder bile among Nigerians. E Afr Med J 1986;63:507–10.

Adelike AD. Experience with cholelithiasis in patients with sickle cell disease in Nigeria. Am J Pediatr Hematol Oncol 1985;7:261–4.

Cotton PB. Endoscopic retrograde cholangiopancreatography and laparoscopic cholecystectomy. Am J Surg 1993;165:474–8.

Deziel DJ, Millikan KW, Economou SG, *et al*. Complications of laparoscopic cholecystectomy: A national survey of 4,292 hospitals and an analysis of 77,604 cases. Am J Surg 1993;165:9–14.

McSherry CK. Cholecystectomy: the gold standard. Am J Surg 1989;158:174–8.

Ndosi BN. Biliary lithiasis in Dar Es Salaam. Australas Radiol 1987;31:292–4.

Neoptolemos JP, Carr-Locke DL, Fossard DP. Prospective randomised study of preoperative endoscopic sphincterotomy versus surgery alone for common bile duct stones. BMJ 1987;294:470–4.

Parekh D, Lawson HH, Kuyl JM. Gall stone disease among black South Africans. S Afr Med J 1987;72:23–6.

Pausawasdi A, Pausawadsi S, Mahaweero W. Clinical study of gallstones in Thai patients. J Med Ass Thai 1979;62:227–34.

Segal I, Walker ARP, Couper-Smith J. The prevalence of gallstones in urban black women. S Afr Med J 1985;68:530.

The Southern Surgeons Club. A prospective analysis of 1518 laparoscopic cholecystectomies. N Engl J Med 1991;324:1073–8.

Ti TK, Yuen R. Chemical composition of biliary calculi in relation to the pattern of biliary disease in Singapore. Br J Surg 1985;72:556–8.

Cholangitis

Lau WY, Fan·ST, Yip WC, Wong KK. Surgical management of strictures of major bile ducts in recurrent pyogenic cholangitis. Br J Surg 1987;74:1100–2.

Leung JWC, Chung SCS, Sung JY, *et al*. Urgent endoscopic drainage for acute suppurative cholangitis. Lancet 1989;i:1207–9.

Li AKC, Chung SCS, Leung JWC, Mok SD. Recurrent pyogenic cholangitis: an update. Trop Gastroenterol 1985;6:119–31.

Toouli J. Surgery of the biliary tract. Edinburgh: Churchill Livingstone, 1993.

Hepatoma

Dewar GA, Griffin SM, Ku KW, Lau WY, Li AKC. Management of bleeding liver tumours in Hong Kong. Br J Surg 1991;78:463–6.

Muhammad I, Mabogunje O. Spontaneous rupture of primary hepatocellular carcinoma in Zaria, Nigeria. J R Coll Surg Edinb 1991;36:117–20.

21

Pancreatitis

Pancreatitis is rare in many tropical countries (central Africa and Papua New Guinea), its incidence depending on alcohol consumption and the prevalence of gallstones. However, it is common in Kerala, South India, and parts of East Africa where tropical pancreatitis was first described. Acute pancreatitis is particularly common in South Africa; a large series of pancreatic psuedocysts was reported from Durban, where acute pancreatitis is a common cause of acute abdominal pain. Alcoholic pancreatitis is common in Australian Aborigines, and gallstone pancreatitis in South-East Asia. Fifty-nine cases of *Ascaris*-induced acute pancreatitis were reported from Kashmir, India in 5 1/2 years.

Acute pancreatitis

Aetiology and pathophysiology

Acute attacks may be isolated incidents, recurrent or superimposed on chronic pancreatitis. The pathophysiology of acute pancreatitis is poorly understood but involves ischaemia of acinar cells, disruption of cell membranes due to lysolecithin from phospholipase activity, and enzymatic digestion of adjacent tissues by proteases, lipases and elastases. Inflammatory cells accumulate, and oedema, haemorrhage or necrosis may spread through tissue planes. Peritoneal exudate, rich in pancreatic enzymes, accumulates in the lesser sac or even the peritoneal cavity as a whole. Absorption of inflammatory mediators, kinins and activated peptides of the complement and coagulation cascades may result in gross systemic effects, including respiratory, circulatory and renal failure. Jaundice may develop secondary to the systemic response and as a result of oedema around the common bile duct.

Acute pancreatitis may subside, progress to necrosis or be complicated by a psuedocyst or an abscess. Recurrent attacks may occur due to ductal disease or to persistence of the underlying cause. The commonest causes are alcohol and gallstones. Other causes are listed in Table 21.1.

357

Table 21.1   Causes of pancreatitis.

Common
  Alcohol
  Gallstones

Less common
  Trauma – blunt or penetrating trauma and abdominal surgery
  Duct obstruction
    Pancreas divisum
    Juxtapancreatic intestinal duplications
    Periampullary cyst or diverticulum
    Annular pancreas
    Ascaris worms
    Afferent loop syndrome
    Tumours

Rare
  Scorpion venom (*Tirtius trinitatus*)
  Anorexia nervosa, bulimia
  Hypercalcaemia:
    Hyperparathyroidism
    Sarcoidosis
    Malignancy
  Hyperlipoproteinaemia
  Viruses:
    Mumps
    Cocksackie B, ECHO, Epstein–Barr, hepatitis A, B
  Bacteria – *Mycoplasma pneumoniae*
  Vascular causes:
    Aortography, cardiopulmonary bypass, vasculitis, hypotensive shock
  Drugs:
    e.g. thiazides, azathioprine, tetracyclines, frusemide, valproate, oestrogens,
      corticosteroids, sulphonamides

Clinical presentation

The typical presentation is acute epigastric pain, which may radiate through to the back, particularly to the left. Nausea and vomiting are common. Generalised peritonitis may develop rapidly with tenderness and rigidity, but because the pancreas is retroperitoneal, tenderness and rigidity may not be marked. Distension may occur as a result of either paralytic ileus or pancreatic ascites. Pancreatic ascites may be diagnosed by aspiration of dark fluid with a high amylase content.

Diagnosis

The diagnosis is made by measuring the serum or urine amylase. The levels are markedly elevated in the first 24–48 h, when diagnostic levels are 3–4 times the laboratory upper limit of normal. Unfortunately many other causes of acute abdominal pathology including perforation, intestinal obstruction and cholecystitis may also raise the serum amylase though rarely to such high levels as pancreatitis. There is no relation between the level of serum amylase and the severity of the attack. Amylase is excreted in the urine so that urinary amylase is worth measuring, especially if the peak of serum amylase may have been missed. Urine amylase strips are available as a screening test.

Ultrasound examination enables visualisation of the pancreas and may detect pancreatic oedema and lesser sac collections. Pseudocyst formation occurs in about 10 per cent of cases. However the pancreas may be difficult to visualize due to bowel gas interposition so that CT scanning is then the best means of demonstrating the integrity of the pancreas.

Whenever doubt remains concerning whether pancreatitis is responsible for an acute abdomen, laparotomy is advised to exclude other causes. In this situation diagnostic laparotomy seems to confer little morbidity and ensures that a surgically treatable condition is not missed.

Grading of severity and prognosis

The severity of the attack and the prognosis depend upon a number of features described by Ranson and Imrie (Table 21.2). When adequate laboratory services are available these prognostic indicators should be recorded on admission and at 48 h. If laboratory services are poor, a severe attack must be determined from the general condition, vital signs, leukocyte count, glucose and urea levels, development of organ failure and presence of pancreatic ascites.

Management

Fluid replacement and resuscitation, analgesia and intestinal rest are the mainstays of treatment. Intravenous fluids, nasogastric drainage and opiate analgesia should be given. Pethidine is preferred to morphine because it does not cause spasm of the sphincter of Oddi. Initially the inflammation is sterile so antibiotics can be reserved for patients with infection. Other medical therapies including steroids, glucagon and trasylol have not been shown to confer significant benefit in clinical trials.

The degree of respiratory impairment is often greater than can be predicted clinically so that oxygen therapy, physiotherapy and close monitoring of respiratory rate, pattern of breathing, colour and blood gases is advisable. An X-ray of the chest may show a small left-sided pleural effusion or basal atelectasis. Deterioration can be rapid so that mechanical ventilation is often necessary for severe cases. Organ failure carries a high mortality, especially in the tropics.

Table 21.2 Prognostic features in acute pancreatitis.

Ranson (New York)	Imrie (Glasgow)
On admission	
Age > 55 years	
WBC > 16 000 per mm³	
Blood glucose > 10 mmol/l	
LDH > 350 units/l	
sGOT > 250 units/l	
Within 48 hours	
Hct fall > 10%	WBC > 15 000 per mm³
PaO_2 < 8 KPa	PaO_2 < 8 KPa
Urea rise > 4 mmol/l	Urea > 16 mmol/l
Fluid sequestration > 6 litres	LDH > 600 units/l
Base deficit > 4 mmol/l	AST > 200 units/l
	Plasma albumin < 32 g/l
	Uncorrected Ca < 2.0 mmol/l
Other indicators of severity	
Dark coloured pancreatic ascites indicates severe attack	
α_2-macroglobulin < 1.5 g/l indicates necrosis	
Development of organ failure (respiratory, renal, cardiac) confers high mortality	

WBC, white blood cell count;
LDH, lactate dehydrogenase;
sGOT = ALT, olanine aminotransferase;
AST, aspartate aminotransferase
Hct, haematocrit

Blood glucose homeostasis must be monitored. Hyperglycaemia may not develop until there is pancreatic necrosis but will require an intravenous insulin–dextrose–potassium infusion. Those with prolonged starvation due to complications or ileus need parenteral nutrition if this is available.

Biliary ascariasis

Ascaris lumbricoides worms in the bile or pancreatic ducts (Figure 21.1) should either be treated expectantly without wormicides until the worm returns to the gastrointestinal tract. Extraction of the worm by ERCP and Dormier basket can sometimes be achieved.

The role of surgery

The role of surgery is limited to laparotomy where the diagnosis is in doubt or to manage complications of pancreatitis.

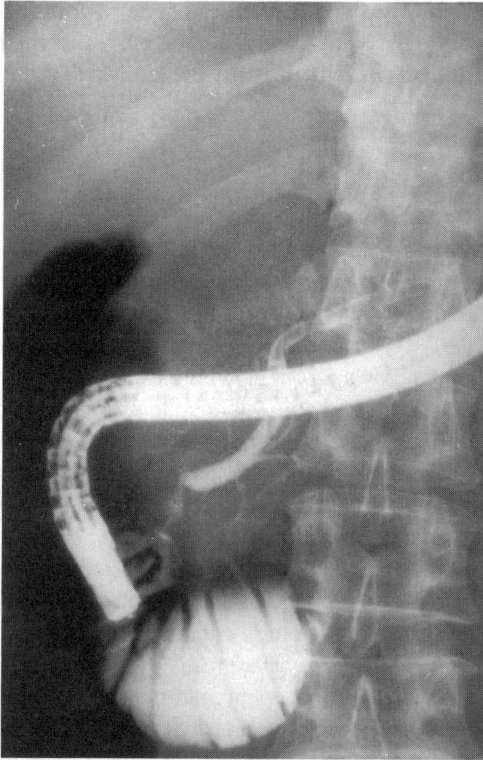

Figure 21.1   Endoscopic retrograde pancreaticogram in a Chinese patient with pancreatitis showing *Ascaris lumbricoides* in the pancreatic duct. This worm was extracted using a Dormier basket (courtesy of Mr SCS Chung).

Peritoneal lavage

Peritoneal lavage may be diagnostic but has also been proposed as a form of postoperative irrigation therapy. Drains are inserted in the lesser sac, paracolic gutters and pelvis so that the peritoneal cavity can be irrigated intermittently. It has not been shown to improve the outcome significantly but is worth considering where renal failure develops and haemodialysis or haemofiltration is not available. In such cases peritoneal diasylate can be used as the irrigation fluid which may help to maintain metabolic balance.

Pancreatic necrosis

Some surgeons advise scooping out the pancreatic phlegmon with or without total pancreatectomy and inserting drains to the lesser sac. Surgery of this nature requires experience and should not be undertaken lightly. Total pancreatectomy early in the disease is more prone to complication and mortality than waiting a few more days for the necrotic pancreas to be soft enough to scoop out. Multiple debridements and packing are often necessary.

Case history 1

A 38-year-old Chinese female was admitted with an 8-h history of acute epigastric pain radiating to the back. She had vomited twice but her vital signs were stable. There was no gas under the diaphragm on an erect chest X-ray and the serum amylase was 1260 units/l. Within a few hours she developed tachypnoea and hypotension. Her PaO_2 was 11.0 KPa and she was treated with intravenous saline, colloids and oxygen. Despite an improvement in blood pressure her general condition deteriorated over the next few hours and she was transferred to the intensive care unit for mechanical ventilation. For the next 48 h she was stable and then she had further episodes of hypotension which required fluids and inotropic support. Because she had paralytic ileus, parenteral nutrition was commenced. On day 7 she developed hyperglycaemia necessitating insulin therapy. Ultrasound of the pancreas was inconclusive because of bowel gas interposition so she had a computed tomography (CT) scan which showed areas of the pancreas to be poorly delineated. A few days later laparotomy was undertaken and the entire pancreas was found to be necrotic. There were no stones in the gallbladder or biliary tree. The pancreas was scooped out by hand and gauze dissection and the pancreatic bed packed. She had four further laparotomies every second or third day to further debride the pancreatic bed until it was clean. Although she had septicaemia she improved after each debridement and change of packs. Once her condition stabilised the packing and relaparotomies were stopped.

Abscess formation

External tube drainage is indicated for an established abscess. Aspiration under ultrasound or CT scan control may be tried in specialised centres. Abscesses or infected psuedocysts may extend behind the right or left colon and require drainage in the loin or iliac fossae. Repeated drainage may be necessary.

Psuedocyst

A psuedocyst is an enzyme-rich collection of pancreatic fluid, usually in the lesser sac. It has no epithelial lining, the walls being derived from fibrous tissue, peritoneum, retroperitoneum or serosa of adjacent viscera. An acute psuedocyst arises as a result of duct disruption during a severe attack of acute pancreatitis and tends to resolve. Chronic psuedocysts arise from obstructed and deformed ducts, normally as a result of chronic pancreatitis with acute exacerbations and regress less readily. Psuedocysts are more often diagnosed now that ultrasound scanning is widely available and occur in at least 10 per cent of cases of pancreatitis. Their clinical presentation includes:

1. persistent vomiting due to a large mass pressing on the stomach and duodenum;
2. an epigastric mass which is smooth, usually slightly tender and often fluctuant; rarely, a psuedocyst may present in the left iliac fossa;
3. biliary obstruction;
4. erosion of a blood vessel which necessitates surgery or embolisation to stop the bleeding;
5. secondary infection with deterioration in the patient's condition; or,
6. failure to improve and persistent fever or leukocytosis after an attack of acute pancreatitis.

Case history 2

A 25-year-old male prisoner was admitted with persistent vomiting. On examination he was dehydrated, febrile and there was an ill-defined mass in the epigastrium, which was moderately tender. The rest of the abdomen was soft. His white blood count was elevated. Endoscopy was normal except there was an impression of a mass behind the stomach. Ultrasound scanning showed a pancreatic psuedocyst. Further questioning revealed he had been beaten and kicked in the abdomen during police interrogation. He was resuscitated, treated by nasogastric suction and observed. Over the next week he failed to improve so a cystogastrostomy was carried out. A few days later he was able to resume a normal diet.

Treatment

A pseudocyst that is not causing severe symptoms can be observed and its size followed with ultrasound examination. Surgery is only necessary for complicated or large persistent psuedocysts. Internal drainage is indicated for uninfected, mature psuedocysts. An anastomosis is made between the cyst and the stomach, jejunum or duodenum, the site depending on the actual anatomy of the cyst. Internal drainage can sometimes be achieved endoscopically rather than by open operation. External drainage is preferable for thin-walled or infected cysts.

Cystadenoma and cystadenocarcinoma

Occasionally pancreatic tumours may be cystic. Cysts that do not resolve should be aspirated and biopsied.

Chronic pancreatitis

Pathology

This term encompasses a variety of conditions causing chronic inflammation. Destruction of the gland with atrophy results in permanent loss of exocrine and endocrine function. It is characterised by pain, diabetes, and pancreatic malabsorption (diarrhoea, steatorrhoea). There are three main types:

1. Chronic obstructive pancreatitis: duct obstruction results in chronic pancreatitis distal to the block with almost normal pancreatic tissue more proximally.
2. Chronic calcifying pancreatitis: irregular, lobular spotty foci of calcium within the gland. Atrophy, stenosis of minor ducts and dilatation of major ducts are features. Surgical relief of obstruction is often effective.
3. Minimal change pancreatitis results in severe intermittent or continuous pain, often following an attack of acute pancreatitis. The gland appears normal but there are microscopic lesions of the acini. Surgery is seldom effective.

Tropical pancreatitis

Tropical pancreatitis is characterised by a triad of upper abdominal pain, diabetes and pancreatic calcification in the absence of a history of alcohol ingestion. These three features are not always present. It was first described in East Africa and 10 per cent of diabetics in East and West Africa have pancreatic calcification. The highest incidence is found in the south Indian state of Kerala. The aetiology is unknown.

Clinical presentation

It presents with persistent, chronic and sometimes severe abdominal pain, often associated with diabetes and significant weight loss. A plain abdominal X-ray may show calcification and sometimes pancreatic duct calculi up to 4.5 cm in diameter. A small proportion may be jaundiced due to pancreatic fibrosis around the distal end of the common bile duct. Tropical pancreatitis is associated with the development of malignancy. The combination of age above 40 years, short duration of symptoms, mass lesions on ultrasonography and main pancreatic duct obstruction on endoscopic retrograde cholangiopancreatography (ERCP) is associated with a high risk of malignancy in Kerala.

Management

Diabetes should be controlled and is the most important factor influencing survival. Malabsorption requires supplementation with pancreatic enzymes. However, the low fat content of the diet in south India is probably responsible for steatorrhoea not being a common complaint there.

Surgery is indicated for intractable pain only where pancreatic duct dilatation and calculi are present. Surgery may be difficult so, if possible, should be preceeded by preoperative ductal assessment by ERCP or direct pancreatic duct cannulation under ultrasound guidance. A long pancreaticojejunostomy (Puestow) is the operation of choice if there is a dilated duct. Stones must be cleared from the main duct. A transduodenal sphincteroplasty may sometimes be added. A distal pancreatectomy alone may be effective in the few cases where disease is limited to the distal pancreas. A chronic pancreatic psuedocyst should be drained into the most appropriate part of the gastrointestinal tract (p 362). The presence of malignancy makes a good outcome from surgery unlikely unless the tumour is small and resectable.

Further reading

Acute pancreatitis

Huizinga WKJ, Baker LW. Treatment of persistent and complicated pancreatic psuedocysts. J R Coll Surg Edinb 1992;37:373–6.

Khuroo MS, Zargar SA, Yattoo GN, *et al. Ascaris*-induced acute pancreatitis. Br J Surg 1992;79:1335–8.

Reynaert MS, Dugernier T, Kestens PJ. Current therapeutic strategies in severe acute pancreatitis. Intensive Care Med 1990;16:352–62.

Vitale GC. Intervention endoscopic retrograde cholangiopancreatography: state of the art. J R Coll Surg Edinb 1992;37:289–98 & 357–68.

Chronic pancreatitis

Mabogunje OA, Lawrie JH. Surgery for chronic pancreatitis in Zaria, Nigeria. World J Surg 1990;14:45–7.

Ramesh H, Augustine P. Surgery in tropical pancreatitis: an analysis of risk factors. Br J Surg 1992;79:544–9.

Russell C. Chronic pancreatitis. Surgery (Medicine group) 1992;247–50.

Sarles H. Chronic pancreatitis and diabetes. Baillières Clin Endocrinol Metab 1992;6: 745–75.

Thomas PG. Observations and surgical management of tropical pancreatitis in Kerala and southern India. World J Surg 1990;14:32–42.

22

The Acute Abdomen in Children

The term 'acute abdomen' defines a clinical picture that includes the sudden recent onset of abdominal pain and tenderness, either localised or generalised, suggesting a clinical diagnosis of peritonitis. This in turn may have several causes of which inflammation of the peritoneum is the final common pathway.

Peritonitis

Bacterial peritonitis may be a primary infection but is more commonly secondary to a disorder of the gut or female genital tract such as intestinal perforation or inflammation of an abdominal viscus. Non-bacterial peritonitis may be due to the presence of blood, urine, or any other noxious agent within the peritoneal cavity.

Pathophysiology

In response to inflammation the peritoneum produces a massive fluid exudate which may be purulent, and the omentum, appendices epiploicae and loops of bowel become oedematous and tend to localise the stimulus by the formation of adhesions and the creation of intraperitoneal abscesses.

Pain is an important feature. Pain of visceral origin which is appreciated through the autonomic nervous system is poorly localised but is regionalised according to the embryological derivation of the affected viscus. Thus visceral pain of foregut origin is referred to the epigastrium, that of midgut origin to the umbilicus and that of hindgut origin to the hypogastrium.

When the peritoneum becomes affected, pain is appreciated through somatic nerves allowing accurate localisation. Thus the early pain of appendicitis – the visceral pain of appendiceal obstruction – is felt at the umbilicus as the appendix is of midgut origin. When inflammation reaches the peritoneum the pain is accurately localised in the right iliac fossa. The pain is thus thought to have moved from the umbilicus to the right iliac fossa – a classical point of history in appendicitis.

Clinical signs and symptoms

As a result of peritoneal inflammation there is a reflex spasm of the muscles of the abdominal wall. This protective reflex spasm is termed 'guarding'. It may be difficult to distinguish between voluntary contraction of the abdominal wall in an anxious patient and involuntary guarding unless the patient is somehow distracted. Guarding may be sufficient to fully justify the description of 'board-like' rigidity.

Rebound or percussion tenderness are encountered when the parietal peritoneum is inflamed. In this regard the umbilical hernia provides an invaluable window into the abdomen. At this site the skin and parietal peritoneum are in apposition and the tenderness of peritonitis is easily demonstrated by gently tapping the apex of the hernia. Where peritonitis is not present, a finger inserted through the hernial ring can clearly palpate the abdominal viscera.

In patients with a patent processus vaginalis inflammation will track down into the scrotum and may present as an acute hydrocele, or mimic a testicular torsion. The converse is also true, if at exploration of the scrotum the tunica is found to contain pus then laparotomy must follow. Inflammation of the peritoneum inhibits peristalsis resulting in an adynamic ileus, either local or general. This in turn contributes to the abdominal fullness frequently seen as well as to vomiting and the resultant fluid deficit.

Acute abdominal symptoms may occasionally be due to extra-abdominal causes. Cardiac, oesophageal and pulmonary diseases may all present with upper abdominal pain. Metabolic disorders such as diabetes mellitus and porphyria may also present with abdominal pain as the dominant symptom. Retroperitoneal inflammation, e.g. urinary infection or perinephric infection, psoas abscesses and occasionally tetanus may produce signs similar to those of the acute abdomen. Perhaps the most frequent extra-abdominal association is with upper respiratory infections which are frequently associated with abdominal pain, presumably due to enlargement of the gut-associated lymphoid tissue. Such mesenteric adenitis may only be diagnosed at exploration for a presumed appendicitis.

In addition to local signs and symptoms within the abdomen, the patient with peritonitis will show signs of fluid deficit, toxaemia and often the symptomatology of the precipitating disorder. Occasionally special investigations may be necessary before surgery, but it must be emphasised that the diagnosis of peritonitis is a clinical responsibility and this cannot be delegated to X-rays, white cell counts or any other index.

Neonatal peritonitis

Signs of peritonitis in the neonate are difficult to elicit and diagnosis is often delayed. Symptoms may be non-specific and simply suggest 'sepsis'. Should no obvious source be found elsewhere, the abdomen must fall suspect despite clinical innocence. By the time local signs (staining of the flanks, abdominal wall oedema, umbilical flare) develop, the pathology is far advanced. Radiography is more useful in this age group where the cause of peritonitis commonly related to gut ischaemia either due to enterocolitis or volvulus.

Management

Almost without exception the diagnosis of peritonitis infers the need for resuscitation with a view to surgery. The only exception is the rare patient in whom a confident diagnosis of primary peritonitis has been made and in whom the response to antibiotic therapy has been complete and sustained.

As the precise diagnosis of the primary cause is often impossible before operation, preparation for theatre must encompass all the likely diagnoses. Thus in addition to fluid resuscitation, antibiotics effective against bowel organisms, particularly Gram negatives, should be used in conjunction with an anti-anaerobic agent. As Gram positive cover is also required it is useful to chose an agent also effective against *Salmonella typhi*. A suitable regime for many areas would include ampicillin, and aminoglycoside and metronidazole. This latter in addition to being active against all obligate anaerobes is also an effective amoebicide. A reasonable alternative is a combination of penicillin and chloramphenicol which has a serious but rare toxicity. Some of the newer cephalosporins and ampicillin/clavulanic acid combinations also have broad spectra of activity including most pathogenic anaerobes.

Circulating blood volume must be restored before operation and fluid resuscitation must continue until the urine output is restored. The minimum acceptable urine volume is 1 ml/kg per hour, every hour, and monitoring this requires an indwelling urethral catheter. Urine output is generally a more useful guide to fluid replacement than pulse or blood pressure alone.

Pain is a distressing symptom and has significant morbid sequelae. The signs of peritonitis cannot be masked by analgesia, the symptoms however can be relieved. As no useful purpose is fulfilled by having the patient suffer pain, analgesics, preferably intravenous, form an important aspect of preoperative management. Similarly vomiting is distressing to the patient and this can be obviated by the passage and regular aspiration of a nasogastric tube.

In areas of endemic ascariasis patients will vomit worms irrespective of the cause of their vomiting. Thus the appearance of worms in vomitus does not by itself justify a diagnosis of complicated ascariasis. Similarly, in many cultures it is traditional to administer a herbal or other enema to patients with abdominal symptoms. The enema must not be blamed for the symptoms of the primary disease.

Practice points
• *Peritonitis implies:*
  – *Fluid loss*
    a. *into peritoneal cavity*
    b. *within bowel*

- *Electrolyte losses*
- *Paralytic ileus*
- *Bacteraemia/septicaemia*
- *Pain*

Practice points
- *Resuscitation requires:*
  - *Intravenous drip*
  - *Nasogastric tube*
  - *Urethral catheter*
  - *Intravenous antibiotics*
  - *Analgesia*

Primary peritonitis

In the First World primary peritonitis is rarely seen, due no doubt to the aggressive use of antibiotics in the management of infections, particularly of the upper respiratory tract. In such areas primary peritonitis is confined almost exclusively to the immunosuppressed child, classically with the nephrotic syndrome. In tropical countries by contrast primary peritonitis can account for up to 5 per cent of all admissions for peritonitis. It is more common in girls.

Pathophysiology

In primary peritonitis the infecting agent originates most commonly from the respiratory tract or female genital tract. The infection is usually due to a single species of organism – *Pneumococcus*, *Haemophilus influenzae* or *Escherichia coli* – rather than the mixed flora of secondary peritonitis. The pus is never malodorous. The faeculent smell of the peritonitic abdomen indicates the presence of anaerobic organisms which are of gut or genital tract origin and therefore indicative of secondary peritonitis.

Clinical presentation

If the patient is immunosuppressed for whatever reason a presumptive diagnosis can be made. Many patients are however only diagnosed at laparotomy performed for peritonitis of unknown origin. Even where clinical suspicion is high, if the response to conservative treatment is equivocal or poorly sustained, surgery will be necessary as even immunosuppressed patients may develop peritonitis secondary to intestinal pathology. Clues that might suggest a diagnosis of primary peritonitis include a high fever, concurrent or recent respiratory infection, female gender or a local 'epidemic'. Otherwise the signs and symptoms are non-specific: diffuse abdominal pain, guarding and rebound tenderness.

Management

Resuscitation should proceed as if the patient were being prepared for surgery. If sufficient free fluid is present to permit safe diagnostic paracentesis, the diagnosis may be confirmed by the finding of a Gram-positive monoculture, and the absence of odour. Intravenous antibiotics will elicit a rapid improvement in clinical signs and symptoms. Should this response be equivocal or poorly sustained then surgery can be performed without delay. This of course implies careful monitoring.

Surgery

Surgery will frequently be undertaken with no specific diagnosis established. It is therefore appropriate to make an incision through which the whole abdomen may be examined. In small children an epigastric transverse incision fulfils this requirement. In older children a longitudinal incision may be necessary, but this is rare under the age of 8 years.

Thin, watery, odourless pus is strongly suggestive of primary peritonitis but a full laparotomy is still essential to exclude a primary lesion. If none is found, appropriate specimens are taken for culture and the peritoneal cavity lavaged with warm saline. Incidental procedures e.g. appendicectomy should never be performed. Subsequent antibiotic therapy can be guided by the results of cultures.

Practice points
- *Primary peritonitis is relatively common in the Third World.*
- *It is caused generally by a single organism.*
- *Pus is thin, watery and does not smell.*
- *A thorough exploration must be made to exclude a primary lesion.*

Appendicitis

Appendicitis can no longer be regarded as rare in the Third World, and has become in many areas the commonest cause of peritonitis. Delayed presentation, associated disorders, particularly malnutrition in children as well as occasionally the lack of surgical or anaesthetic expertise conspire to make the mortality of appendicitis in tropical areas distressingly high.

Pathophysiology

In the vast majority of patients with appendicitis the initial event is obstruction of the appendiceal lumen. Frequently this is due to hypertrophy of the lymphoid tissue within the wall, or to a luminal concretion or faecalith. In the tropics, in addition to faecaliths, fruit pips, and other ingested material, pin-worms, round worms, schistosomes and amoebae have all been associated with acute appendicitis. Following luminal obstruction there is an accumulation of mucus within the lumen, bacterial proliferation and eventual necrosis of the wall secondary to the tension within.

The omentum, small bowel and appendices epiploicae respond by attaching to the sick organ and attempt to localise the infection which results from necrosis. When successful the resulting phlegmon may present as an appendix mass, which may progress to, or be a form of, appendix abscess. When unsuccessful, and the thin omentum in children has been blamed for the relatively poor ability of children to localise the inflamed appendix, then rupture into the free peritoneal cavity with the development of generalised peritonitis results.

Clinical features

During the phase of visceral obstruction pain is felt in a midgut distribution – at the umbilicus. When the peritoneum is inflamed the pain is accurately localised to the right iliac fossa (see above).

The tip of the appendix is usually retrocaecal but may lie in any position. Contiguous inflammation of any number of structures may attempt to confound the clinician.

Thus psoas spasm drawing attention to the hip joint may be seen in retrocaecal appendicitis, urinary frequency with pyuria in pelvic appendicitis, and diarrhoea may result if the appendix is in contact with the terminal ileum.

Tenderness over the right iliac fossa is a fairly constant finding with associated rebound tenderness. Guarding prevents the clear definition of a mass in many patients but a sensation of fullness may be recognised.

Systemic signs include a low fever, rarely over 38.5°C, halitosis and a furred tongue. Symptoms vary enormously but anorexia is almost constant. Headache and high fever must raise suspicion of typhoid fever, or some other non-appendiceal pathology.

Due to the variability of signs and symptoms clinical diagnosis is often erroneous. Careful clinical observation will detect many who do not need surgery, but it is better to operate and be sure than to delay surgery in one who needs it.

Management

The management of acute appendicitis is emergency appendicectomy, and the patient must be made fit for surgery. Fluid replacement is often urgently required. Once the diagnosis is made analgesics should be given, and prophylactic antibiotics started (metronidazole or cefoxitin).

Surgery

With the patient under general anaesthetic and paralysed, examine the abdomen again. Under anaesthesia a mass may be palpable which was previously concealed.

The incision depends upon the diagnosis. If the diagnosis is of appendicitis and the signs were restricted to the right iliac fossa, then a grid iron muscle-splitting incision is adequate. However if the diagnosis is one of peritonitis of uncertain origin then a laparotomy incision is indicated. Having located the appendix, secured its mesentery, ligated the base and excised the organ, it is unnecessary to invaginate the stump in the traditional way, and transfixion ligature of the base is adequate. Lavage of the peritoneal cavity with saline completes the procedure.

Appendix abscess

Drains are rarely indicated but may be used to drain large periappendiceal abscesses. It is not in fact essential to remove the appendix in such cases. Drainage of the abscess is the life-saving procedure, the appendicectomy can be done later. Drainage is only appropriate in a localised abscess. One cannot drain the peritoneal cavity. The decision to suture the subcutaneous tissue and skin rests upon assessment of the degree of contamination during surgery. It is perfectly safe to leave the superficial layers of the wound open and dressed with tulle gras.

Normal appendix

If the appendix is found to be normal at exploration it is essential to examine other organs that may account for the clinical picture. By retracting the lower border of the wound it is easy to examine the ovaries, tubes and uterus; occasionally torsion of an ovarian cyst or tumour, salpingitis or ectopic pregnancy may be found. It is important to seek a Meckel's diverticulum which is found in 2 per cent of the population some 50 cm from the ileocaecal valve. Such a diverticulum may be the source of diverticulitis or perforation of a peptic ulcer. In any event it should be removed.

The nodes of the ileal mesentery and retroperitoneum should be assessed if mesenteric adenitis is suspected. If nothing is found and the peritoneal cavity is clean the wound may be closed and extra-abdominal causes for the presenting symptoms sought. If nothing is found through an iliac fossa incision but there is pus or other evidence of mischief within the peritoneal cavity, then the iliac wound should be closed and a formal laparotomy made.

Intussusception

Intussusception results from disordered intestinal motility such that the proximal bowel invaginates into the distal bowel (Figure 22.1). In Western countries most patients are under one year of age and intussusception is associated with hypertrophy of lymphoid tissue in the bowel wall, either as a result of a respiratory infection or weaning diet. In the Third World this subset of patients is also seen but is equalled in number by older children in whom the primary disorder is an acute diarrhoeal illness. Lead points such as Meckel's diverticulum, polyps or other tumours are rare. In tropical countries presentation is usually delayed resulting in cumulative management difficulties. Further the differential diagnosis is much broader and encompasses such disorders as ascariasis, amoebiasis, dysentery and herbal enemata.

Pathophysiology

As the proximal bowel passes into, and along the distal bowel, firstly the lymphatic, then the venous drainage are obstructed resulting in oedema and

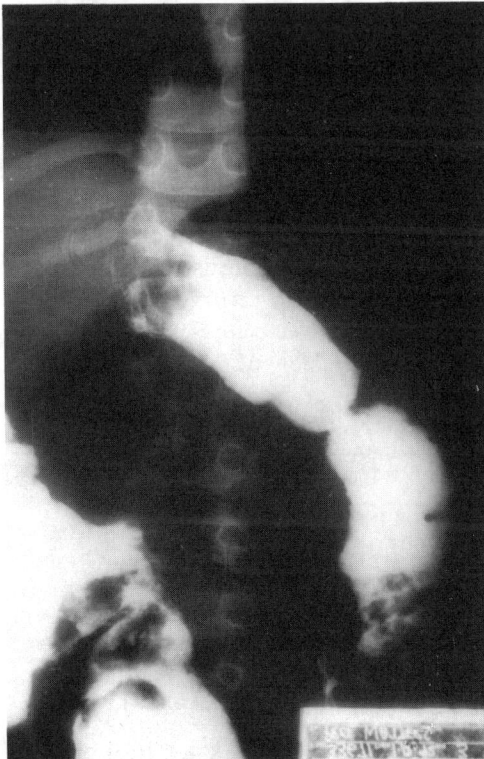

Figure 22.1 Barium enema showing an intussusception extending to the mid-transverse colon.

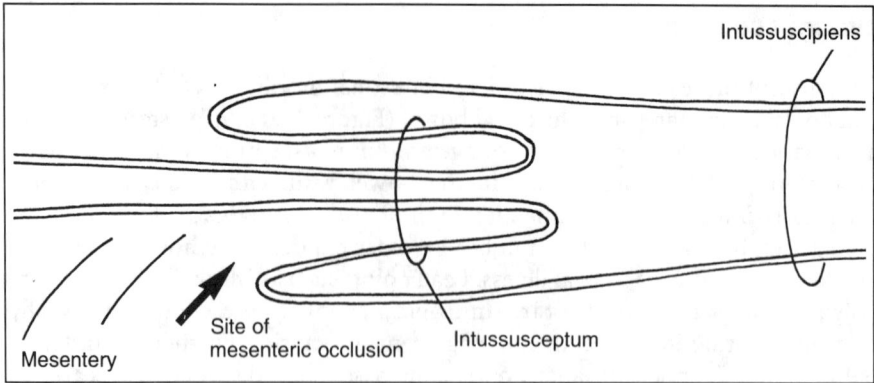

Figure 22.2 Anatomy of an intussusception.

congestion of the intussusceptum within the intussuscepiens which prevents reduction (Figure 22.2). This mucosal congestion results in blood and mucus escaping into the lumen of the distal bowel and this is classically passed as 'red currant jelly' stools, although bleeding from intussusception may be anything from torrential haemorrhage to none at all.

Ultimately microcirculatory occlusion occurs and the intussusceptum becomes gangrenous. However as the venous and lymphatic drainage from the gangrenous bowel is occluded the patient may be deceptively well. Only when reduction is attempted will organisms and bacterial toxins flood into the portal circulation with resulting endotoxaemia and septic shock.

Because the terminal ileum contains a major portion of the gut-associated lymphoid tissue it is a common site of origin of intussusception. In children over 2 years in whom the aetiology is probably different, more than 50 per cent originate in the transverse colon. The intussusceptum may extend a variable distance along the distal bowel often protruding per anum where it must not be confused with rectal prolapse (see below). Occasionally the intussusception involves only the small bowel (Table 22.1).

Table 22.1   Site of intussusception in 77 children.

	Under 2 years	Over 2 years	Total
Ileocolic	37 (80%)	11 (35%)	48 (62%)
Colocolic	5 (11%)	17 (55%)	22 (29%)
Enteroenteric	4 (9%)	3 (10%)	7 (9%)

Clinical presentation

In babies the clinical triad of intestinal colic, reflex vomiting and rectal blood loss is frequently seen. The colic may be dramatic. The baby pales, screams and draws up the legs. This lasts for several minutes before the spasm passes, the screaming stops and the child may go to sleep. Vomiting may occur, not because of intestinal obstruction but on a reflex basis. Blood may be passed rectally and there is usually a mucoid stool.

In older children the illness often begins with diarrhoea. This may suddenly cease with the onset of colic and vomiting which may be difficult to distinguish from the colic of enterocolitis. The patient may be dehydrated from the diarrhoeal illness in addition to the vomiting.

Examination at all ages may reveal a sausage-shaped slightly tender mass. Failure to palpate the mass does not exclude an intussusception as it may be hiding under the costal margin or liver. The mass must be distinguished from a bolus of ascaris worms. Usually this is easy on clinical or plain radiological grounds, but if doubt persists a contrast enema is urgently indicated to rule out an intussusception.

In 25 per cent of patients the intussusceptum is palpable on rectal examination and this should never be omitted. Because the presentation may be similar to amoebic colitis any patient with blood in the stool deserves proctoscopy to assess mucosal ulceration.

An intussusception prolapsing per anum can be differentiated from a rectal prolapse by passing a finger alongside the projecting mass into the rectum (see also Figure 23.3). This will be impossible to achieve in rectal prolapse. Additionally as an intussusception is tethered on one side by the mesentery it tends to prolapse in a curve towards that side.

Diagnosis

A contrast enema may be both diagnostic and therapeutic, although it is generally less therapeutically successful in the tropics than in temperate regions. This may in part be due to the later presentation of children in tropical areas. Dilute barium sulphate should be used but not Gastrografin because the latter may cause dehydration.

As contrast permeates between the intussusceptum and intussuscepiens it outlines the mucosal pattern of the intussusceptum as a coil-spring. By elevating the bag of contrast medium to a maximum height of 1.5 m the intussusception may slowly reduce, and this can be watched on the X-ray screen. Reflux of contrast into the terminal ileum along with the passage of flatus and improvement in the child's symptoms confirm reduction. Air is an effective reduction agent, and a modified sphygmomanometer can be used to apply up to 100 mmHg pressure to the apex of the intussusception and reduction similarly monitored radiologically.

Management

Before any therapeutic manoeuvres are attempted the child must be fully resuscitated. This may require large volumes of plasma and crystalloid to restore urinary output. Antibiotics should be started in anticipation of bacteraemia following reduction. The only absolute contraindication to air or contrast reduction is evidence of perforation or peritonitis. If however no progress is made in any 10-min period of attempted reduction, surgery is necessary.

Surgery

The abdomen is opened, usually through a right-sided transverse incision which can be extended as necessary. The lesion is defined and gentle pressure applied to the apex of the intussusception to slowly reduce it. Hurrying will result in serosal tears, or worse, of the intussuscipiens. Pulling on the invaginated bowel will simply avulse it. The apex of the reduced intussusceptum is often oedematous and thickened. This is not a lead point and does not need to be removed.

Ischaemic bowel or a genuine lead point such as Meckel's diverticulum requires resection and primary anastomosis. It is quite unnecessary to fix the caecum or perform any other manoeuvres to prevent recurrence.

Post-operative care

Meticulous monitoring is required to maintain fluid balance. Antibiotics against gut flora should be continued. There is a 2 per cent risk of recurrence following non-operative reduction but a much smaller risk following surgery.

Practice points
- *Non-operative reduction is sometimes successful despite a long history.*
- *Contraindicated if peritonitis or frank perforation present.*
- *Operate only after full resuscitation.*
- *Squeeze out an intussusception, never pull it.*
- *Don't perform incidental procedures.*
- *Anticipate endotoxaemia.*

Special situations

1. Intussusception occasionally occurs after a laparotomy, particularly with retroperitoneal dissection. Such intussusceptions are usually enteroenteric and not demonstrated on enema studies. Diagnosis is usually made at a second-look operation following persistence of postoperative ileus. Surprisingly these lesions rarely become ischaemic, despite the delays in diagnosis, and simple reduction is all that is needed.
2. Chronic intussusceptions occur without intestinal obstruction, and symptoms may be present for weeks. Although the bowel is clearly viable in this situation, operative reduction is often made necessary by adhesions between the intussusceptum and the neck of the intussuscepiens.

Such patients allegedly have an increased incidence of lead points, particularly lymphomata.

Typhoid perforation

Typhoid fever is endemic in many areas of the Third World being associated with poor sanitation and contamination of water supplies. The disease is seen occasionally in First World areas among travellers, and epidemics are periodically seen throughout the world.

Surgical interest in typhoid centres upon perforation of the gut which is seen in 2–3 per cent of cases in children, and intestinal bleeding which is seen less often. It must be emphasised that these are complications that occur in a patient already debilitated by the systemic effects of the primary disease. The reduction in mortality following perforation over the past decade from 60 per cent to < 10 per cent, has been almost entirely due to recognition of this fact and the placement of due emphasis on prompt recognition of perforation, aggressive resuscitation and early surgery.

Presentation

Intestinal perforation may occur at any stage of the disease in any patient but is most commonly seen in the second or third week of illness. An 'acute abdomen' may be the presenting complaint or perforation may occur in a child already on treatment. In this latter group the import of complaints of abdominal pain may be underestimated. Any sudden deterioration in the condition of a child being treated for typhoid, particularly if associated with abdominal pain must raise suspicion of perforation. The mortality of delay in diagnosis is high enough to recommend operative diagnosis in cases of doubt.

Investigation

Half of the patients with perforation will show radiological evidence of free air. Half of the patients will not. The diagnosis of perforation is clearly a clinical responsibility, and it is important to note that absence of pneumoperitoneum does not exclude intestinal perforation. Similarly whilst leucopaenia may suggest typhoid fever, perforation may be associated with a white cell count that is normal or high.

Patients may show laboratory evidence of the primary disease such as deranged hepatic function, Widal tests or blood cultures and cognisance must be taken of pre-existing organ dysfunction during preparation for theatre, but there is no laboratory index of perforation.

Resuscitation

Although the surgery for typhoid perforation is rarely extensive, an investment in preoperative preparation pays dividends. Antibiotic cover must encompass not only *Salmonella typhi* but also the intestinal flora that are now released into the peritoneal cavity. Circulating volume must be restored and freeze-dried plasma may be indicated to correct any pre-existing deficit of hepatic clotting factors.

Surgery

Perforation occurs through ulceration of a lymphoid aggregate within the ileal, or rarely caecal wall. The intervening bowel is usually healthy and well able to withstand suturing. Thus excision of the affected Peyer's patch with direct repair of the ileum, oversewing of near-perforations which present as dark patches on the adjacent bowel and peritoneal lavage with saline is all that is required. Diversion, bypass or resection of lengths of bowel are generally unnecessary however obviously if multiple perforations are clustered in a short length of bowel it may be expedient to resect that length rather than perform multiple excisions. Wound infections can be minimised by leaving the superficial layers of the wound unsutured.

Post-operative care

Despite having a laparotomy these patients still have typhoid fever and not surprisingly complications are frequent. Chest infection occurs not only as part of the septicaemia but also follows inadequate pain relief.

Antibiotics are continued, despite which intraperitoneal abscesses are occasionally seen and these, in addition to the possibility of reperforation through a suture line or through another lymphoid aggregate, justify an aggressive attitude to reoperation if clinical progress is not maintained. Intestinal fistulae are rare and as they generally originate in the distal ileum, can be treated non-operatively.

Recurrence or relapse of typhoid can be seen in about 5 per cent of patients.

Bleeding

Typhoid causes ulceration of the mucosa of the ileum in particular and it is not surprising that bleeding occurs. That it does not stop is perhaps more remarkable. In many patients this reluctance to stop bleeding is clearly due to an acquired thrombocytopaenia or a deficiency of hepatically derived clotting factors secondary to typhoid hepatitis. These parameters must be corrected before any thought is given to operative intervention.

Occasionally exsanguinating haemorrhage will mandate intervention, and despite the volume of blood being passed it may be difficult to identify the source. Angiography is of limited value, often revealing an unhelpful diffuse 'blush'. Occasionally the surgeon may have no alternative to a blind right hemicolectomy. This should not be undertaken lightly as it is in this group of patients that the long-term sequelae of loss of the terminal ileum will be most clearly manifest.

Amoebiasis

Entamoeba histolytica is a common commensal of the alimentary tract in the Third World. Although the presence of encysted amoebae in the stool is held by the WHO to represent amoebiasis, clinicians refer only to invasive amoebiasis as indicative of a disease state.

Amoebae are commensals in the caecum and right colon and encyst as they pass to the left. Under undefined circumstances they may invade the mucosa producing an amoebic dysentery or mucosal colitis which rarely attracts surgical attention due to its dramatic response to metronidazole.

Pathophysiology

The fundamental lesion of amoebiasis is an occlusive vasculopathy affecting small vessels in the target organ. In the liver this results in liquefactive necrosis which manifests as hepatic 'abscesses'. In the colon full thickness, or transmural, necrosis results in perforation. To describe the surgical expression of this disease as 'perforation' is perhaps misleading as the operative findings are usually of a varying length of dead colon which has ceded its ability to retain organisms. The striking feature of the colonic pathology is the attraction of the omentum which initially attempts to seal the leakage and may in fact revascularise the necrotic colon. This has an important bearing on operative management. It also affects the presentation as the omentum wrapping around the diseased bowel effectively retroperitonealises the disease and prevents contamination of the peritoneal cavity until late in the disease process. Thus signs of peritonitis may not be seen until the pathology is advanced.

The cause of the initial vasculopathy may be related to the development of anti-neutrophil cytoplasmic antibodies which are known to be associated with hepatic amoebiasis and other forms of vasculopathy.

Presentation

Any child, but particularly any malnourished child, with a current or recent history of copious diarrhoea, prostration and abdominal pain must be suspected of suffering from amoebic colitis. The stool is often mucoid and contains blood causing confusion with intussusception (see above). Occasionally the stool contains large sloughs of rectal mucosa or rarely a mucosal cast of the rectum and colon.

Hepatic amoebiasis may co-exist in 20 per cent of patients. Because the omentum effectively confines the disease initially to the retroperitoneum, abdominal signs may be unconvincing and amount to little more than tenderness on deep palpation. It must be emphasised that progression of the disease from mucosal colitis to transmural necrosis and ultimately free perforation may be undramatic and close clinical monitoring is required to detect the gradual deterioration.

In endemic areas all patients presenting to a surgical service with diarrhoea or blood in the stool are entitled to expect proctoscopy to evaluate the rectal mucosa. If no ulcers are present at this site then amoebiasis can be dropped down the table of differential diagnoses.

Investigation

Following proctoscopy, the cardinal diagnostic finding is of haematophagous amoebae on microscopy of fresh stool. The finding of encysted forms is irrelevant. Confirmatory tests such as gel diffusion tests are rarely available at the time decisions have to be made, and have unfortunately high false-negative rate.

Radiographs may support a diagnosis of transmural colitis by showing a fixed loop of colon on serial films. In the acute phase contrast studies are hazardous and usually show no specific changes.

Management

Patients with amoebic colitis are invariably critically ill with severe fluid and electrolyte derangements. Children show signs of severe malnutrition with sufficient frequency to suggest that the association may not be random.

Fluid replacement is essential. Broad-spectrum antibiotics are required in the face of peritoneal contamination with colonic flora, and an amoebicide, such as metronidazole is essential. During resuscitation the patient's condition may so improve that emergency surgery becomes unnecessary. However in the presence of free perforation, clinical deterioration or a failure to maintain clinical improvement during resuscitation, surgery is mandatory. A flow chart outlining the principles of management is illustrated in Figure 22.3.

Surgery

When laparotomy is planned for suspected amoebic colitis, the anaesthetised patient should be placed on the operating table in the Lloyd-Davies position allowing access to the perineum for bowel irrigation. It is prudent to insert a

Severe amoebic colitis suspected
Diarrhoea, Acute abdomen

↓

Proctosigmoidoscopy
Multiple tissue and slough biopsies
Stool examination or preservation
plain abdominal radiographs

Evidence of perforation
(e.g. Extraluminal gas)

No evidence of perforation

↓

24 h resuscitation

Urgent resuscitation

Metronidazole IV
Antibiotics IV

Metronidazole IV
Antibiotics IV   → To exclude
Blood culture   typhoid

Not improved   Improved

↓

Contrast enema at
6 weeks to assess
extent of strictures

Phase I - Laparotomy
  - Resection/exteriorisation
  - On-table colonic irrigation
  + Ileostomy decompression

Patent or minor stenosis   Stricture

↓

Phase II - Closure of ileostomy only

Laparotomy resection
and anastomosis

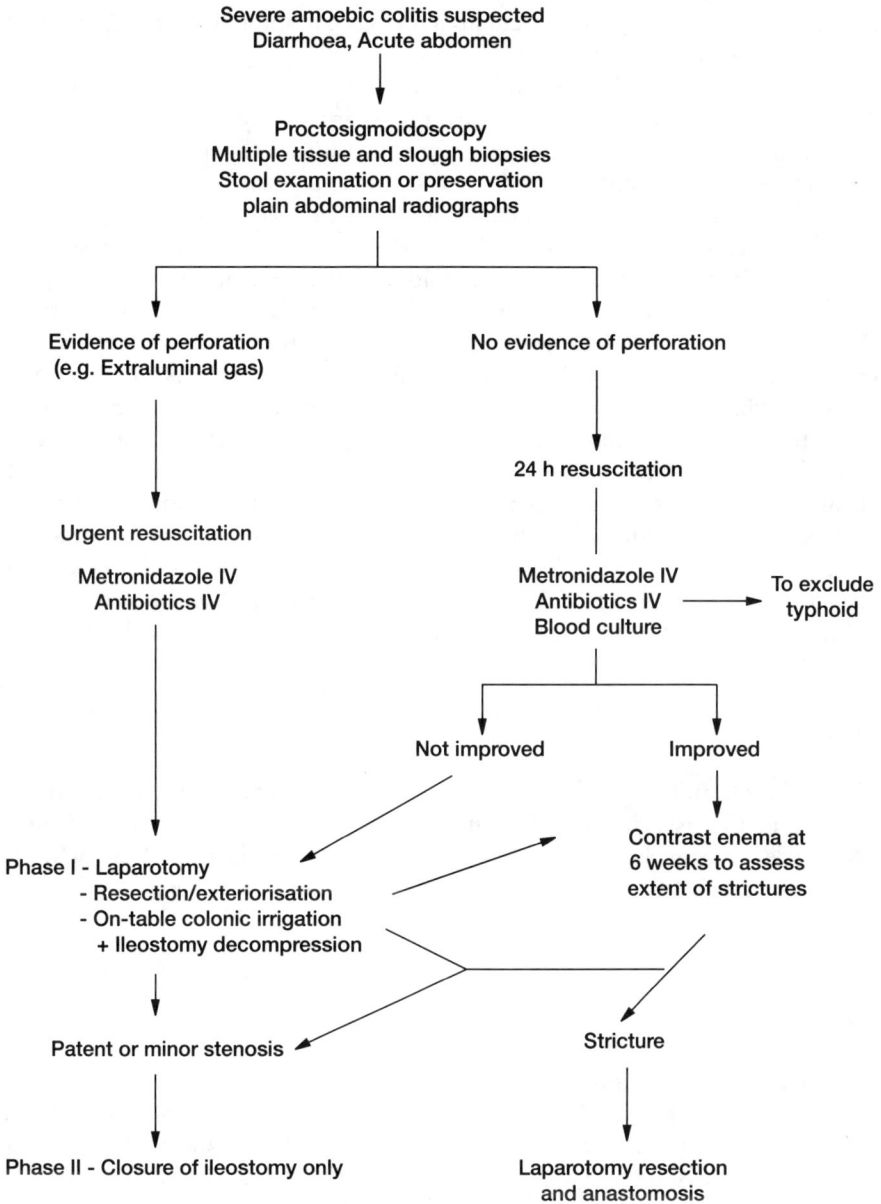

Figure 22.3 The management of amoebic colitis.

suitable tube, approximately 2 cm in diameter, per anum, before surgery starts in order to collect the effluent.

On opening the abdomen the diseased colon will be obscured by omental 'wraps'. It is important not to disturb the wraps in any way, and it is unnecessary to expose the underlying colon to confirm transmural colitis. The adherence of the omentum to the area is ample evidence.

If the disease is limited in extent and can be encompassed by a standard colonic resection, then this should be carried out. Anastomosis is never indicated and it is necessary to create a colostomy and mucus fistula.

If the whole colon is involved resection carries a prohibitive mortality. Under these circumstances, without in any way disturbing the omental wraps, a loop of ileum is intubated using a large Foley catheter. This is passed into the caecum where the balloon is inflated. Copious quantities of warm saline are used to irrigate the colon until the effluent is gin-clear. If the irrigant leaks out into the peritoneal cavity, the leakage points must be temporarily secured with clamps or simple sutures to permit effective irrigation. Provided the omental wraps have been undisturbed, the reduction in contamination by lavage allows healing to proceed. The ileotomy is exteriorised to bypass the colon and maintain decompression. The colon can be re-evaluated and strictures dealt with at 6 weeks when the patient is well.

Prognosis

There is still an appreciable mortality from fulminant amoebic colitis in children and the associated malnutrition compounds perioperative difficulties. Many deaths are related to intractable oedema which, like the colitis itself, may have its basis in the development of anti-neutrophil cytoplasmic antibodies.

Ascariasis

The ascaris worm is familiar to all who have treated patients in the tropics, and infestation is so prevalent in these areas that it is a rare patient indeed who is unaffected. Thus ascariasis can be associated with any disorder, but is not necessarily the cause of that disorder. The ascaris worm however is rightly held responsible for a number of abdominal syndromes several of which may present with an 'acute abdomen'.

The worm is acquired by the ingestion of ova previously deposited in areas of poor sanitation. Children playing in these areas pick up soil under finger nails and elsewhere and transfer the ova to their alimentary tract. Ova can also be ingested along with salads or uncooked vegetables grown in areas where 'night soil' is used as a fertiliser.

After a complex life-cycle within the host the adult worms take up residence in the small bowel. Each female produces ova in prodigious numbers, and children can quickly acquire a massive worm load. Patients excreting 50 000 ascaris ova per gram of stool are by no means uncommon. Surgical problems relate to the mass of worms as well as to their migration from the gut into the hepatobiliary and pancreatic ductal systems.

Complications

Probably the commonest complication of ascariasis, and the least acknowledged is malnutrition. The parasites exist by stealing the patient's food, and when present in large numbers this loss can be significant. Surgical problems include:

- bolus obstruction,
- intestinal volvulus,
- hepatobiliary ascariasis and
- acute pancreatitis,

all of which may present acutely. That these are more frequently seen in children reflects the 'dose:mass' ratio. In adults complications are most commonly seen among puerperal women who have had pica in the last trimester of pregnancy.

Bolus obstruction

A congregation of worms is particularly liable to obstruct the intestine of a small child. Left to their own devices the worms in such an obstructing bolus will disentangle themselves. This can be encouraged by an antispasmodic. The natural history of bolus obstruction treated by resting the bowel and an antispasmodic is resolution by the morning after admission. Deviation from this norm requires explanation. Either the original diagnosis was incorrect or there has been progression.

If the worms in such a bolus are killed by the administration of a vermicide, or perhaps worse paralysed by the administration of a piperazine-like compound, they clearly will be unable to disentangle themselves and an emergency can be precipitated.

A bolus of dead worms may require operative removal in the face of non-resolving obstruction. More seriously the tension in the bowel wall over the bolus may cause an anti-mesenteric necrosis of the bowel necessitating resection. It is therefore important to withhold specific vermicides until the obstruction has been relieved.

The progression of simple bolus obstruction to a complete or strangulating obstruction can occur despite adequate primary treatment and justifies the hospitalisation and close observation of such patients. The risk of volvulus occurring in such a patient is sufficient to include radiological re-evaluation in patients who fail to settle within 24 h.

Volvulus

A bolus of worms can act as the bob of a pendulum allowing twisting of a loop of small bowel to occur. This may occur while the patient is under observation for bolus obstruction and appears to be encouraged by the use of vermifuges.

If the diagnosis is made early surgery can be performed before necrosis of the bowel occurs. Early diagnosis depends on suspicion, recognition of deviation from the norm for bolus obstruction and radiological evidence of a complete obstruction.

Frequently patients present *de novo* with an 'acute abdomen' and the diagnosis may not be suspected before surgery.

Surgery

In patients with ischaemic volvulus it is important to resect the necrotic loop without untwisting it. If the bowel perfusion appears questionable then detorsion and a period of waiting with the patient ventilated with 100 per cent oxygen and the bowel wrapped in warm swabs is essential to determine viability.

If the bowel proves to be viable extraction of the worms via an enterotomy is necessary. Attempting to push worms into the colon is extremely traumatic to the bowel and does not ensure that they will stay there. Worms will not emerge through a properly constructed suture line, but if any doubt remains, piperazine can be instilled into the lumen above and below the enterotomy to discourage the adventurous.

Hepatobiliary ascariasis

The migration of worms into the hepatobiliary ductal system may be associated with cholangitis and abscess formation within the liver parenchyma. Under such circumstances the patient may present with the signs and symptoms of an 'acute abdomen'. More usually patients complain of biliary colic with signs confined to the right upper quadrant.

Approximately 25 per cent of patients admitted with simple worm bolus obstruction will harbour worms in the biliary tree, often asymptomatically.

The definitive diagnosis will be made with ultrasound or intravenous cholangiography. Management is usually non-operative, waiting for the worms to emerge under their own steam. Killing the worms in the biliary ducts may lead to stricture formation, hepatic granulomata or provide a nidus for stone formation. Surgery is reserved for:

- unresolving cholangitis, despite antibiotics,
- unremitting pain,
- acute pancreatitis and
- persistence of the worms beyond an arbitrary 6-week period.

Worm pancreatitis

In the Third World, certainly among children, ascariasis is the commonest cause of acute pancreatitis. A transient hyperamylassaemia is seen in many patients with hepatobiliary worms, presumably due to oedema or spasm of the sphincter of Oddi. True pancreatitis is due to a worm impacting in the main pancreatic duct with disruption of the distal gland. Operative management often includes distal pancreatectomy.

Sickle cell disease

Sickle cell anaemia is the commonest haemoglobinopathy, and perhaps the commonest serious inherited disorder in Africa. Apart from the signs of chronic haemolytic anaemia the disease is characterised by intermittent crises, or vaso-occlusive episodes. These may be stimulated by hypoxia, cold, dehydration or a remote infection.

When vaso-occlusion affects the mesenteric or abdominal visceral vessels signs of an 'acute abdomen' will present. The spleen is commonly affected with multiple infarcts eventually reducing the functioning splenic mass.

Diagnosis rests upon a history of sickling and identification of the precipitating factor.

Pigbel: enteritis necroticans (see pages 326–9)

23

Anorectal Disorders

Anal canal anatomy and physiology

Anal epithelium

The anal canal is 4 cm in length and lined in its lower part by skin (keratinising squamous epithelium) without hair or sweat glands. The upper part is lined by mucosa (columnar epithelium) (Figure 23.1). The junction between skin and mucosa is called the mucocutaneous junction and separates columnar epithelium from squamous, the autonomic nervous system from the somatic and the portal venous system from the systemic. The transitional zone is called the

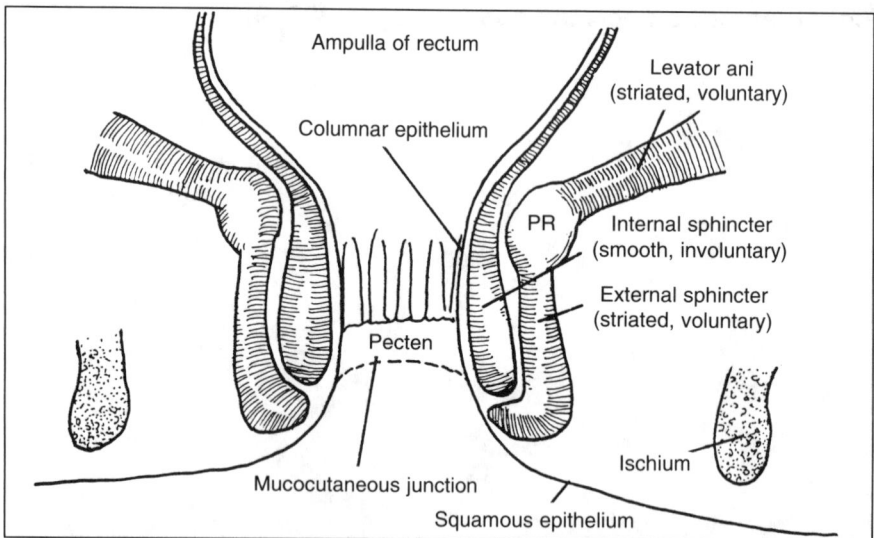

Figure 23.1 Anatomy of anus. Note the anus is normally closed at rest by the action of the internal sphincter and the anal (haemorrhoidal) cushions. This figure shows the external sphincter as one continuous muscle rather than subcutaneous, middle and deep bundles. The internal sphincter may be lower than the mucocutaneous junction under anaesthesia. PR = puborectalis muscle.

386

pecten and is lined by non-keratinising squamous epithelium. From the mucosal surface one can see anal columns with valves at their lower end. Above these valves lie the openings of anal glands which originate in the submucosa. When they become blocked they can act as the source of perianal sepsis.

Anal sphincters

The internal and external anal sphincters encircle the anal canal and are essential for normal continence.

Internal sphincter

The internal sphincter is a smooth, non-striated, involuntary muscle in continuity with the muscle of the rectum, responsible for anal tone at rest. It is innervated by the pelvic parasympathetics (S 2, 3, 4) which cause it to relax in response to dilatation of the rectum. This response is called the rectoanal reflex and is absent in Hirschprung's and Chagas' diseases, and may be absent or impaired in muscular disorders such as scleroderma. Damage to the pelvic parasympathetic nerves during childbirth, or pelvic surgery such as hysterectomy, may result in a failure of the anus to relax (anismus), thus causing chronic constipation.

External sphincter

The external sphincter is a striated, voluntary muscle innervated by the inferior branch of the internal pudendal nerve (S 2, 3, 4). It is responsible for continence, when one has the urge to defecate, until a socially acceptable place and time are found. This is dependent on cortical control via an intact spinal cord. It can be assessed by asking the patient to contract his anus. At the upper end of the external sphincter lies the levator ani muscle, which fans out across the pelvis to form the pelvic floor. The puborectalis sling is the medial part of this muscle which is felt as a thick, firm band looping around the anorectal junction (S 2, 3, 4). Continence is also dependent on the anal canal being kept closed at rest by the three anal cushions and an anorectal angle of about 60–105° (Figure 23.2).

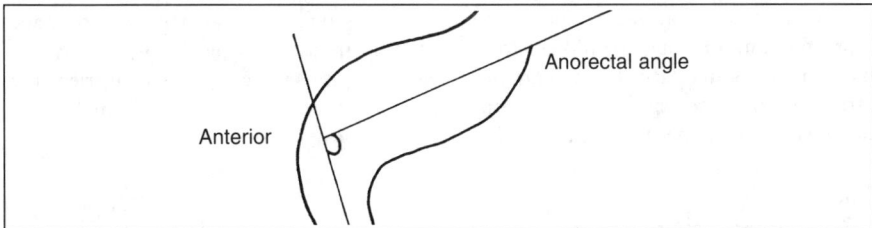

Figure 23.2 The anorectal angle. The normal angle is between 60 and 105°. The anorectal angle may be increased in rectal prolapse and incontinence.

Neurovascular supply and lymphatic drainage

Blood supply and lymphatics

The upper part of the anal canal is supplied by branches of the superior rectal artery. Venous drainage is to the portal system and the lymphatics drain to the internal iliac nodes.

The lower part is supplied by branches of the inferior rectal artery. Venous drainage is to the systemic circulation and lymph drains to the superficial inguinal nodes.

Innervation

The lower, skin-lined part is supplied by branches of spinal nerves originating in the sacral roots of the cauda equina (internal pudendal nerves – S 3, 4). This part has sensation. The upper anal canal is innervated by the autonomic nervous system (sympathetic nerves from L 1, 2 and pelvic parasympathetics) and has no sensation.

Clinical assessment

Patients with anorectal problems usually come to the outpatient clinic. The key to accurate diagnosis is to take a brief but detailed history of the presenting problem. The history should be followed by careful examination of the abdomen and then the anorectum in good light, which involves inspection, digital palpation and proctosigmoidoscopy. Privacy, light, a torch, an examination couch and a proctoscope are needed. The proctoscope should be cleaned in water, detergent and disinfected in Cidex (2 per cent glutaraldehyde). Most conditions can be diagnosed and treated without special investigations. Most wrong diagnoses are the result of inadequate or rushed examination. Special investigations that may be indicated include barium enema, sigmoidoscopy and biopsy.

In centres large enough to have an anorectal laboratory where there are large numbers of patients with complex anatomical or physiological disorders of continence, other special investigations may be indicated such as anorectal manometry, electrophysiology, colonic motility studies and defecating proctography with measurement of the anorectal angle. Endoanal ultrasound is being increasingly used to stage anorectal tumours but is unlikely to be available in most tropical hospitals where malignancy is still relatively uncommon. In many hospitals in developing countries only barium enema and rigid sigmoidoscopy may be available but these will enable the diagnosis to be made in most tropical patients.

Practice point
• *The commonest reason for making the wrong diagnosis is failure to carry out adequate anal examination including inspection, palpation and proctoscopy.*

Clinical presentation

Pain and discomfort

Severe pain

When perianal pain is severe and thus the dominant symptom, one of three diagnoses is likely: a perianal haematoma (thrombosed pile), acute anal fissure or perianal abscess. Take a history of the development of symptoms. A history of intermittent bright red blood or prolapse suggests haemorrhoids, sharp pain of sudden onset commencing with passage of hard stool suggests anal fissure and increasing pain over a few days often associated with fever suggests perianal abscess. All of these conditions can be diagnosed by inspection. A perianal haematoma (thrombosed pile) or fissure can be seen without rectal examination by parting the buttocks and anal skin. In the case of a perianal abscess, induration, inflammation, tenderness and/or fluctuation are usually evident from inspection and palpation. In the case of a submucous abscess within the anal canal rectal examination is excruciating but the canal may still feel normal and nothing will be seen until examination under anaesthesia is performed. It is often kinder with severe anal pain to defer rectal examination until the patient is under anaesthesia.

Discomfort

Anorectal **discomfort** rarely occurs without some other symptom being the major problem. A careful examination including proctoscopy will normally diagnose the cause, which will include haemorrhoids, skin tags, chronic fissure, rectal prolapse and fistula *in ano*.

Proctalgia fugax

One other painful condition of uncertain origin is proctalgia fugax characterised by fleeting sharp spasms of anal pain. This condition cannot be diagnosed until a full examination has been performed under anaesthesia to exclude all other treatable causes.

Bleeding

Bleeding per rectum may be due to anal pathology or disease higher in the gastrointestinal tract. Ask about the colour of the blood: is it bright red, suggesting an anorectal cause; or dark red, suggesting a colonic cause? Ask where the blood was noticed, whether on the toilet paper, in the toilet, on the outside of the stool or mixed in the stool. Fresh blood in the toilet or on the toilet paper suggests an anal cause for bleeding. Blood on the outside of the stool may also originate from the anus, but blood mixed in the stool suggests rectal or colonic pathology. The causes of bleeding per rectum are shown in

Table 23.1   Causes of bleeding per rectum.

Anal bleeding

Fresh blood, often on the toilet paper, in the toilet or on the outside of the stool

Haemorrhoids
Fissure *in ano* (pain the dominant symptom if acute)
Rectal prolapse (prolapse the dominant symptom)
Proctitis (associated with mucus and often exudate)
Solitary rectal ulcer (rare)
Anorectal polyp
Carcinoma anus or rectum

Colorectal bleeding

Blood fresh or dark, on the outside or mixed in the stool depending on level and the rate of bleeding.

Infection (diarrhoea the dominant symptom)
  Amoebiasis
  Shigella
  Proctocolitis (cytomegalovirus, syphilitic, gonococcal etc.)
Inflammation (diarrhoea usually the dominant symptom)
  Crohn's disease, ulcerative colitis
  Radiation enteritis/proctitis
  Psuedomembranous colitis
Intussusception (abdominal pain and sometimes a mass)
  May originate from small or large bowel (see pp 373–7).
Degenerative disease
  Diverticulitis (pain, altered bowel habit – diarrhoea or constipation, bleeding not usually dominant unless profuse)
  Angiodysplasia and vascular malformations (bleeding dominant)
Neoplasia
  Benign or malignant polyps
  Colorectal cancer

Table 23.1. All patients with rectal bleeding should have a proctoscopy performed. Sigmoidoscopy is essential for those over the age of 40 years or where the bleeding is persistent and the diagnosis is in doubt.

Practice points

- *Do not necessarily accept an anal cause for rectal bleeding until pathology in the rectum and colon has been excluded. In the tropics although colorectal cancer is less frequent than in developed countries many patients with this condition are under 40.*
- *One diagnosis not to miss is intussusception, particularly in children (see p 373). The classical symptoms are cramping abdominal pains, passage of dark red blood per rectum, and sometimes an abdominal mass. However, the presentation can be variable and the diagnosis is often missed if it is not considered and confirmed by a barium enema (Figure 22.1).*

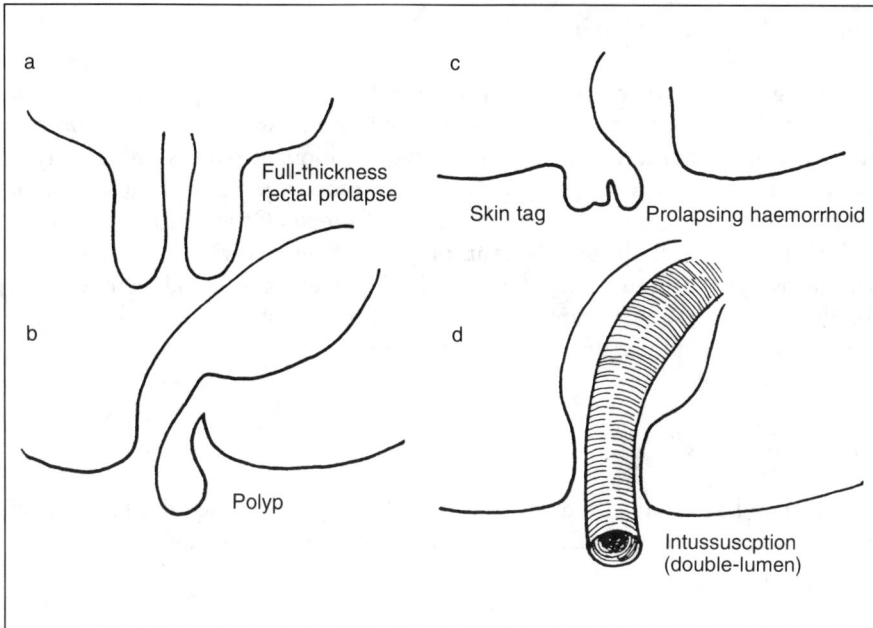

Figure 23.3   Different pathologies presenting with prolapse.

Mucus and slime

Mucus and slime suggest inflammation or infection. A villous adenoma or rectal tumour may occasionally produce copious amounts of mucus so that the passage of mucus is the dominant symptom. Infection is diagnosed by stool microscopy and culture, inflammation and tumours by sigmoidoscopy and biopsy. Some pathogens, particularly in immune-deficient states, may only be detected by rectal biopsy.

Prolapse

The patient usually complains of something 'coming down' or 'protruding' with a bowel motion. The prolapse may reduce spontaneously or need digital reduction. The commonest cause is prolapsing haemorrhoids, particularly in young adults. Rectal prolapse is more common at the extremes of life. In a young child the mother will complain about rectal prolapse which is usually full thickness. It is important to differentiate between rectal prolapse and the rare case of an intussusception prolapsing through the rectum (Figure 23.3). In the former there is only one lumen but in the latter there is a lumen around the intussuscepting bowel. Intussusception usually presents with abdominal pain and passage of dark red blood per rectum. In the elderly, rectal prolapse may be associated with discomfort, bleeding, mucus or discharge. Rectal or anal polyps may also present by prolapsing through the anus.

Lower abdominal pain

Cramping midline lower abdominal pain, relieved by passing stool is termed tenesmus. This is a non-specific symptom that may be associated with colorectal infection, inflammation or neoplasia. Lower abdominal pain is an indication for rectal examination, proctoscopy, sigmoidoscopy and biopsy. Stool microscopy and culture should also be performed. Other causes of lower abdominal pain include bladder pathology, salpingo-ovarian pathology and prostatitis. History and examination, including pelvic and rectal examination, should indicate the structure involved. Specific investigations include urine microscopy and culture and pelvic ultrasound.

Skin disorders

The anal and perianal skin may be affected by any generalised dermatological problem. Contact dermatitis may be caused by local medicines and applications.

Itching

Where the skin problem is confined to the perianal area the commonest complaint is itching (pruritus). Itching may also be caused by mucous discharge from the anus or pus from a fistula *in ano*. Always consider fungal infection and take scrapings for microscopy and culture. Purplish discoloration and induration of the skin may occur in association with inflammatory bowel disease (Crohn's). Vaginal discharge may also irritate the perianal region.

Sinuses

Discharging sinuses may be tubercular in origin or may represent a fistula *in ano* (see below). Hidradenitis suppuritiva may also affect the perianal skin and presents with multiple pustules and sinuses.

Skin tags

Some patients have anal skin tags associated with a fissure *in ano* (midline posteriorly) or haemorrhoids (3, 7, 11 o'clock). These tags may become oedematous, inflamed and painful. They may make cleaning the anus difficult after defecation and harbour faecal matter which stains the underwear.

Warts

Where anal intercourse is practised anal warts are a common manifestation of sexually transmitted disease. These warts are caused by human papilloma virus (HPV) and may be florid, making identification of the anal opening difficult.

Table 23.2 Causes of anorectal ulceration.

Trauma
Anal fissure
Solitary rectal ulcer

Infection
Pyogenic infection associated with immune deficiency
Amoebic colitis
Herpes simplex
Syphilis
Cytomegalovirus
Tuberculosis
Haemophilus ducreyi
Chlamydia
Primary HIV

Neoplasia
Squamous carcinoma anus
Kaposi's sarcoma
Adenocarcinaoma

Inflammation
Ulcerative colitis
Crohn's disease

Ulcers

Determine how long the ulcer has been present, whether it is painful, its progression and describe it carefully. Ulcers with raised edges may be malignant; ulcers with undermined edges or fistulous tracts may be due to chronic inflammation such as tuberculosis or inflammatory bowel disease. The causes of anal ulcers are shown in Table 23.2. Anal ulcers should be biopsied and material sent also for bacteriological and viral studies if possible.

Disorders of continence

In patients who complain of incontinence it is important to take an accurate history. Incontinence may be of flatus or stool. Continence may only be impaired if there is watery stool or it may be constant. History of surgery or injury to the anorectal area should be asked about. Anal dilatation to six or eight fingers may have damaged the anal sphincters or damage may have been caused by operations that aimed to lay open an anal fistula. Rectal prolapse may damage the pelvic floor and anal sphincters as may genital prolapse in females. Difficult or multiple deliveries may tear or stretch the anorectal musculature or result in a pressure or traction injury to the pelvic parasympathetic nerves (S 2, 3, 4).

Incontinence in children

Incontinence in children (encopresis) may be secondary to social or psychological problems. Normally a child is continent of faeces by the age of 3 years and certainly by 5 years. The clinical approach is to first exclude neuromuscular causes and then fully assess the child's social and psychological background.

Incontinence in adults

In cases of incontinence, examination should start with inspection. Good examination may partially compensate for lack of special investigations. Are there any scars or sinuses? Look carefully at the anus. A patulous anus suggests laxity of the internal sphincter. Ask the patient to bear down. Does the anal mucosa prolapse? Is there any genital prolapse? Scratch the anal skin. Does it contract normally? Then perform digital examination. Feel for the tone at rest (internal sphincter) and ask the patient to squeeze on your finger (external sphincter). Assess the anal canal length. Proctoscopy will reveal any other or associated local pathology such as anterior rectal prolapse or haemorrhoids.

When available, other special investigations for incontinence include anorectal manometry, measurement of the anorectal angle (radiologically) and in cases where there may be neuromuscular damage, electrophysiology may help to determine whether the muscles or nerves are responsible.

Stricture

Occasionally difficulty in defecation may be due to a stricture. Biopsy will be necessary to elucidate the cause of the stricture which may be congenital, a complication of previous surgery, inflammatory or malignant.

Specific disorders

Anorectal infection

The **abscesses** are described according to their anatomical site: gluteal, ischiorectal and perianal. Perianal abscesses may be submucosal, subcutaneous (or subsphincteric) or intersphincteric (Figure 23.4). Ischiorectal and perianal abscesses may spread to the pararectal space. Pararectal abscesses may originate from pelvic appendicitis or pelvic inflammatory disease.

Patients with inflammatory bowel disease (ulcerative colitis and Crohn's disease) and HIV infection are prone to develop anorectal sepsis. The commonest complication of perianal infection is fistula *in ano* with or without recurrent abscesses. More severe complications include septicaemia, necrotising fasciitis and Fournier's gangrene. Rarely the anorectal sphincters may be damaged by necrosis in associated with a neglected perianal abscess (see Case history 1).

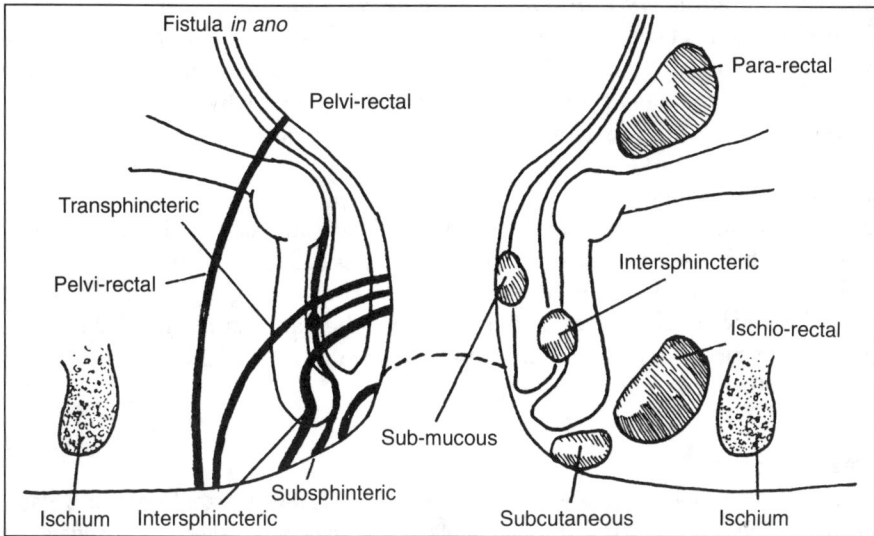

Figure 23.4 The surgical anatomy of anorectal infection (right side of figure) and fistula *in ano* (left side of figure).

Management

Examination under general anaesthesia

Patients with perianal abscesses require incision and drainage under general anaesthesia. This procedure should be combined with a thorough rectal examination, including proctoscopy. Some patients have submucosal abscesses within the anal canal and have no external signs of abscess, only great pain and fever. A Parks' speculum (anal retractor with three attachable blades) aids assessment of anal canal pathology.

Incision and drainage

The incision should be large enough to allow the cavity to heal from the inside out. If the skin heals over while the cavity is still discharging slough there may be a recurrent abscess. Some recommend a cruciate incision, and then cutting off the corners. The important principle is to allow free drainage. The abscess cavity is normally left open and the dressings are changed twice daily.

Patients should be encouraged to take baths twice daily at the time of dressing change. Some abscess cavities bleed profusely after drainage; this bleeding can be controlled by packing with gauze. The gauze should be removed within 12–24 h since it may act as a plug preventing drainage. The time taken for healing depends on the size of the abscess cavity but is normally 1–3 weeks. Continuing discharge from a perianal abscess wound for a longer time suggests there is an underlying fistula. A fistula *in ano* is usually treated once the acute sepsis has settled. Antibiotics are not normally required unless there is evidence of systemic sepsis, spreading soft tissue infection or immune deficiency.

Incision, curettage and primary closure under antibiotic cover

This method has been shown to be as effective as incision and drainage alone in a number of studies. Data on its effectiveness in developing countries are scarce but there seems no reason, in selected patients, why the advantages of fewer dressings and less pain should not be obtained.

Fournier's gangrene

Fournier's gangrene requires **excision** of all necrotic skin and subcutaneous tissue combined with broad-spectrum antibiotics including penicillin. Repeated debridement may be required and neglected Fournier's gangrene may extend into the abdominal wall or down into the subcutaneous tissue of the thigh. About half the cases of Fournier's gangrene are due to neglected perianal sepsis and the others to periurethral sepsis.

Case history 1

A 24-year-old oriental female presented with high fever and anal pain of 3 days' duration. The examining doctor was unable to see any abnormality on inspection and could not do a rectal examination because of the pain. Upon examination under anaesthetic he found a huge submucous abscess which had already caused considerable necrosis of the lower anal sphincter on the right side. He cleaned out the abscess cavity and commenced broad-spectrum antibiotics. Further drainage was required after 48 hours because the temperature remained high. Thereafter the patient improved and continence was preserved. In this case faecal diversion by colostomy was not required but had the abscess persisted or continence been lost a colostomy would have been advised.

Fistula in ano

A fistula is an abnormal communication between two epithelial lined surfaces. In the case of fistula *in ano* the abnormal communication is between the skin and anorectal mucosa. The fistula presents as an opening in the perianal area, which discharges pus and may have granulation tissue protruding from it. There may be an associated perianal abscess or a history of recurrent perianal abscesses. Fistulae *in ano* may be classified as high or low depending on whether the track passes below or above the puborectalis at the upper edge of the external sphincter (Figure 23.4). The direction and height of the track can only be assessed by passing a probe through the fistula under anaesthesia with a good light and an anal speculum.

Low fistulae are described according to their anatomical route: subsphincteric, intersphinteric or transphincteric (Figure 23.4). These are treated by laying open the fistula and allowing the tissues to heal from the base of the wound out to the surface. Sometimes the fistulous track can be completely excised (fistulectomy) as a core rather than laying open a wide area. Recurrent fistulae should be treated by an experienced surgeon and histology should be obtained to exclude tuberculosis and inflammatory bowel disease.

High fistulae are difficult to treat and require careful assessment by a senior surgeon in order to avoid rendering the patient incontinent (see Case history 3). The high fistula may be termed a pararectal or pelvirectal fistula.

Practice points
- *Goodsall's rule (Figure 23.5) states that a fistulous opening lying anterior to the equator of the anus passes directly in a radial fashion into the anus. A fistulous opening lying posterior to the equator curves round to enter the midline posteriorly. Knowledge of this rule helps identify the fistula track under anaesthesia.*
- *Always take a biopsy of a fistula* in ano, *particularly if it is recurrent.*

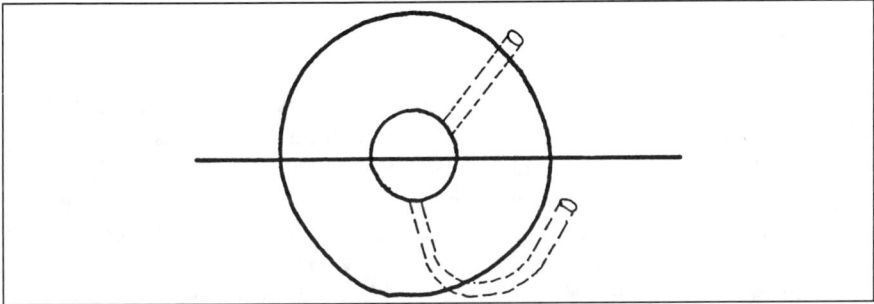

Figure 23.5 Goodsall's rule: A fistula *in ano* anterior to the equator passes radially into the anal canal, whereas one posterior to the equator passes in a horseshoe pattern.

A fistula should always be biopsied as a rare cause is tuberculosis. In countries where inflammatory bowel disease is common, Crohn's disease or ulcerative colitis may need to be controlled by medication before attempting surgery. Recurrent fistulae should not be definitively treated without histology. Since anorectal sepsis and fistula *in ano* are common in HIV disease, it is wise to avoid large anal wounds if the patient is severely immunocompromised because they are unlikely to heal. Colloid carcinoma of the anus may rarely present with a fistula, and rarely an adenocarcinoma or squamous carcinoma may arise in a chronic fistulous tract.

Case history 2
A 37-year-old male Zambian presented with recurrent perianal abscesses. Close questioning revealed that although the incision wound appeared to heal each time there remained a small 'boil' which intermittently became tender before discharging a small amount of pus and appearing to heal. Examination revealed a small opening on the right buttock near the anal margin. At examination under anaesthesia the opening was probed and found to enter the anal canal below the puborectalis muscle. The tract was laid open and after the wound healed the fistula never recurred.

Case history 3

A senior surgeon from the University Teaching Hospital was visiting a rural mission hospital 100 km from the capital. There he was shown a patient who had a recurrent anal fistula after multiple operations in his own teaching hospital. Under anaesthesia the fistulous tract was probed and extended above the puborectalis into the rectum. The fistulous tract was cored out up to the levator ani. The rest of the tract was vigorously curretted and then two Number 1 nylon sutures were inserted up the tract, into the rectum and out of the anus. These were tied tightly leaving a bridge of tissue between them of about 2–3 mm. The surgeon instructed the mission hospital doctors to divide the bridge of tissue between the sutures after 4 weeks. This they did, the wound healed without recurrence and the patient's continence was preserved.

Haemorrhoids

Normally the anal canal has three vascular cushions at 3, 7, and 11 o'clock which help keep the canal closed at rest. Constipation, often associated with eating a refined, low-fibre diet, is a common cause but persistent diarrhoea may also aggravate or cause haemorrhoids. Haemorrhoids are prolapsing anal cushions and not varicosities of the anal canal. Varicosities (a disorder of veins) of the anal canal occur only rarely in portal hypertension.

Haemorrhoids present with bright red bleeding, prolapse, discomfort and mucous discharge. Pain is only severe if thrombosis occurs. Haemorrhoids can usually only be diagnosed by using a proctoscope. On inspection of the anal skin, external skin tags in the 3, 7 and 11 o'clock positions may suggest the presence of internal haemorrhoids. (The tags are redundant anal skin created by persistent haemorrhoidal prolapse and the tag is left behind after the internal haemorrhoid has returned to the anal canal.) Treatment depends on the degree of prolapse but all patients should be advised to take a high-fibre diet.

Classification and treatment

Haemorrhoids are classified and often treated according to the extent of prolapse:

First degree

Prolapse down the anal canal but not out of it. This type can only be recognised by proctoscopy (Figure 23.6) and commonly presents with bright red bleeding per rectum. Treatment is usually by injection sclerotherapy.

Second degree

Prolapse out of the anal canal but reduce spontaneously. The patient often complains of prolapse but may also have bleeding and discomfort. Treatment is by rubber-band ligation.

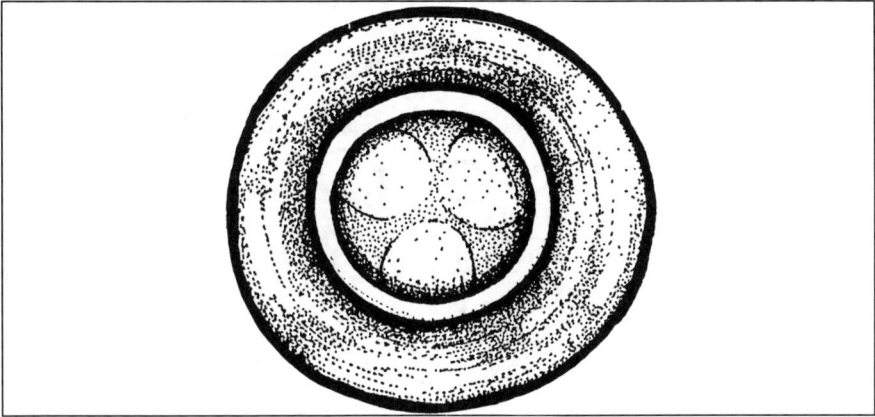

Figure 23.6 Haemorrhoids prolapsing into the proctoscope in the 3, 7 and 11 o'clock positions.

Third degree
Prolapse and require digital reduction to return the haemorrhoid to the anal canal. Treatment is by rubber-band ligation or haemorrhoidectomy.

Thrombosed pile
A third degree haemorrhoid may sometimes become congested and thrombosed. It is extremely painful and incision of a thrombosed pile with expression of the clot relieves the pain. This procedure can normally be performed with local anaesthesia in a casualty department and should not require general anaesthesia unless the diagnosis is in doubt.

Irreducible haemorrhoids
Irreducible haemorrhoids should be admitted and require reduction under anaesthesia. The reduction should be maintained by elevating the foot of the bed and inserting an anal pack.

A thrombosed external pile
The term describes a perianal haematoma with thrombosis within the skin lined, external skin tag part of the haemorrhoid. Pain is agonising but easily relieved by evacuating the clot under local anaesthesia.

Skin tags (Figure 23.7)
If troublesome, these can be excised, but this is often unnecessary if other measures are successful in controlling the internal haemorrhoids.

Practice points
- *Haemorrhoids are diagnosed with a proctoscope.*
- *Always exclude other pathologies in patients with rectal bleeding by performing sigmoidoscopy or barium enema, or both before assuming the*

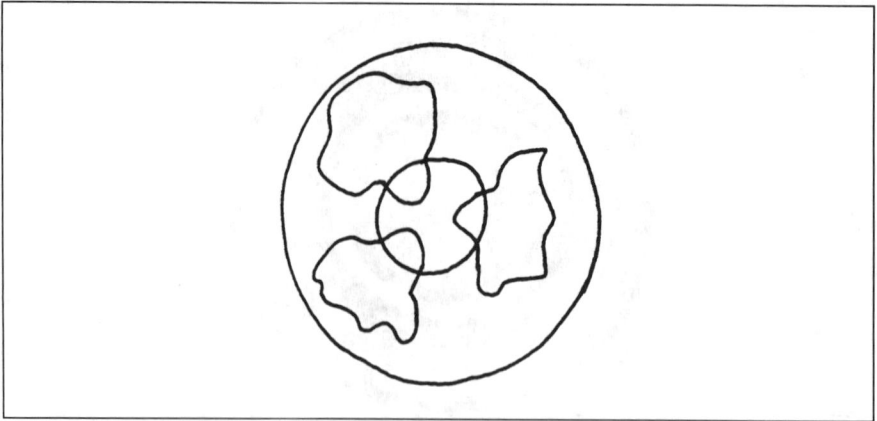

Figure 23.7   Anal skin tags associated with haemorrhoids in the 3, 7 and 11 o'clock positions.

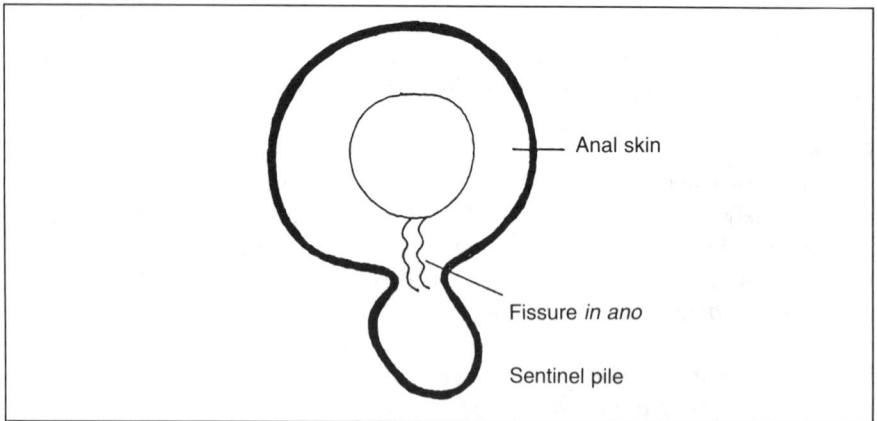

Figure 23.8   Posterior fissure *in ano* with sentinel pile.

blood is coming from haemorrhoids. Do not miss a rectal or colonic neo-plasm.

- *All patients with haemorrhoids should be encouraged to take a high-fibre diet sufficient to achieve soft, formed bowel motions daily. Constipation and straining are the commonest causes. Fifty per cent of patients can be treated by a high-fibre diet alone and definitive treatment may be unsuccessful if constipation persists.*

Fissure in ano

A fissure is a linear tear in the skin-lined part of the anal canal (Figure 23.8). It is usually caused by passage of a hard stool but fissures are more common in patients with inflammatory bowel disease. Since this area is in the lower third, skin-lined part of the anal canal, the fissure can be recognised by inspection on parting the anal skin. Digital examination is not necessary to diagnose a fissure. The common site is the midline posteriorly and there is often a sentinel pile (skin tag) just distal to the fissure. The patient presents with pain and bleeding. Pain is intense in an acute fissure. In childbirth a woman may suffer an anterior anal fissure. Homosexuals may also develop fissures after anal intercourse.

Treatment

Many fissures heal within a month of a high-fibre diet the aim of which should be to eliminate constipation and produce at least one well-formed but soft stool per day. If pain is severe it is kinder to treat the fissure urgently by anal dilatation (4–5 fingers) or internal sphincterotomy (cutting the lower half of the internal sphincter). Anal dilatation and sphincterotomy both aim to cause limited damage to the internal sphincter thus reducing anal spasm and pain. The fissure then heals. Non-healing or unusual looking fissures should be biopsied, particularly if sexually transmitted diseases are suspected. A chronic fissure may require excision.

Anal canal stricture

Causes

The causes of strictures of the anorectum include:

1. Congenital anomalies (sometimes with a fistula to the vagina in the female or bladder/urethra in a male). Although these are normally recognised in the neonatal period because of failure to pass meconium, less severe abnormalities may not be discovered until later in life.
2. Complications of surgery or radiotherapy.
3. Malignancy.
4. Endometriosis of the rectovaginal septum.
5. Chronic inflammationary diseases including inflammatory bowel disease and tuberculosis.

The underlying pathology must be determined by biopsy.

Treatment

Benign strictures
Inflammatory strictures often respond to regular dilatation. There is no better anal dilator than the daily passage of a well formed stool. Initially a benign stricture should be dilated under anaesthetic and the patient supplied with a dilator to take home and perform twice daily dilatations.

Malignant strictures

Abdominoperineal resection is usually necessary because patients in the tropics rarely present with early lesions. Often anal canal malignancy is visible on presentation or the tumour is causing large bowel obstruction. Anorectal neoplasia is discussed below.

Anorectal neoplasia

Polyps

Clinical presentation

Polyps either present with bleeding or prolapse, or they will be discovered on proctoscopy. The polyp must be biopsied to determine whether it is benign or malignant. If there are multiple polyps, polyposis coli, an inherited disorder with a high incidence of malignancy, should be excluded by an endoscopic examination and barium enema. In patients over 40 years of age further investigation to look for other polyps or malignancy is always advisable. Polyps over 2 cm in size have a high chance of being malignant and it is likely that most adenocarcinomas of the colon and rectum develop in polyps.

Treatment of polyps

Anorectal polyps can normally be excised from within the lumen of the anorectum using a Parks' speculum or operating sigmoidoscope. Polyps higher in the colon can be excised colonoscopically or, if this is not available, by open operation. Care should be taken to completely excise the base of the polyp and achieve adequate haemostasis. A neoplastic polyp should be carefully followed up.

Case history 4

A 34-year-old Melanesian male presented with rectal bleeding. The company doctor performed proctosigmoidoscopy and saw multiple polyps. He biopsied some of these in the outpatients. One biopsy showed malignancy in the polyp but not invading the base. The patient was referred to the teaching hospital for barium enema and possible surgery. Repeat sigmoidoscopy showed four or five polyps in the distal rectum but the sigmoid colon was clear to 30 cm. The repeat biopsies suggested non-neoplastic inflammatory polyps. Barium enema was normal. The surgeon then excised all the remaining polyps per rectum and, after confirming each was non-neoplastic, elected to observe the patient by regular sigmoidoscopy and barium enema. It appears the company doctor excised a solitary malignant polyp completely. Although the diagnosis of polyposis coli was reasonable at first, this is the second case of so-called polyposis coli in the tropics which the author has noted to be due to inflammation not neoplasia, since the polyps have regressed under observation. Fortunately the patient was spared abdominoperineal resection and a permanent colostomy.

Tumours of the anal canal

Tumours present with bleeding, stricture or prolapse. Rarely anal neoplasia may cause infection or fistula formation. Always examine the inguinal lymph nodes because malignant tumours from the lower anal canal metastasise there.

Benign tumours

These include polyps, warts or condylomata accuminata and papillomas which may be sessile or pedunculated.

Malignant tumours

In the upper canal adenocarcinoma similar to that arising in the rectum may develop. Lymphatic spread is to the internal iliac nodes. Treatment will be abdominoperineal resection if it is resectable. If the tumour is advanced a colostomy may spare the patient from dying from intestinal obstruction. Cryosurgery or diathermy may provide local palliation.

In the lower skin-lined canal squamous carcinoma, basal cell carcinoma (locally invasive only) or melanoma may occur. Spread is to the inguinal nodes. Cloacogenic or basaloid carcinoma is a non-keratinizing squamous carcinoma arising from the pecten near the mucoepidermoid junction. Mucoepidermoid carcinoma may also arise there.

The management depends on the type and stage of the tumour and the patient's general health. Unfit elderly patients with an fungating lesion may respond to diathermy ablation or a colostomy when there is obstruction.

Colorectal carcinoma

This tumour causes a sixth of cancers in the USA and Europe and is responsible for one-sixth of cancer-related deaths. It is commonest in the sixth and seventh decades. Predisposing factors include a high-fat diet, red meat and long intestinal transit time. Patients with polyposis coli develop colorectal cancer in the fourth and fifth decades of life and those with ulcerative colitis for more than 20 years have a high incidence. Most cancers probably develop in an adenomatous polyp which has grown to 1–2 cm in size.

Most countries in the tropics have only 5 per cent of their population over the age of 60 years and a fatty, low residue diet with plenty of red meat is rare. Colorectal cancer is therefore unusual except in Singapore, Hong Kong and other more developed parts of South-East Asia with an elderly, affluent population. In the poorer developing countries in sub-Saharan Africa colorectal cancer often presents under the age of 40 years. The epidemiology of colorectal carcinoma in Africa is discussed further on pp 183–4.

Pathology

The tumours tend to be annular, polypoid or ulcerated lesions. Dukes' classification allows an assessment of prognosis.

A   confined to the mucosa
B   confined to the wall of the colon
C_1 metastases in the pericolic lymph nodes
C_2 metastases in the inferior mesenteric nodes
D   metastases in the liver or elsewhere

Stage D was never described by Dukes himself. The 5-year survival rates are 90, 60, 30 and less than 10 per cent for stages A, B, C and D respectively. Unfortunately at least 50 per cent of patients in the West and most patients in the tropics present with advanced stage C or D adenocarcinomas. Other prognostic features have been described by Jass who scores four factors: limitation of growth to bowel wall, the tumour margin, the presence of peritumoural infiltrate and the number of lymph nodes with metastasis.

Clinical presentation
Patients in the tropics often come late with complications such as large bowel obstruction or perforation. Colorectal carcinoma is commoner on the left side of the colon in both the tropics and developed nations. Early symptoms include change in bowel habit, blood or mucus in the stool and abdominal pain, including tenesmus. Right-sided lesions may present with anaemia, weight loss and sometimes an abdominal mass. If there is no abdominal mass abdominal examination is usually unremarkable. Rectal examination will enable tumours in the lower 8–10 cm of the anorectum to be palpated.

Investigations
Faecal occult blood will be positive in ulcerated or bleeding tumours. Rigid sigmoidoscopy will enable direct visualisation of the tumour in the distal 25 cm. Flexible sigmoidoscopes may reach the descending colon but colonoscopy is the only certain way to visualise the whole of the colonic lumen. Colonoscopes may not be available where colorectal carcinoma is rare. Barium enema examination will then have to be relied on to visualise what cannot be seen on sigmoidoscopy. A good double-contrast enema in a well-prepared bowel will give a good outline of the mucosal surface of the colon. Unfortunately a barium enema performed by an inexperienced doctor may demonstrate only large lesions.

   One pitfall to beware of in biopsy is that if the actual tumour is missed and the biopsy samples the adjacent bowel there may be coexistent schistomisasis or amoebiasis present in endemic areas. Always try to visualise the whole large bowel when you suspect colorectal carcinoma and do not accept a diagnosis of parasitic or bacterial infection if you did not clearly see the site of biopsy. It is better to repeat the sigmoidoscopy and biopsy if there is doubt.

Management
Colorectal cancer requires surgical excision. Tumours more than 7–8 cm from the anal verge can usually be resected without the need for a permanent colostomy. Coloanal anastomosis, or low rectal anastomosis using a stapling gun, spare many patients a colostomy.

Abdominal perineal resection is indicated for resectable, low rectal and anal tumours. About 10 per cent of tumours present with liver metastases. A solitary liver metastasis can be resected in a specialised unit. Chemotherapy and radiotherapy may be offered to selected patients but contribute little to the management strategy in countries where colorectal carcinoma is still relatively rare.

Rectal prolapse

In infants the prolapse is usually full thickness and requires reduction by the mother whenever it occurs. The condition normally resolves without complication within a few months. Surgery is rarely necessary but a temporary Thiersch wire can be inserted for 2–3 months if the rectum cannot be reliably and repeatedly reduced by the mother.

In adults prolapse may be partial or full-thickness. Elderly patients with weak pelvic floors are prone to this disorder. As the tissues stretch the anorectal angle becomes more obtuse (approaching 180°) so that the rectal tissue can prolapse through the anus (Figure 23.3). Partial-thickness prolapse is anterior and can sometimes be treated by avoidance of constipation, injection sclerotherapy or banding. Full-thickness prolapse may be associated with incontinence of faeces or flatus and requires operative repair (rectopexy using, most commonly, Ivalon sponge). In elderly unfit patients a Thiersch wire (formerly stainless steel, now No. 2 nylon suture) may be inserted around the anal sphincter, tightening it so that it only admits a finger.

Anterior mucosal rectal prolapse may sometimes cause a rectal ulcer due to trauma to the anterior rectal mucosa.

Solitary rectal ulcer

Occurs on the lower anterior rectal mucosa, often apparently spontaneously. It may present with bleeding and discharge per rectum. Management includes biopsy to exclude other causes, treating any anterior rectal prolapse and advising the patient to avoid constipation, straining and self-digitation.

Inflammatory bowel disease

Both Crohn's disease and ulcerative colitis are rare in the tropics. However, cases have been reported from Southern Africa, and the Indian sub-continent. Patients with inflammatory bowel disease may present with weight loss, bloody diarrhoea and mucus, or associated joint, skin or eye inflammation, intestinal obstruction, anorectal problems (fissure or fistula), or toxic dilatation of the colon. The diagnosis is made by colonoscopy or sigmoidoscopy, biopsy and barium enema. Treatment is largely medical using topical or systemic steroids to induce remission and sulphasalazine (Salazopyrine) to maintain remission. Complications such as intestinal obstruction or toxic dilatation of the colon may require emergency surgery. A detailed description of inflammatory bowel disease and its treatment is beyond the scope of this book but it needs to be considered in the differential diagnosis of proctitis or persistent anorectal pathology.

Case history 5
An expatriate male in his early thirties who had lived for 10 years in the tropics presented with a 2-month history of bloody diarrhoea with mucus and pus, and cramping lower abdominal pains (tenesmus) relieved by defecation. Procto-sigmoidoscopy revealed red and ulcerated anterior and lateral rectal mucosa but beyond the rectosigmoid junction the appearance was normal. Rectal biopsies re-vealed intense inflammation and the tropical pathologist wrongly suggested amoebic inflamation despite failing to identify haematophagous trophozoites. There was no improvement on metronidazole so he was rebiopsied and the specimen sent to a neighbouring country where the diagnosis of ulcerative colitis was made. He was treated by prednisolone (Predsol) enemas and sulphasalazine (Salazopyrine). In Zambia the author regularly saw Asian patients with inflammatory bowel disease.

Anorectal HIV disease

Patients with HIV infection are prone to develop perianal sepsis, ulcers and proctocolitis. The causes for these conditions will be diagnosed by taking samples for bacteriology and histology. Treatment is then directed towards the cause. Anorectal neoplasia has been reported in HIV sufferers, including lymphoma, squamous carcinoma, carcinoma *in situ* and Kaposi's sarcoma. Anorectal surgery should be minimised in the presence of immunedeficiency as it may lead to non-healing wounds which are worse than the original condition treated.

Warts (condylomata acuminata)

Anal warts in HIV positive patients may grow rapidly and spread to involve the anal mucosa. They may be large and not respond to conventional therapy such as podophyllin. They may undergo neoplastic transformation. Diathermy and excision is necessary for florid growths. Recent experience with ultrasonic dissection has been promising in obtaining reduced wound trauma in an area which may heal poorly.

Sexually transmitted diseases of the anorectum

These diseases occur in both HIV-positive and HIV-uninfected individuals. The principal infections are included in Table 23.3. Patients present with

Table 23.3 Anorectal problems in HIV infection.

Sepsis
    Abscess
    Fistula
    Fournier's gangrene

Ulceration
    Primary syphilis
    Fissure *in ano*
    Herpes simplex
    Cytomegalovirus
    Tuberculosis
    HIV (primary)
    Haemophilus ducreyi
    Chylamydia
    Neoplasia

Neoplasia
    Warts (HPV induced)
    Lymphoma
    Kaposi's sarcoma
    HPV-related intraepithelial neoplasia
    Squamous carcinoma

Proctocolitis
    Gonorrhoea
    Chlamydia
    Herpes simplex
    Cytomegalovirus
    Campylobacter
    Cryptosporidia
    Isospora belli
    Amoebiasis
    Shigella
    Giardia

ulceration, fissures, and proctocolitis. The key to diagnosis is to biopsy the affected area and send stool and exudate for microbiological analysis. Always consider the possibility of coexistent HIV infection. Treatment should be directed to the specific cause.

Pilonidal sinus and pilonidal abscess

A sinus is a blind track opening on to one epithelial lined surface. The sinus may be congenital or acquired and lies in the natal cleft between the buttocks. It typically occurs in hairy Caucasians and is rare in the tropics. Pilonidal sinuses can occur in the hands of hairdressers. Abscesses may be recurrent and are due to hairs and other concretions being driven down the sinus tracks. A pilonidal abscess should be treated by incision and drainage. Once the infection has settled the sinus track can be excised and the resulting defect closed by an advancement flap or allowed to heal by secondary intention.

Disorders of continence

The treatment of incontinence is a highly specialised area of surgery, rarely necessary in the tropics and requiring complex anatomical and physiological assessment. It is beyond the scope of this text so that the following paragraphs contain only a very brief outline.

Incontinence

General measures include advice about avoiding diarrhoea and performing timed rectal evacuation by using low enemas and suppositories. Pelvic floor exercises may strengthen weak musculature. Specific treatment is directed towards the cause: repair of the sphincters by postanal repair may be indicated if damaged but functioning muscle fibres can be demonstrated. Rectal or genital prolapse should be treated surgically to prevent further sphincter and pelvic floor damage.

Constipation

General measures include advice about ensuring a soft and bulky stool by means of a high-fibre diet. Suppositories and enemas are often abused by patients with chronic constipation but they may be necessary to keep the bowels opening regularly. Some patients may benefit from sphincterotomy if there is a failure of the internal sphincter to relax (e.g. spinal injury or paraplegia). Occasionally short-segment Hirschprung's disease at the anorectal junction may have been missed. In these cases the rectoanal reflex will be absent. Myotomy may then cure the patient. Patients with faecal impaction in a chronically dilated large bowel will require evacuation of faeces to allow, if possible, the bowel motility to recover. In gross cases this may sometimes require a temporary colostomy. Sigmoid resection to shorten the large bowel has proved unsuccessful in treating chronic constipation. In the chronic phase of Chagas' disease difficulty with defecation may develop due to loss of bowel motility and the development of megacolon. This is discussed on pp 316–17.

Congenital anomalies

Most congenital anomalies are diagnosed in the first few hours or days of life. Anorectal atresia with or without fistula, imperforate anus and Hirschprung's disease are discussed in Chapter 24 and normally require early or urgent surgery.

Rarely, difficulty with defecation or a pelvic mass may be due to an anterior sacral meningocoele or sacrococcygeal teratoma. The latter is normally clinically obvious at birth. The mass is palpable on rectal examination. A postanal dermoid cyst or dimple may also occur.

Further reading

Forrest APM, Carter DC, MacLeod IB, editors. Principles and practice of surgery. 2nd ed. Edinburgh: Churchill Livingstone, 1990.

Goligher JC. Surgery of the anus, rectum and colon. London: Baillière Tindall, Saunders, 1984.

Mann CV, Russell RCG, editors. Bailey and Love's short practice of surgery. 21st ed. London: Chapman and Hall, 1992.

Naader SB, Archampong EQ. Cancer of the colon and rectum in Ghana: a five year prospective study. Br J Surg 1994;81:456–9.

Ojo OS, Odesanmi WO, Akinola OO. The surgical pathology of colorectal carcinomas in Nigerians. Trop Gastroenterol. 1992;13:64–9.

Probert CS, Mayberry JF, Mann R. Inflammatory bowel disease in the rural Indian subcontinent: a survey of patients attending mission hospitals. Digestion 1990;47: 42–6.

Drugs and treatments for anorectal problems

Phenol in almond oil: Used for injection sclerotherapy of haemorrhoids. 2–3 ml is injected submucosally into each pile at or near the anorectal ring. Prolapsing anterior rectal mucosa may also be treated by submucosal injection.

Rubber band ligation: By applying a rubber band over the neck of a haemorrhoid it is strangulated and sloughs off in about 10 days. It is a suitable method for prolapsing haemorrhoids but the rubber band must be applied to the mucosal component of the haemorrhoid (which is painless). Rare complications include septicaemia and bleeding.

Cidex: Two per cent glutaraldehyde, which is suitable for disinfection of surgical instruments that cannot be autoclaved. Disinfection needs to be 'long enough and strong enough'. For proctoscopes and sigmoidoscopes that have been thoroughly cleaned (all contaminant matter removed before disinfection) 20 min is probably long enough to prevent transmission of bacterial infection, HIV or hepatitis B and C. Cidex is commonly used to disinfect fibreoptic endoscopes after thorough cleaning. The duration of disinfection varies from centre to centre. Twenty minutes was recommended by an interim report from the British Society of Gastroenterology. Subsequent studies have shown this time can be shortened, probably to 5 min providing cleaning of the instrument is excellent. Cidex has a shelf-life of about 4 weeks.

Podophyllin: Used to paint warts which it then burns. Repeated applications may be necessary after ensuring that any dead tissue from the previous application has been excised. Treatments should be repeated at least weekly if one is enthusiastic to cure the patient. Large areas of florid warts are not suitable for podophyllin treatment.

High-fibre diet: Fibre is the roughage that is naturally contained in husk of corn or mealies. Refining flour, rice or maize removes much of the roughage. City life-styles with over-refined foods are associated with many so-called 'Western' diseases such as diverticular disease, carcinoma of the colon, constipation, gallstones, hiatus hernia and diabetes. Although lack of fibre may be only one factor there is no doubt that patients with anorectal problems do best if constipation is avoided and they have at least one soft (as opposed to hard), but formed bowel motion per day. Westerners often add bran to their diet and there are numerous modern foods supplemented with bran such as Kellog's All Bran and bran breads. In the tropics, patients can be encouraged to eat at least two pieces of fruit per day and plenty of green vegetables that have not been overcooked. They need to eat enough to achieve their soft, formed bowel motion daily and most patients manage with natural foods. Try to avoid elective operations until the patient has proven he or she can take a high fibre diet. Patients need to learn to be involved in their own management because often, particularly in the cities, it is the high fibre diet that will prevent recurrence rather than any surgical treatment for haemorrhoids or fissure.

Ivalon sponge: A synthetic polymer used for rectopexy in full-thickness rectal prolapse. It is inert and so rarely becomes infected. When it is placed around the rectum at the rectosigmoid junction, fibrosis is encouraged which keeps the rectum fixed in the pelvis during straining. Marlex mesh is an alternative agent and if nothing is available the rectum could be mobilised and replaced with or without fascia lata.

Thiersch wire: Stainless-steel wire is placed around a patulous anus to prevent rectal prolapse. The wire should be tied tight enough to just allow the index finger to fit in the anal canal. Because the ends of the wire can cause discomfort Thiersh wire procedures are now done with No. 2 nylon or Prolene. This procedure is not as effective at preventing full thickness rectal prolapse in elderly Caucasians. However it may be adequate as a temporary measure in the infirm or very young and may suffice for some adult patients in the tropics.

24

Congenital Abnormalities of the Gastrointestinal Tract

Congenital abnormalities of the gastrointestinal system are by no means rare. In the UK the incidence of bowel atresia is around 1 in 330 neonates. In a study in Port Moresby, Papua New Guinea, 14 gastrointestinal abnormalities were detected in 10 000 deliveries (around 1 in 700). Variations exist in the patterns of congenital malformations seen in different parts of the world, and while it is difficult to give exact incidence rates for many tropical and non-industrialised areas, abnormalities of the gastrointestinal tract are relatively common and in some areas some types of abnormality appear to occur more frequently than in Western populations. Thus while not presenting as everyday problems for those working in general paediatric or surgical units, congenital abnormalities of the gastrointestinal tract are sufficiently common to necessitate medical officers being familiar with the presentations and management of the most common. With early diagnosis (sometimes even *in utero*) and appropriate management, many children born with these abnormalities can have both a normal life expectancy and a normal quality of life. Missed or delayed diagnosis and inappropriate management may lead to major morbidity in some, and death in others.

Congenital abnormalities of the gastrointestinal tract may occur as part of a multisystem disorder, associated with major chromosomal abnormalities such as the trisomies 13, 18, and 21, or forming part of other recognisable syndromes. Some, such as Hirschprung's disease and pyloric stenosis show a multifactorial inheritance pattern. The importance of environmental influences in their aetiology is unclear and the factors that cause failure of the normal orderly development of the embryonic and fetal bowel remain unknown. The majority of congenital gastrointestinal abnormalities occur sporadically.

Common presentations

As in any other area of medicine, a careful history is the most important part of the diagnostic process. The time at which symptoms and signs appear is

411

often crucial to understanding the anatomical pathology. An important clue to the possibility and site of intestinal obstruction in a baby is a history of polyhydramios in the mother. Table 24.1 relates the major abnormalities of the bowel to the time of onset of symptoms and signs.

Practice point
- *Polyhydramnios in the mother suggests the possibility of duodenal or upper small bowel obstruction in the fetus. Pre-natal ultrasonography may confirm the diagnosis.*

Table 24.1 Congenital abnormalities of the bowel in relation to time of presentation and symptoms and signs.

Clinical presentation	Abnormality
Obvious at birth	
Abnormal or absent anus	Imperforate anus or fistula
Abdominal defect	Gastroshisis (no sac for bowel)
	Exomphalos (bowels in sac)
Within minutes of birth	
Hypersalivation	Oesophageal atresia, TOF
Respiratory distress	Diaphragmatic hernia
Within the first 6 hours of birth	
Hypersalivation	Oesophageal atresia, TOF
Respiratory distress	TOF, diaphragmatic hernia
Vomiting	Upper GI atresia, bands
Abdominal distension	Upper GI atresia, intrauterine perforation
Between 6 and 24 hours of birth	
Vomiting	
Abdominal distension	Duodenal or midgut atresia or volvulus
Failure to pass meconium	neonatorum, meconium plug, Hirschprung's
24 Hours of birth to 4 weeks of life	
Constipation, vomiting	
Abdominal distension,	
Abdominal mass	Hirschprung's disease
Pain	duplications, malrotation
GI bleeding	
Coughing	TOF, evantration of the diaphragm
Chest infection	
2–6 Weeks after birth	
Projectile vomiting	Hypertrophic pyloric stenosis
Regurgitation of feeds	Gastro-oesophageal reflux

TOF = tracheo-oesophageal fistula

Anatomical abnormalities obvious at birth

While the 'gross' abnormalities such as exomphalos and gastroschisis are immediately obvious at birth, the commonest abnormality in this group, imperforate anus, will only be discovered on examination of the perineum. Since early diagnosis and early management are imperative, the importance of routine inspection of the perineum of all newborn babies cannot be overstressed. The term 'imperforate anus' is often applied loosely to cover the whole spectrum of anorectal abnormalities. The finding of an imperforate anus should alert the examiner to look for a cutaneous fistula anterior to the anal dimple (including the vaginal introitus or scrotum) and to look for the passage of meconium *per vaginam* in girls and *per urethram* in males. The latter signifies an associated fistula between the bowel and the genitourinary system. Such a fistula, if large, may prevent the early onset of abdominal distention.

A skin covered mass over the sacrococcygeal area, present at birth, is likely to be either a myelomenigocele (or related neural tube anomaly) or a sacrococcygeal teratoma. There is no immediate urgency to deal with these, and both conditions are best dealt with in a specialised surgical unit if possible. The sacrococcygeal terratoma may extend into the pelvis and present major problems for the most experienced surgeon. Rectal examination must be performed.

Vomiting

Persistent vomiting is a common feature of the newborn and in the first few hours of life may often indicate nothing more serious than swallowed irritants such as meconium, maternal blood, or mucus. Nevertheless all babies with vomiting must be carefully assessed. Such assessment includes the time of onset, the content, character, and frequency of the vomiting, and the degree of abdominal distension. The overall appearance of the baby is most important, since vomiting in a baby who has toxaemia and is weak and ill is likely to indicate neonatal sepsis or volvulus neonatorum, whereas babies with intestinal obstruction, at least in the first few hours before the onset of deydration and electrolyte imbalance appear relatively well. Repeated vomiting of milk, or clear gastric secretions, with distension limited to the upper abdomen in a baby who is generally well is suggestive of duodenal atresia. However 85 per cent of duodenal obstruction occurs distal to the bile duct entry so that the vomiting is often bile-stained. The presence of forceful peristalitic waves across the upper abdomen may suggest pyloric stenosis but this condition most commonly presents between the third and eighth week of life.

Practice point
- *Vomiting in a baby who is weak and ill and has toxaemia is likely to indicate neonatal sepsis or volvulus neonatorum, whereas babies with intestinal obstruction, at least in the first few hours before the onset of deydration and electrolyte imbalance, appear relatively well.*

Bile-stained vomiting

Bile-stained vomiting should always suggest the likelihood of intestinal obstruction and is almost always associated with abdominal distension. In general the earlier the onset of the bilious vomiting and abdominal distension, the higher the level of obstruction. Thus an ileal atresia or band may present within the first 12 h, whereas a high rectal atresia may not become apparent for 24 h. Bile stained vomiting may also be a feature of a septicaemic baby with a functional ileus, a preterm baby with necrotising enterocolitis or a baby with an intrauterine perforation and peritonitis. In these situations, bowel sounds are usually absent.

Blood in the vomit

Swallowed maternal blood is the commonest cause of a baby vomiting blood in the first 24 h of life. The babies appear perfectly well, and the vomiting is usually relieved by a stomach washout. Persistent bloody vomiting indicates intestinal bleeding which if severe may produce the signs of blood loss and hypovolaemia, demanding urgent resuscitation. Any doubt as to the origin of the blood can be resolved very simply by mixing a dilute solution of the blood in water with 1 per cent sodium hydroxide (Apts test). Fetal haemoglobin does not denature with alkali – and stays pink – in contrast to adult haemoglobin which becomes brown. Bleeding of infant origin, confirmed clinically or on testing, while uncommon, raises the possibilities of medical causes including haemorrhagic disease of the newborn and other haemorrhagic conditions and the less commonly occurring surgical causes such as 'peptic' bleeding, duplication of the bowel, and haemangioma.

Vomiting and crying

Vomiting associated with crying should alert the doctor to check for obstructed inguinal hernia. While not strictly a congenital abnormality, inguinal hernia may be present at birth and if so there is a high risk of bowel obstruction. Vomiting and crying may also be a feature of congenital volvulus secondary to malrotation of the bowel. Intussusception as a cause of crying and vomiting is uncommon in the newborn, usually presenting later at between 5–18 months, or in a more chronic form in older children. Also consider the possibility of testicular torsion in an infant with vomiting and crying.

Persistent and unexplained vomiting

In a neonate with persistent and unexplained vomiting, the possibility of a hidden infection such as in the urinary tract or meninges should be considered as should the possibility of the rare inborn errors of metabolism such as galactosaemia glycogen storage disease, and errors of amino acid and fat metabolism, many of which are associated with hypoglycaemia. Abdominal masses causing gastric compression may also cause persistent vomiting.

Regurgitation of feeds persisting beyond the neonatal period may indicate the possibiity of gastro-oesophageal reflux, particularly if the child has a history of recurrent respiratory infections and is failing to thrive.

Abdominal distension

Distension at birth

Abdominal distension present at birth should alert the doctor to the possibility of an intra-abdominal mass or intrabdominal fluid. Abdominal masses include duplication cysts of the bowel, with or without volvulus. A mass arising from the pelvis in a baby girl should raise the possibility of vaginal atresia and hydro(metro)colpos. Cystic malformations of the kidney and hydronephrosis may be easily palpable, while Wilms' tumour, hepatoblastoma, and other tumours of childhood, both benign and malignant may be present in the newborn. In a sick-looking newborn baby with a silent, fluid-filled abdomen, consider the possibility of intrauterine perforation with peritonitis. Meconium ileus should also be considered in countries where cystic fibrosis occurs.

Distension occurring after birth

It is useful to remember the guideline that distension resulting from high intestinal obstruction presents within the first 12 h of life, whereas that arising from lower obstruction becomes obvious later. As in the case of vomiting, the differential diagnosis always includes neonatal sepsis, which is usually accompanied by non-specific signs of toxicity.

Abdominal distension due to congenital agangliosis of the large bowel (Hirschprung's disease) may present within the first 24 h, or at any stage up until 6 months of age.

Practice point
• *Distension resulting from high intestinal obstruction presents within the first 12 h of life, whereas that arising from lower obstruction becomes obvious later.*

Delay in passing meconium

Most newborn babies pass meconium within the first 24 h of life. In assessing a baby referred for failure to pass meconium, it should be remembered that some babies pass meconium during the delivery, and subsequently not for more than 24 h.

Where there is an obstructive cause the cardinal signs of obstruction, distension and vomiting will, sooner or later, become apparent. The examiner must always look for early signs of distension. Apart from the anatomical causes of obstruction such as atresia obstruction may be due to a meconium plug, or a functional cause such as inadequate bowel contraction as in Hirschprung's disease. A lubricated thermometer or preferably an unbreakable probe carefully and gently inserted into the rectum will help to determine if there is rectal atresia or may stimulate the passage of a meconium plug. The finding of a meconium plug should alert the doctor to the possibility of cystic fibrosis, particularly in populations where this autosomally inherited condition is common.

Practice point
- *The passage of a small amount of meconium does not exclude intestinal obstruction due to mid- or high-gut problems because in these cases desquamated cells and lower intestinal secretions result in some meconium production.*

Hypersalivation and spilling of feeds

Hypersalivation present from birth almost always indicates the presence of oesophageal atresia in association with tracheo-oesophageal fistula. The baby with this sign should not be fed before being investigated by passing a 10-Fr catheter to exclude the diagnosis of oesophageal atresia. Should the baby be inadvertently fed before the diagnosis is made, rapid onset of spilling the feeds often associated with coughing will suggest the diagnosis.

Practice point
- *Hypersalivation present from birth almost always indicates the presence of oesophageal atresia in association with tracheo-oesophageal fistula.*

Respiratory distress

There are many causes of respiratory distress in the newborn. However, the possibility of diaphragmatic hernia should always be considered in a baby presenting with distress from birth. The scaphoid abdomen, which is supposedly often a feature of this condition, is not always obvious. The most common presentation is that of a term baby with respiratory distress who deteriorates from the time of birth. It is always important, in this situation to exclude a tension pneumothorax.

Eventration of the diaphragm is a less severe problem, and may not be diagnosed for some months or even years – when the child has an chest X-ray for persistent or repeated chest infections.

Diagnosis of the common form of tracheo-oesophageal fistula is usually made in the first few hours of life. The less common forms, however, without oesophageal atresia, present in the first weeks of life with respiratory signs of cough and recurrent chest infections. Respiratory symptoms and signs are also the presenting features of gastro-oesophageal reflux, again, usually presenting in the first few weeks and months of life.

Jaundice

A degree of 'physiological' jaundice is the norm from the second to tenth day of life. 'Pathological' jaundice in the first 2 weeks of life is almost always medical, early onset being associated with conditions of increased haemolysis such as blood group incompatibility, and later onset being associated with infection. In these cases the hyperbilirubinaemia is primarily unconjugated. The much rarer surgical causes of jaundice should be considered in the differential diagnosis of jaundice persisting into the third and subsequent weeks of life, particularly when the hyperbilirubinaemia is of mixed, or predominantly conjugated (direct) type. Biliary atresia and choledochal cyst should be considered in the differential diagnosis in such instances.

Inborn errors of bilirubin metabolism are extremely rare in practice though are commonly included in textbooks. The only one which presents in the neonatal period is Crigler–Najjar syndrome and is diagnosed by detecting high levels of unconjugated bilirubin. Dubin–Johnson and Rotor syndromes result in conjugated hyperbilirubinaemia and present in older children and adolescents. Gilbert's syndrome which presents with recurrent episodes of unconjugated hyperbilirubinaemia occurs in older children and adults.

Investigations

Some congenital abnormalities may now be detected pre-natally by routine ultrasonagraphy. Mothers with polyhydramnios should be carefully scanned for evidence of duodenal or other intestinal atresia in the fetus. The polyhydramnios is due to the inability of the swallowed liquor to pass down the gastrointestinal tract and be absorbed. Knowledge of gastrointestinal defects will enable the child to be born in a centre equipped to deal with the abnormality.

Simple investigations are all that is required to complement a good history and examination in the diagnosis of the majority of congenital abnormalities of the gastrointestinal system. In bowel obstruction a plain film of the abdomen taken in the erect position will show distended bowel with fluid levels. The presence of subdiaphragmatic gas or intra-abdominal calcification confirms intrauterine perforation. In a child with imperforate anus, an inverted film (**invertogram**) may indicate the level of rectosigmoid patency. A chest X-ray will help to exclude the possibility of associated congenital heart disease, and will demonstrate clear lung fields before anaesthesia.

In a newborn baby with respiratory distress a chest X-ray may demonstrate a diaphragmatic hernia (Figure 24.1), though in practice when the baby

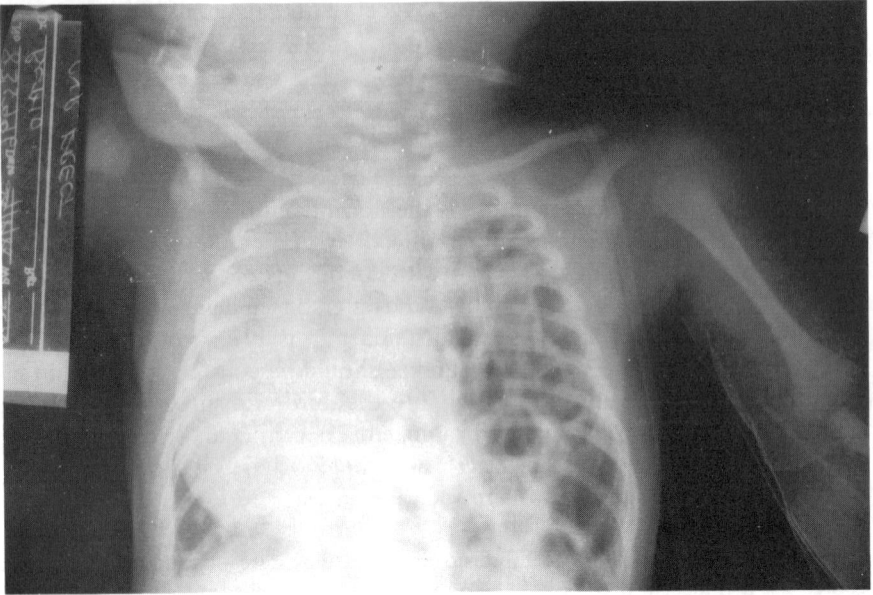

Figure 24.1 Left diaphragmatic hernia in the newborn. The left thorax is filled with stomach and small bowel. The mediastinum is pushed over to the right side and the neonate is in respiratory distress.

is rapidly deteriorating it is often necessary to make the distinction between this condition and tension pneumothorax on clinical grounds by performing a therapeutic and diagnostic chest aspiration to relieve suspected tension.

Practice point
• *In a newborn baby who develops rapidly increasing respiratory distress in the first hour of life, the most likely diagnosis is tension pneumothorax which requires immediate aspiration of the pleural cavity. Diaphragmatic hernia will be diagnosed on chest X-ray but if there is no time to take an X-ray always aspirate the chest.*

In a child with hypersalivation difficulty in passing a nasogastric tube and the demonstration of the tube coiling up in the upper oesophagus on chest X-ray is sufficient to confirm the diagnosis of oesophageal atresia and tracheo-oesophageal fistula. Where the diagnosis is uncertain and no other investigative facilities are available a small amount of dilute barium (but not Gastrografin) can be given and aspirated after the X-ray (Figure 24.2).

Newborn babies, provided they are born to healthy mothers, will have normal biochemistry. If intestinal obstruction is diagnosed early they are unlikely to have major electrolyte disturbance, so the inability to measure urea and electrolytes should not prevent early surgical management. The situation is different if diagnosis is delayed, in which case resuscitation must precede operation.

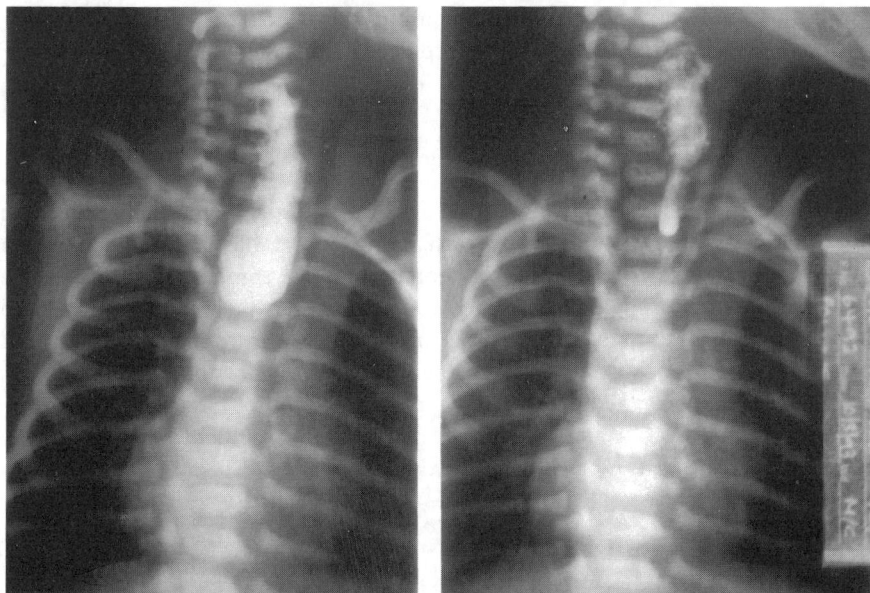

Figure 24.2 Oesophageal atresia in a newborn regurgitating all feeds. Barium swallow is not normally advised and if inadvertently performed all the barium should be aspirated immediately after the film.

Immediate management

Nasogastric tube

When a congenital abnormality of the gut necesitating immediate surgical treatment is diagnosed in the newborn it is imperative to stop oral feeding (if it has started), and to insert a nasogastric tube.

Intravenous fluids

Give intravenous fluid. If the baby is dehydrated it will be necessary to correct electrolyte and fluid balance. Otherwise, maintenance fluid should be given. This consists of 5 or 10 per cent dextrose for the first 48 h of life, and thereafter 0.18 per cent normal saline in 4.3 per cent dextrose, with 1 g potassium chloride per litre or similar solution.

Maintenance rates suitable for most situations are as follows:

Day 1	60 ml/kg
Day 2	90 ml/kg
Day 3	120 ml/kg
Day 4	150 ml/kg
Day 5+	150 ml/kg

This regime takes into account small amounts of fluid loss (10–20 ml/kg per day). Larger amounts should be replaced with normal saline.

Keeping the baby warm

It is vital that the baby is always kept warm. Even in the tropics babies become hypothermic with often disastrous consequences. Portable incubators are often not available in the tropics. When a neonate must be transferred for definitive surgery the baby can be wrapped in cotton or orthopaedic wool or wrapped up in cooking tinfoil to preserve heat. It is important to ensure the head is covered by a simple gauze hat as the head represents a large proportion of the neonate's body surface area. Vacolitres of warmed intravenous fluids can be used as home-made hot water bottles but ensure that the temperature is carefully controlled and that the bags do not leak.

Practice point
- *When transferring a neonate for surgical correction of a gastrointestinal problem always insert a nasogastric tube. Keep the child warm during transfer.*

Oxygen

If you suspect diaphragmatic hernia oxygen therapy should ideally be given via an endotracheal tube to avoid distending the stomach and exacerbating the respiratory distress. If oxygen is given via a nasal canula make sure there is a patent nasogastric tube in place to minimise gastric distension.

Antibiotics

If the possibility of peritoneal soiling at operation is present, or if there are signs of respiratory involvement following aspiration, broad-spectrum antibiotic cover should be given. One regimen used in Papua New Guinea prescribes ampicillin 30 mg/kg 12 hourly in the first week and 6 hourly in subsequent weeks plus gentamicin 2.5 mg/kg 12 hourly.

Nutritional support

If there is a likelihood of prolonged postoperative starvation (e.g. after repair of exomphalos, or gastroschisis) preparations for partial or complete intravenous feeding should be made.

Definitive management of specific abnormalities

The congenital obstructive lesions of the alimentary tract will be considered in anatomical order and then a miscellaneous group of the defects of parietes, biliary tract and other rare malformations will be discussed.

Oesophageal atresia

Surgical correction is the only hope of survival in patients with oesophageal atresia with or without tracheo-oesophageal fistula.

Pathology

In 85 per cent of the cases there is an oesophageal atresia with a fistula between the distal oesophagus and the trachea (Figure 24.3).

Diagnosis

The child who blows bubbles in the newborn period and has an obvious difficulty in swallowing his saliva probably has an obstruction of the oesophagus. The most likely reason is oesophageal atresia. Any feeds mistakenly given are regurgitated. However, the diagnosis should ideally be made before a feed or at any rate before a second feed. The essential feature is the inability to swallow which antenatally results in polyhydramnios in 20 to 25 per cent of affected pregnancies. The diagnosis can be established or excluded by passing

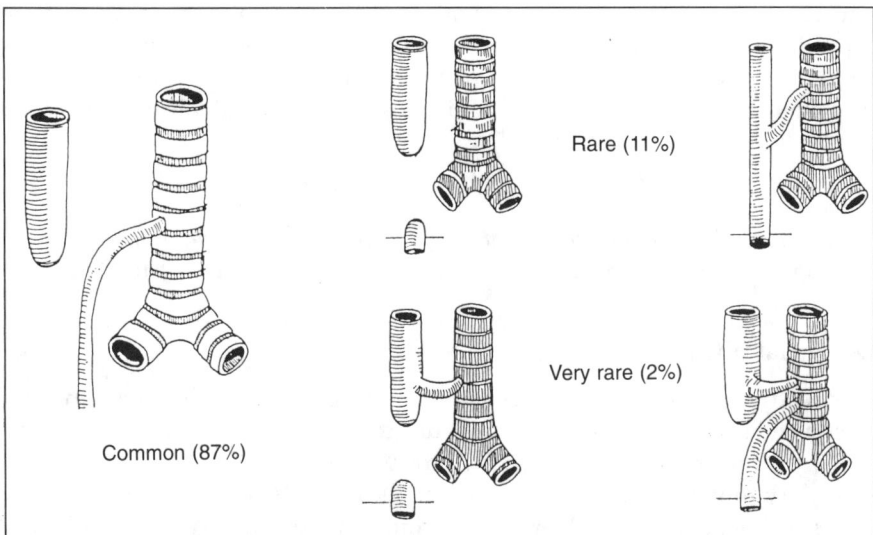

Figure 24.3 Pathological anatomy of oesophageal atresia and tracheo-oesophageal fistula.

a 10-Fr tube. Its progress will be arrested 10–12 cm from the gums in oesophageal atresia. It is not normally advisable to use contrast media as this may spill over into respiratory tract. Where there is doubt about the diagnosis dilute barium should be used and aspirated after the procedure (Figure 24.2).

Management

The infant should be transferred to a centre where surgery can be undertaken. It is important to suck the oesophagus and nasopharynx to keep it empty. The infant should be kept warm during transfer. Antibiotics, correction of fluid and electrolyte abnormalities and chest physiotherapy are essential to improve the baby's general condition.

The aim of the surgery is to divide the fistulous connection between trachea and oesophagus and achieve a primary anastomosis of the oesophagus. This is possible in the majority of the cases. Good exposure is achieved through a right lateral thoracotomy through the fourth intercostal space. The upper pouch can be easily identified by passing in a catheter through the nose. If the lower segment is not obvious it can be found by tracing the vagus nerve. Survival depends on the general condition of the infant, the nature of the defect and facilities and skill of the surgical team.

When a primary anastomosis is not possible or unsafe, delayed primary anastomosis or late oesophageal replacement can be done. An oesophagostomy to keep the upper oesophagus clear of secretions and a gastrostomy for feeding are then essential.

Congenital atresia and stenosis of the bowel

The baby has persistent vomiting with the degree of abdominal distension depending on the level of obstruction. The passage of a small amount of meconium does not exclude a high or a mid-gut obstruction. A high index of suspicion is required to make the diagnosis of intestinal obstruction. Frequently its diagnosis is delayed.

Practice point
* *Persistent vomiting in a newborn baby is usually due to one of three causes: intracranial haemorrhage, severe infection and intestinal obstruction.*

Duodenal obstruction

Obstructive lesions of the duodenum are more common than oesophageal atresia and can be from intrinsic causes due to atresia, stenosis or a valve which may be complete or incomplete and extrinsic causes due to midgut volvulus secondary to malrotation or duodenal duplications. Associated abnormalities occur in about 50 per cent. Down's syndrome is present in 30 per cent of North American cases.

Diagnosis

It is common to find polyhydramnios in the mother. The baby has persistent vomiting which may be either bile-stained or clear. The abdomen is not grossly distended except in the upper abdomen. A plain film of the abdomen showing the 'double-bubble trouble' appearance clinches the diagnosis (Figure 24.4). It may not show after gastric aspiration or continuous vomiting. It is important to remember that duodenal obstruction in infancy can also be caused by volvulus of the mid-gut and congenital bands and that annular pancreas may be associated with atresia.

Management

The treatment of choice is retrocolic duodenoduodenostomy. If the duodenum is grossly dilated it should be reduced by imbrication. The dilated proximal duodenum takes a varying period of time to function. The baby can thus suffer dehydration and electrolyte imbalance. In order to avoid this complication and improve the chances of cure a temporary gastrostomy to decompress the stomach and a feeding jejunal tube from stomach through the anastomosis is essential. The gastric aspirate can then be returned through the jejunal tube.

Jejunal and ileal atresia

The obstruction may occur at any level. Bile stained vomiting is accompanied by generalised abdominal distension if the site of obstruction is in the distal

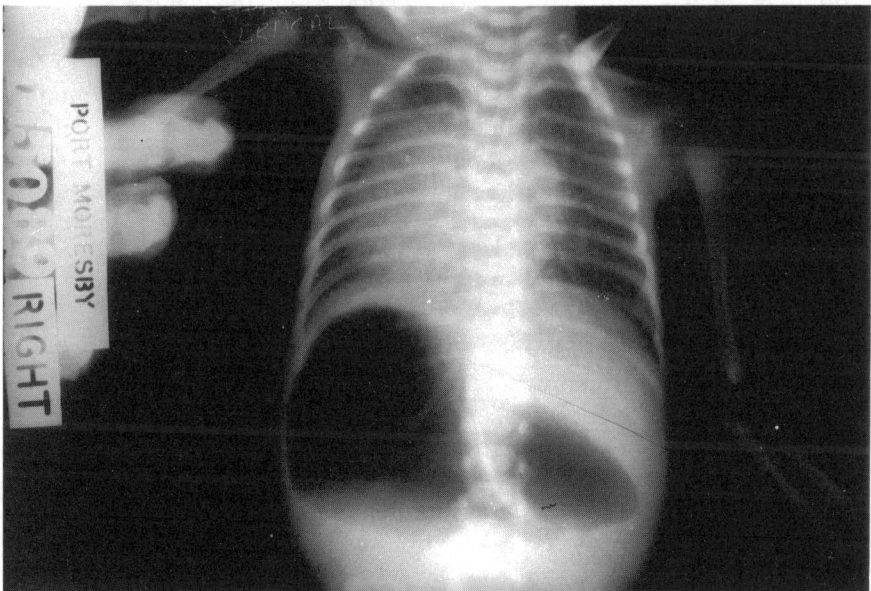

Figure 24.4 'Double-bubble' appearance of duodenal atresia in a neonate with dextrocardia and situs inversus. Normally the larger of two bubbles (the stomach) lies on the upper left hand side of the abdomen. The finding of one congenital anomaly should alert the clinician to the possibility of others.

jejunum or ileum. Multiple fluid levels are evident on an erect X-ray. The proximal loop can be grossly dilated and may perforate. The various types are shown in Figure 24.5. Surgical management involves resection of the atresia and the grossly dilated segment of bowel with continuity restored by end-to-end anastomosis. Always check the patency of the distal lumen in case there are multiple atresias. This can be done by flushing the distal bowel with saline. Multiple atresias require multiple resections and anastomoses. Ileus may sometimes be prolonged in the postoperative period so that nutritional support may be required.

Malrotation and volvulus of the midgut

Volvulus is twisting of the bowel upon its own axis or the axis of its mesentery. Midgut volvulus is usually caused by abnormal re-entry of the bowel during its developmental return to the abdominal cavity. The caecum remains in the right hypochondrium and a peritoneal band is found running from the caecum to the right side of the abdomen across the second part of the duodenum. This is the transduodenal band of Ladd which may obstruct the duodenum following the volvulus. Most commonly the volvulus occurs just distal to the bands.

Diagnosis

Symptoms often develop in the neonatal period within the first few days of life but may present later after several months. The early symptom is vomiting followed by distension. The vomitus is at first gastric and later bilious or fecal in nature. The volvulus may be intermittent so causing recurrent symptoms. Malrotation and volvulus should be suspected in any infant who develops intestinal obstruction after an uneventful postnatal period or when symptoms of obstruction are intermittant. A plain film will show dilatation of the stomach and duodenum.

Management

The involved intestine may become gangrenous and profound shock and death can result. Hence laparotomy is urgent. The volvulus is untwisted usually in an anticlockwise direction, Ladd's bands are divided and the base of the mesentery widened. The caecum and the ascending colon are placed on the left side of abdomen. No attempt is made to restore the normal arrangement. If gangrene of the bowel has already occurred, resection and anastomosis is done and the chances and quality of survival depend on the length of the remaining gut.

Congenital hypertrophic pyloric stenosis

Typically the first born male child is commonly affected. Usually this condition

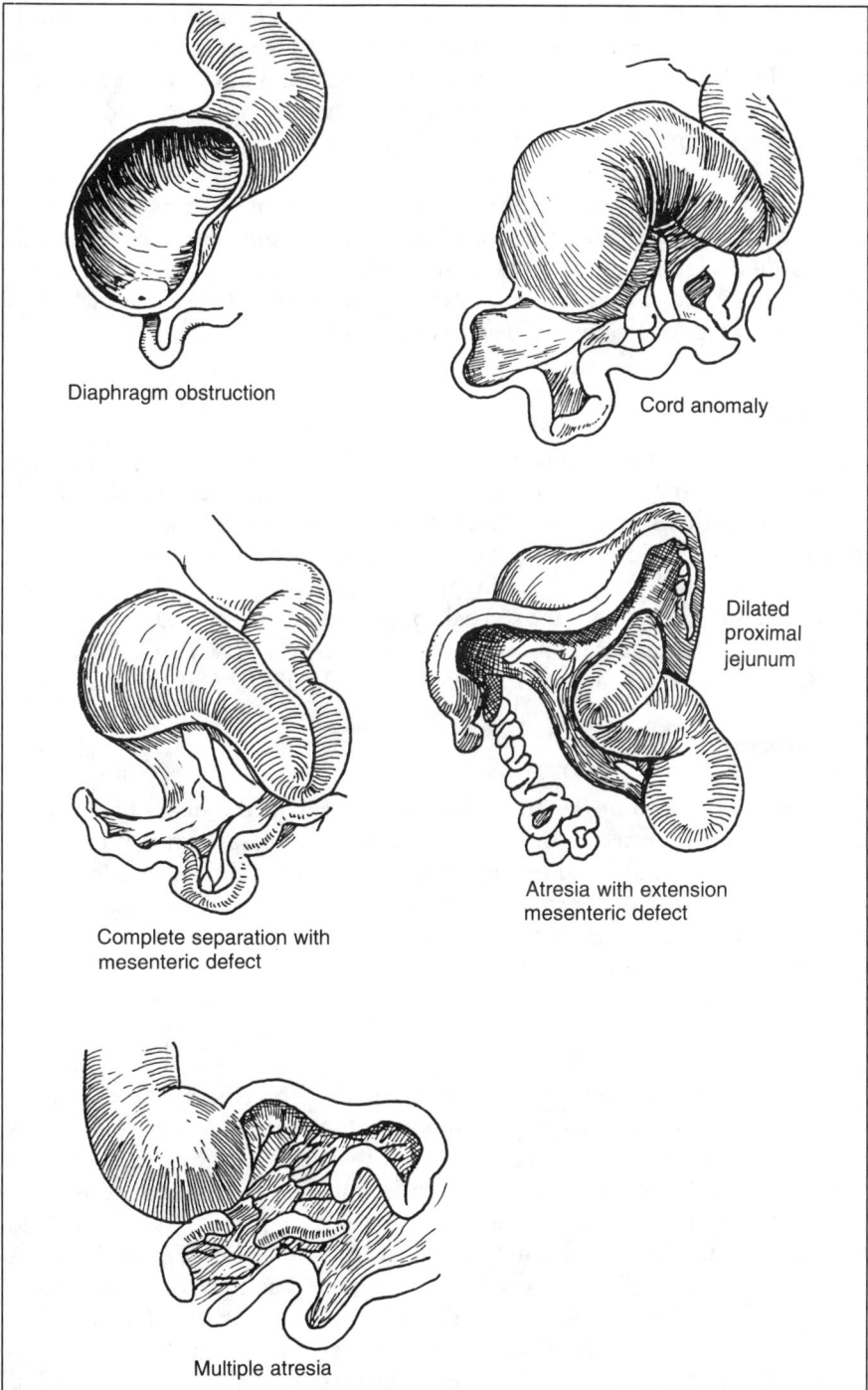

Diaphragm obstruction

Cord anomaly

Complete separation with
mesenteric defect

Dilated
proximal
jejunum

Atresia with extension
mesenteric defect

Multiple atresia

Figure 24.5   Different types of small intestinal atresia.

presents between the third week and sixth week with projectile vomiting which is never bile stained. After feeding visible peristalsis may be seen running from left to right. Palpation of the hypertrophic pylorus as an olive sized mass to the right of the xiphisternum just under the liver edge during a test feed clinches the diagnosis. Untreated loss of gastric secretions leads to dehydration and metabolic alkalosis and hypokalaemia. The child becomes miserable and lethargic. If clinical features of pyloric stenosis are present but a pyloric tumour cannot be palpated, the use of a small amount of radiographic contrast will reveal a dilated stomach, and 'string sign' when an X-ray of the abdomen is taken after 15 min. Ultrasound can also be used to identify the mass which is usually palpable with careful repeated examination.

Management

Correction of dehydration and electrolyte imbalance is necessary before operation. Pyloromyotomy (Ramstedt's operation) is the treatment of choice. Where a skilled anaesthetist is not available the operation can be done under local anaesthetic. The abdomen is opened by a transverse incision over the right rectus muscle which is split. The hypertrophied pylorus is held between the thumb and index finger and the serosal coat is incised and the muscle coat split open down to the mucosa without perforating the mucosa. Feeds are started after 6 h. The survival rate after this operation should be 100 per cent.

Hirschprung's disease

The disease is due to an absence of ganglion cells in the distal bowel. The length of bowel affected varies but the defect extends proximally from the anorectal junction and distal rectum to the descending colon or even rarely to the right colon and distal parts of the small intestine. In most cases the narrow, aganglionic segment begins at the pelvirectal junction. Proximally the obstructed large intestine is enormously dilated and hypertrophied.

Diagnosis

The passage of meconium is delayed and often scanty. Abdominal distention and vomiting are early features. The abdominal distension may be so severe as to cause respiratory embarassment. Waves of visible peristalsis can be appreciated. On rectal examination the rectum is empty. If the affected segment is short and low a ring of constriction can be felt. A plain film shows gross distension of the large and small bowel with fluid levels (Figure 24.6). A barium enema will delineate the contracted segment and proximal distension (Figure 24.7). Preliminary washouts should be avoided as these may decompress the distended colon. Rectal biopsy is essential at multiple levels to examine for ganglion cells and to detect increased cholinesterase activity if Hirschprung's disease is present. Suction mucosal biopsies of the rectum can be done if facilities are available.

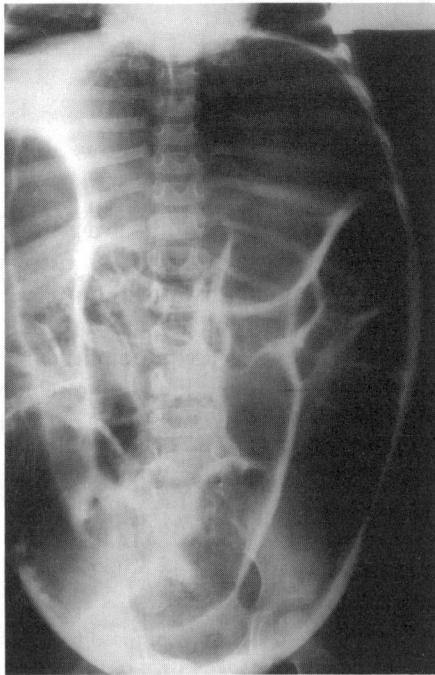

Figure 24.6   A 4-year-old female presenting with gross colonic and small bowel distension due to untreated Hirschprung's disease.

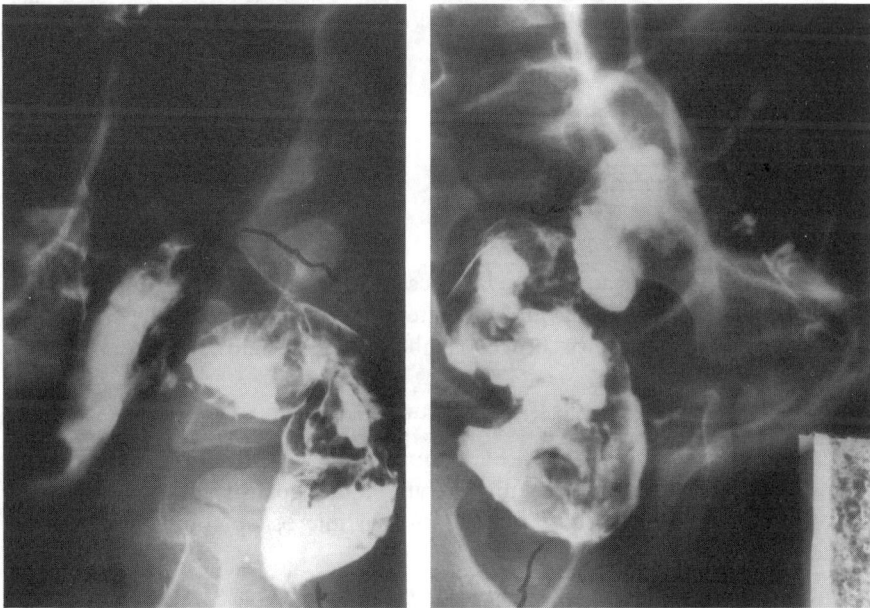

Figure 24.7   Barium enema showing constricted (aganglionic) and dilated (ganglion cells present) segments of the colon in the same 4-year-old female with untreated Hirschprung's disease.

Management

The aims of management are:

1. immediate relief of obstruction by colostomy;
2. anastomosis of ganglion-containing normal bowel to the anal canal once the baby is a few months old.

Relief of obstruction by colostomy is urgent as severe enterocolitis may develop, especially in long standing cases. The extent of the disease can be assessed at this time. Biopsy of normal (distended) bowel, the transitional zone and site of colostomy should be performed. The colostomy is then placed on the most distal ganglionic segment. A longitudinal full thickness biopsy is taken involving both the aganglionic and ganglionic segment. The distal and proximal site is marked by tags. Definitive surgery is performed when the baby is healthy, thriving and an experienced surgeon is available. The bowel should be well prepared with normal saline with soap enemas. Tap water in the enemas may cause water intoxication, electrolyte imbalance and could be fatal.

In the **Soave** operation the rectum is divided above the pelvic floor and the mucosa is cored out. The aganglionic segment is resected and the ganglionic segment is pulled into the muscular tunnel of the rectum and anastomosed to the anus. In the **Duhamel** procedure the aganglionic segment is removed down to the pelvic floor and the rectum is divided and closed at this level. The sacral hollow is opened up and the ganglion containing segment is brought down and into the stretched anus after making a transverse incision. The colon is fixed by loose sutures into the rectum and a crushing clamp is used to crush the spur between the colon and rectum. The clamp becomes loose once the spur separates.

Anorectal malformations

Classification

There is no universally accepted classification for imperforate anus. Broadly they are divided into 'high', 'intermediate' and 'low' anomalies depending on whether the termination of bowel is above, at or below the pelvic floor (Figures 24.8 and 24.9).

In males they may be classified (Figure 24.8) as:

1. High: anorectal agenesis with or without urinary fistula, rectal atresia.
2. Intermediate: rectobulbar urethral fistula, anal agenesis without fistula.
3. Low: anocutaneous fistula, anal stenosis or microscopic anus and ectopic anus.

In females the classification (Figure 24.9) includes:

1. High: anorectal agenesis with or without rectovaginal fistula; rectal atresia (Figure 24.9b).

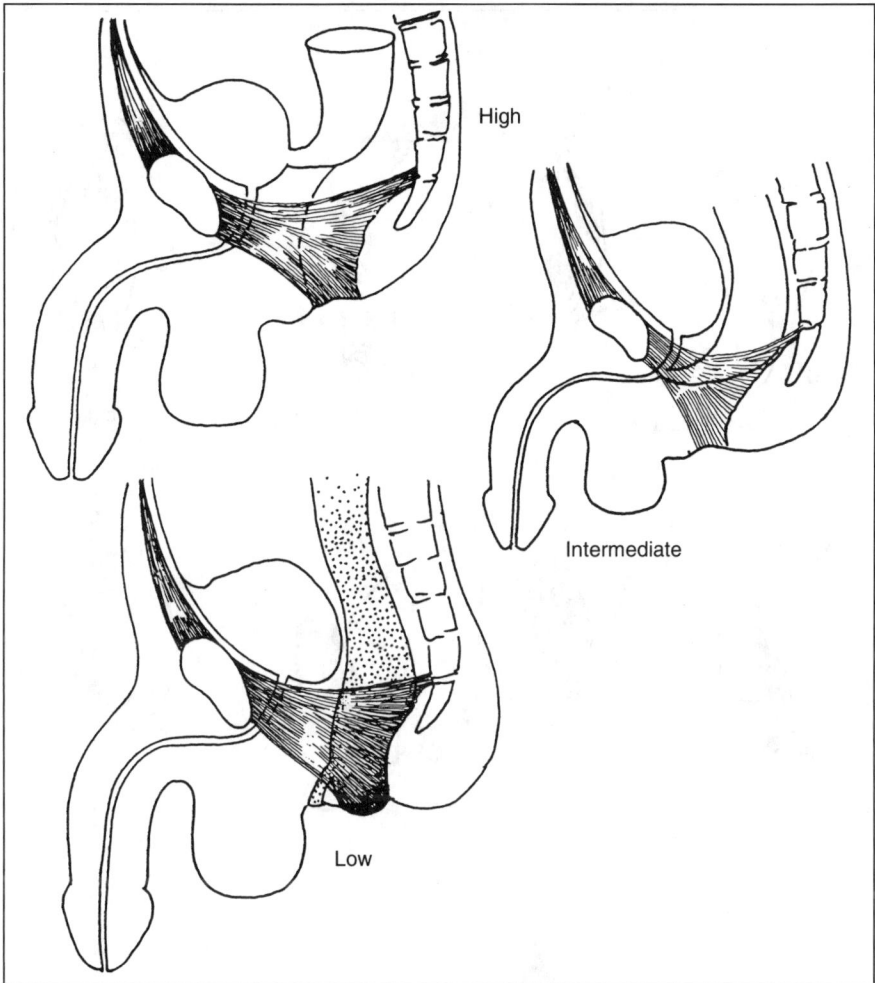

Figure 24.8 Anorectal anomalies in males.

2. Intermediate: rectovestibular fistula, rectovaginal fistula and anal agenesis without fistula.
3. Low: anovestibular fistula (Figure 24.9c(i)).
4. Cloaca: a single perineal hole (Figure 24.9a).

Presentation

Babies with imperforate anus do not show abdominal distension in the first few hours of life. Even if a perineal fistula is present, meconium is often not seen until 16–24 h after birth. Therefore early clinical examination and early invertograms may be misleading so that the final decision about the need for

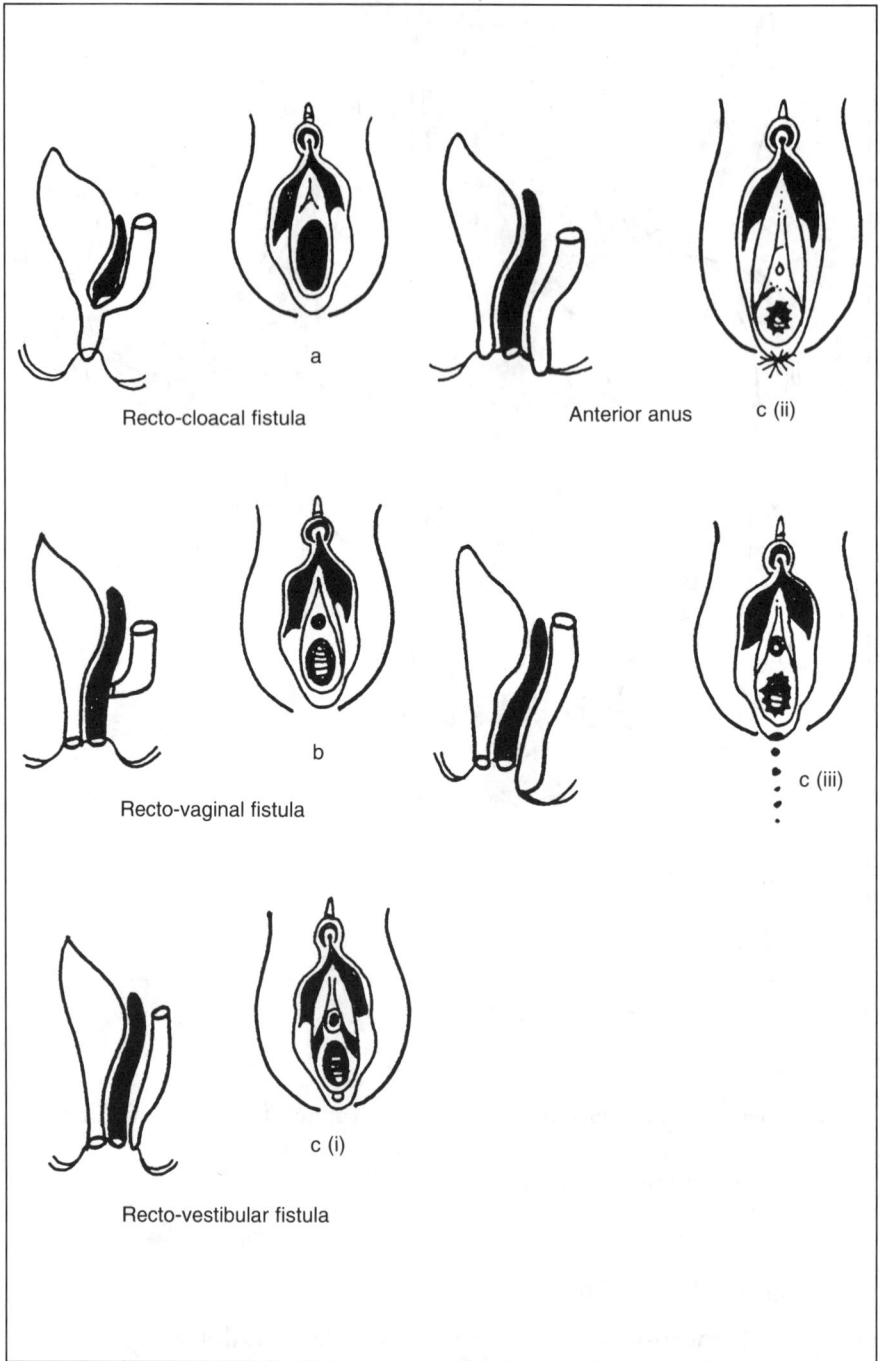

Figure 24.9   Anorectal anomalies in females.

colostomy should be made at 24 h. In the tropics babies often present late with abdominal distension and vomiting. An invertogram is only necessary in the small proportion of cases where clinical examination is equivocal in determining whether the abnormality is low, intermediate or high. Associated urinary tract abnormalities should be excluded by ultrasound examination and are particularly common in females with a cloaca. In females with hydrocolpos there may be a palpable lower abdominal mass. The dilated vagina may compress the trigone of the bladder and interfere with drainage of the ureters.

High anorectal abnormalities

In high and intermediate anomalies the clinical presentations include 'flat or round bottom', meconium in urine, air in the bladder, and more than 1 cm bowel-skin separation as measured by invertogram.

Low anorectal abnormalities

The perineum should be inspected for findings typical of low anomalies which can be treated by local 'cutback' procedures.

1. An anal membrane through which the bluish-green colour of meconium can be seen in a good light.
2. A midline raphae cutaneous fistula.
3. An anterior or stenosed anus.

An **anal membrane** can be incised and the anal canal dilated twice daily after operation. Where the anal tube opens anteriorly as a small **anocutaneous fistula** in the perineum a 'cut-back' procedure is all that is necessary. The canal is probed and a scissor blade inserted. A cut is then made with the scissors in the midline posteriorly to give an anal orifice of about a centimetre. Anal dilatation should then be performed twice daily from the first day after operation. This procedure is not suitable if the anal canal opens in the median raphe of the scrotum, in the vagina or if there is a urethral fistula. An anterior or stenosed anus can be enlarged by a cutback and the size of the canal maintained by twice daily anal dilatation for a minimum of 6 weeks.

Management

High abnormalities

A diverting colostomy is recommended in all cases of imperforate anus except where there is an obvious low anomaly like anocutaneous fistulae and anal stenosis. It is always safer to divert the faecal stream to avoid the risk of infection. A proximal sigmoid colostomy with separated stomas completes the faecal stream, makes it easier to clean the shorter distal colon and facilitates a distal loopogram before definitive surgery. A distal colonic biopsy should be performed to exclude the rare case of co-existent Hirschprung's disease.

Associated urinary tract obstruction should be recognised and treated appropriately.

The best technique for correction of imperforate anus is a posterior sagittal anorectal plasty (PSARP) described by Pena (see further reading). The basic principles are to stay in the midline to avoid any neurological damage, use an electrical stimulator to distinquish sphincters from surrounding structures, strict haemostasis and the operation should be performed by a surgeon familiar with the anatomy of the perineum in the neonate. Postoperatively anal dilatation is mandatory; it should be started 2 weeks after operation and must be performed twice a day by the mother. The colostomy is closed when the anus can be dilated to size 12 Hegar in newborns and infants.

Sacroccoccygeal teratoma

A teratoma that arises from the tip of the sacrum or the front of the coccyx may present at birth or in the first year of life. It may be large enough to obstruct labour. The tumours are obvious at birth. The differential diagnosis includes the much less common anterior sacral meningocoele and other tumours such as chordoma or ganglioneuroma. Malignancy develops in up to 30 per cent of sacrococcygeal teratomas but malignant recurrence is unlikely if the tumour is completely excised in the first month of life. The best treatment is excision in the first few days of life. The prognosis is good.

A pre-sacral teratoma may also present later as a posterior mass on rectal examination or as a cause of urinary obstruction. The diagnosis should not be missed if a rectal examination is done in all children with urinary obstruction. The later the presentation the more likely is malignant transformation.

Abdominal wall defects

Coexistent congenital abnormalities are more common with exomphalos than gastroschisis.

Gastroschisis

The infant is born with a defect in the anterior abdominal wall usually to the right of the umbilicus as a result of failure of development of the abdominal wall. The bowel is exposed, not covered by any membrane and therefore it is thickened and covered with exudate. Atresia and malrotation are the only other frequently associated anomalies.

The prolapsing bowels should be cleaned, without stripping off adherent exudate, and wrapped in clingfilm before transfer to a surgical unit. Broad-spectrum antibiotic therapy should be commenced.

Two options for surgical treatment are available. The first is primary closure after vigorous stretching of the abdominal wall and repositioning of the intestine. This often necessitates mechanical ventilation for days or weeks and such facilities are often not available in the tropics.

The other method is gradual replacement of the bowel into the peritoneal cavity avoiding tension which would interfere with ventilation. A silastic sheet can be sutured to the skin to form a bag around the bowels and the size of the bag progressively reduced by sutures over the next 7–10 days. If there is an associated malrotation the caecum should be placed in the left upper quadrant and Ladd's band divided if present.

Exomphalos

The abdominal contents herniate into the umbilical cord. There is an extra-abdominal mass of intestine and solid organs, commonly the liver, covered by fusion of the layers of the amniotic membrane and the peritoneum. It may vary from a small hernia to a giant one. The defect is at the umbilicus and the peritoneal sac may rupture during or after delivery. Associated cardiac abnormalities and Down's syndrome are more common with exomphalos than gastroschisis.

The management depends on the size of the hernia. Small and moderate lesions can be closed primarily. The limiting factor is impairment of ventilation. Large hernias can be treated by either vigorous stretching of the abdominal wall, replacement of the abdominal contents and ventilatory support, or, non-operatively by painting the sac with silver sulphadiazine or mercurochrome to make it dry and tough. Gradual epithelialisation occurs and the ventral hernia which persists can be formally repaired when the child is older. Silver sulphadiazine is preferred to mercurochrome because of the risk of mercury poisoning. Exomphalos, particularly small ones, may be associated with Meckel's diverticulum which is a persistence of the intestinal portion of the vitellointestinal duct, present in 0.3 to 3 per cent of the population.

Umbilical hernia

Umbilical hernias are almost normal in many populations in sub-Saharan Africa. Umbilical hernias rarely obstruct and there is no urgency for surgical treatment in the first few years of life. Spontaneous closure is common in the first 1–5 years of life and the timing of repair in persistent hernias depends to some extent on parental acceptance of the abnormality after the first birthday.

Umbilical discharge

The most common cause of discharge is an umbilical granuloma which can easily be managed by painting with copper sulphate or silver nitrate. Congenital causes of a discharging umbilicus are a persistent vitellointestinal duct and a persistent urachus. These often do not present until later in life. The nature of the discharge (whether faeculent or watery) will point to the cause and a sinogram will outline the tract. The treatment is excision. Cysts in the base of the cord or at some point in the tract may be associated with either of these conditions.

Cantrell's deformity

There is a midline defect of the epigastrium and lower sternum. Diaphragmatic and cardiac defects may be associated with it. Repair requires extensive reconstruction using the costal cartilages, and reapproximating the rectus abdominis muscles in the midline and is performed at about 2 years of age.

Congenital diaphragmatic hernia

This anomaly is a failure of development of the diaphragm with displacement of abdominal viscera into the chest. The common site is posterolaterally (foramen of Bochdalek) on the left side. A hernia on the right side occurs very rarely.

Diagnosis

The common presentation is respiratory distress developing within the first few minutes or hours of life which is not relieved by oxygen therapy. In a left-sided hernia heart sounds are better heard on the right side of the chest, the apex beat is displaced to the right and there is decreased air entry on the left side of the chest. The abdomen sometimes appears scaphoid and empty. A plain X-ray is usually diagnostic (Figure 24.1), showing loops of bowel in the chest.

Management

The infant who is having respiratory distress soon after birth needs ventilatory support and resuscitation. Ventilation and oxygen therapy by bag and mask may cause deterioration by distending the stomach which is in the left thorax. Endotracheal intubation is indicated and a nasogastric tube should be inserted to minimise gastric distension. Surgery through a transverse upper abdominal incision is indicated as soon as the infant is resuscitated. The bowels are replaced in the abdomen and the diaphragm repaired. If there is an associated malrotation the caecum should be placed in the left upper quadrant and no attempt made to restore normal anatomy. The prognosis depends upon whether there is associated pulmonary hypoplasia. Those with normal lungs usually do well even if the facilities are limited.

Herniation through an anterior defect close to the midline (foramen of Morgagni)

This diaphragmatic hernia rarely presents with respiratory distress in the newborn but rather later in life as an abdominal emergency when strangulation of the contents of the hernia occurs.

Reflux oesophagitis and hiatus hernia

Clinical recognition

A history of persistent vomiting or regurgitation of feeds associated with recurrent episodes of respiratory infection or wheezing and/or evidence of gastrointestinal blood loss in an infant or young child who is failing to thrive should raise the possibility of pathological gastro-oesophageal reflux. Lower oesophageal pH monitoring is the diagnostic method of choice, if available, but requires experience in its interpretation particularly in the first year of life in which reflux is often 'physiological' and self-limiting rather than pathological. A barium swallow usually demonstrates reflux and may also show anatomical abnormalities associated with reflux such as hiatus hernia.

Management

The treatment of gastro-oesophageal reflux is usually conservative in the first instance with thickening of the feeds and positioning the infant upright after feeding in young infants. Antacids and H_2-receptor blockers are added if these simple measures fail. In later infancy pharmacological agents such as metoclopramide directed at increasing the tone of the lower oesophageal sphincter and speeding gastric emptying may be indicated. Surgery in the form of fundoplication is only required for refractory cases or the development of peptic strictures. The management of hiatus hernia is discussed further on pp 291–2.

Choledochal cysts and Caroli's disease

A choledochal cyst is a localised cystic dilatation of all or part of the common duct. Of these 80 per cent present in childhood and the female:male ratio is 4:1. There is no established genetic factor for the disease. Although a choledochal cyst may occur as a single entity, it is often associated with other biliary abnormalities like distal common bile duct stenosis or an anomalous junction of the pancreatic and common bile ducts.

The aetiological factors proposed fall in to two categories, either:

1. reflux of pancreatic enzymes into the bile duct, or,
2. distal obstruction of the common bile duct.

Four forms of choledochal cysts have been described (Figure 24.10). In **Caroli's disease** there are multiple intrahepatic bile duct cysts.

Clinical recognition

Abdominal pain, jaundice and a palpable mass present only in 30–40 per cent of patients. The most comon presentation in infants is prolonged jaundice with pale stools and dark urine; episodic abdominal pain with mild jaundice in children; and in adults right hypochondeal pain, fever, rigors and mild jaundice. A palpable abdominal mass is uncommon in adults. It is essential to differentiate choledochal cysts from biliary atresia and neonatal hepatitis. The diagnosis is usually established by abdominal ultrasound which demonstrates the cyst. Failure to diagnose a choledochal cyst may result in biliary fibrosis, cirrhosis and liver failure.

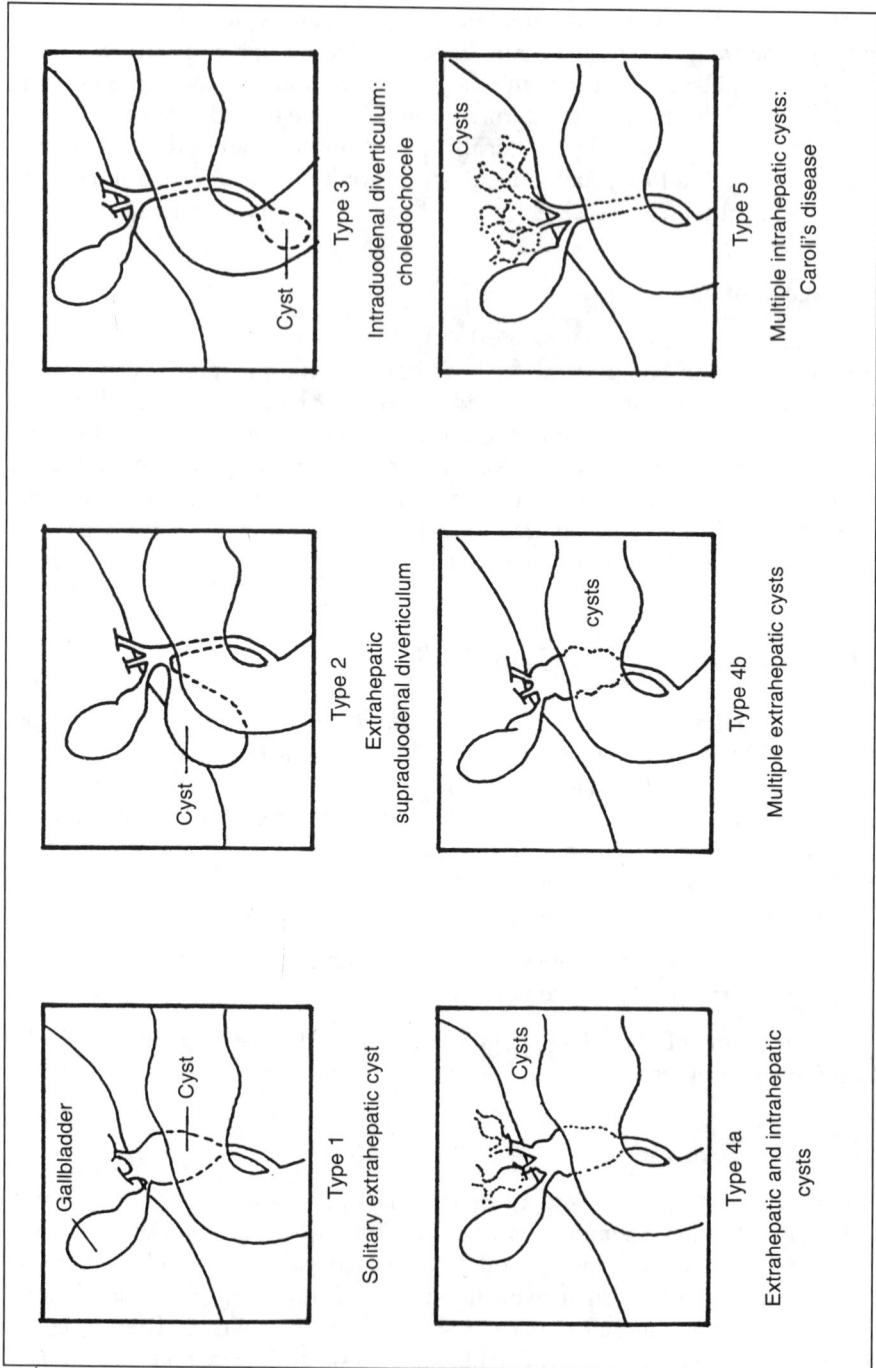

Figure 24.10   Anatomical classification of choledochal cysts.

Management

The original method of cystoduodenostomy or cystojejunostomy are no longer acceptable because of the high incidence of anastomatic stricture since as the cyst wall is fibrous structure it does not reduce after drainage. The current method of choice is excision of the cyst, removal of gallbladder and hepaticojejunostomy. The exact procedure depends on the anatomy of the cyst and any intrahepatic component.

Caroli's disease

The treatment depends on whether the disease is limited to one or both lobes of the liver. Hepatic lobectomy is advised for unilobar disease. Bilobar disease requires a Roux-en-Y cholangiojejunostomy, transhepatic intubation or liver transplantation depending on the extent and the facilities available.

Intrauterine perforation

Intrauterine perforation may occur as a primary entity, or secondary to other pathology such as meconium ileus (see Cystic fibrosis) or volvulus. In primary perforation, the underlying aetiology is thought to be vascular – since the perforation is usually sited at the vascular watershed between the middle and inferior mesenteric artery. The majority of these perforations heal spontaneously – either in the intrauterine or early neonatal life, and surgical intervention is not indicated unless there are signs of secondary infection. Where perforation has occurred secondary to underlying obstruction, surgery is required.

Necrotising enterocolitis

This disease is not a congenital abnormality but may complicate premature birth, Hirschprung's disease or exchange transfusions in the first 2–3 weeks of life. It presents with abdominal distension, vomiting and blood in the stool. The infant is extremely ill and becomes dehydrated and lethargic. Breast milk is protective. The organisms implicated include *Clostridium perfingens, Klebsiella, Salmonella* and *Escherichia coli.*

An abdominal X-ray may show gas in the wall of the bowel and in severe cases gas may also be seen in the portal system (Figure 24.11).

Management

Resuscitation, nasogastric aspiration and systemic antibiotics should be given. If the infant improves there is no need for surgery. Surgery is indicated for perforation or persistent bowel obstruction. Failure to improve after 24–48 h of medical therapy is a relative indication. At surgery the necrotic bowel should

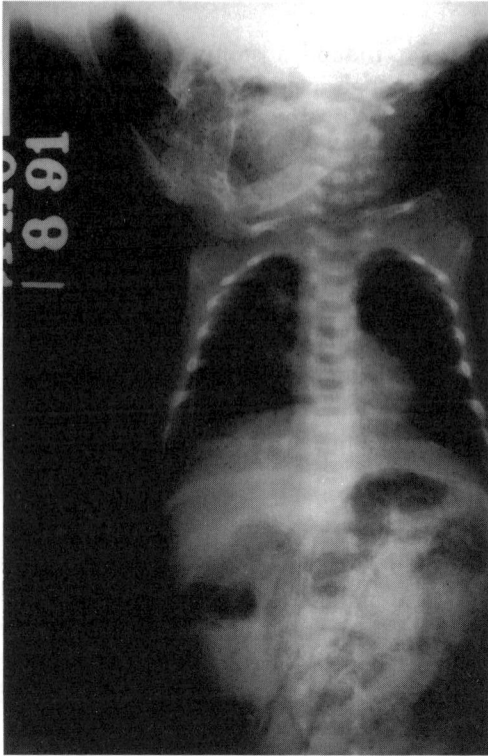

Figure 24.11   Necrotising enterocolitis showing gas shadows in the wall of the bowel.

be resected and an ileostomy performed. The bowel should not be anastomosed at this stage. One potential complication in those who improve is that healing may be associated with stenosis which will require resection.

Cystic fibrosis

Cystic fibrosis is a genetically determined disorder of the exocrine secretory glands, with multisystem involvement. The clinical manifestations are secondary to the production of secretions with abnormal physicochemical properties which results in blockage of glandular and larger lumina. The underlying defect is now known to be an abnormality of the production of a membrane chloride channel – the cystic fibrosis transmembrane regulator – and more than 100 different mutations of the gene-situated on chromosome 7 have been described. The commonest of these is a deletion of three bases (D 508), occurring in approximately 85 per cent of patients.

Cystic fibrosis occurs predominantly in Caucasians – with a frequency of 1 in 2000 to 1 in 2500 births. It is very much less common in non-Caucasians the incidence in Black Americans is 1 in 17 000, and it is said to be even less common in Asian children. No cases have been described so far in Melanesians.

In Caucasian populations the most common presentations involve the gastrointestinal tract and the respiratory tract. Between 10 and 20 per cent of patients present at birth with meconium ileus. The clinical features in 'uncomplicated' meconium ileus are early onset of abdominal swelling, bile stained vomiting and delay in passing meconium. Plain abdominal X-rays show moderately distended small bowel with few, if any fluid levels, and there may be a granular appearance of the bowel contents, resulting from gas bubbles within the meconium. Management of such 'uncomplicated' cases consists initially of a Gastrografin or barium enema to loosen the meconium and allow its evacuation.

Malabsorption occurs in 85–95 per cent of patients with cystic fibrosis, and is often evident almost from the time of birth. Other gastrointestinal manifestations of cystic fibrosis include rectal prolapse and intussusception.

The definitive diagnosis of cystic fibrosis is made by the finding of elevated levels of chloride in sweat. The sweat test is difficult to perform with accuracy and should be done by skilled staff at a referral centre.

Further reading

Congenital anomalies – various articles in: World J Surg 1993;17(3):295–391.

Dryden R, Vince J. Birth defects in Papua New Guinea. UPNG Press, Box 320, University P O, Papua New Guinea 1988.

Kelly DA, Buick RG. Congenital abnormalities of the biliary tree. Surgery (Medicine Group) 1992;10:149–52.

McQuitty JC, Lewis NC. Cystic Fibrosis. In: Rudolph AM, Hoffman JIE, Rudolph CD, editors. Rudolph's pediatrics. 19th Ed. London, Sydney: Appleton and Lange, 1991:1526–33.

Motala C, Ireland JD, Hill ID, Bowie MD. Cholestatic disorders of infancy – aetiology and outcome. J Trop Paed 1990;36:218–21.

Nwako FA. A textbook of paediatric surgery in the tropics. Basingstoke: Macmillan, 1980.

Pena A. Current management of anorectal anomalies. Surg Clin N Am 1992;72(6): 1393–416.

Wright V. Surgical problems. In Robinson NRC, editor. Neonatal intensive care. 3rd ed. London: Edward Arnold, 1993:268–89.

Index

CPSIA information can be obtained
at www.ICGtesting.com
Printed in the USA
JSHW050238040322
23450JS00003B/6